146

CLINICAL

ELECTROENCEPHALOGRAPHY

CLINICAL ELECTROENCEPHALOGRAPHY

THIRD EDITION

L. G. KILOH, M.D., B.Sc., F.R.C.P., D.P.M.
Professor, School of Psychiatry, University of New South Wales

A. J. McCOMAS, B.Sc., M.B., B.S.
Director of Neurology, McMaster University, Hamilton, Ontario

J. W. OSSELTON, B.Sc.
*Senior Lecturer in EEG, Royal Victoria Infirmary and Medical School,
University of Newcastle upon Tyne*

LONDON

BUTTERWORTHS

ENGLAND: BUTTERWORTH & CO. (PUBLISHERS) LTD.
                LONDON: 88 Kingsway, WC2B 6AB

AUSTRALIA: BUTTERWORTHS PTY. LTD.
                SYDNEY: 586 Pacific Highway, 2067
                MELBOURNE: 343 Little Collins Street, 3000
                BRISBANE: 240 Queen Street, 4000

CANADA: BUTTERWORTH & CO. (CANADA) LTD.
                TORONTO: 14 Curity Avenue, 374

NEW ZEALAND: BUTTERWORTHS OF NEW ZEALAND LTD.
                WELLINGTON: 26−28 Waring Taylor Street, 1

SOUTH AFRICA: BUTTERWORTH & CO. (SOUTH AFRICA) (PTY.) LTD.
                DURBAN: 152−154 Gale Street

First Edition   1961
Reprinted   1962
Reprinted   1964
Second Edition   1966
Reprinted   1970
Third Edition   1972

Suggested UDC Number 616·831−073·97

ISBN: 0 407 13602 9

Printed in Great Britain by
Redwood Press Limited
Trowbridge, Wiltshire

CONTENTS

v

FOREWORD

In the eleven years that have elapsed since the publication of the first edition, *Clinical Electroencephalography* has won a firm and secure place as a standard text within its field. It is extensively used by neurologists, psychiatrists, and physicians as well as those who specialize in electroencephalography in all parts of the world. As textbooks are prone, like individuals, to a more or less slow ageing process, determined in part by initial endowment and to some extent by subsequent experience, the question of senescence inevitably arises after the lapse of more than ten years. But the writer finds more indications of an open-minded response to current developments and a readiness to look to the future than tendencies to dwell reminiscently on the past.

Electroencephalographic investigations have played a prominent part in the advances made in the past few decades in our understanding of sleep. As sleep recording is acquiring increasing practical importance, in addition to its value as a research tool in neurology and psychiatry, the authors have incorporated a section on overnight sleep. Similarly, as the monitoring of a whole range of physiological parameters has come to form an indispensable part of intensive care, the authors have incorporated a lucid and balanced statement of applications of the electroencephalogram in this newly arisen therapeutic area. In the case of sensory evoked potentials, the clinical applications are for the present limited but a large literature has grown out of the attempts of investigators in every part of the world to explore the value of this technique for elucidating the problems of a number of psychiatric and neurological disorders. This volume contains an introduction to this expanding literature that successfully avoids sacrificing cogency to compression. The preparation of a work intended to serve as a guide to clinical practice presents different problems from those involved in writing a scientific textbook. The latter must aim at the critical evaluation of existing knowledge and the progress that has been made in constructing a clear and coherent theoretical framework for it. A text intended to be used for clinical practice must on the other hand be aimed primarily at assisting the complex decision-making process that confronts the medical practitioner faced with an individual case with all its facets and ambiguities. Statistical trends have to be related to situations in certain ways unique, the nature of the disorder may be undecided and the laboratory tests intended to shed light on this, including the results of EEG examination, may be equivocal. The findings of one group of observations can be evaluated only in relation to the results of the others and some measure of circularity in reasoning cannot be avoided. Decisions have to be taken, even though the evidence is far from complete. Probabilities have to be weighed, judgements balanced and the exercise demands tact, imagination and flexibility of approach in varying degrees. This text will help the practising clinician in many such situations because the authors' work well exemplifies a number of these qualities.

Newcastle upon Tyne   MARTIN ROTH

PREFACE

We welcome Alan McComas as co-author of this edition. An absence of basic neurophysiology was a deliberate omission in previous editions, but a better understanding of the mechanisms underlying the generation of the EEG demands that this deficiency should now be remedied. Late of Newcastle upon Tyne, Professor McComas is now Director of Neurology at McMaster University.

A chapter on special techniques has been added in an attempt to describe some of the commoner applications of EEG outside routine laboratory recording. The study of sensory evoked potentials and of overnight sleep are rapidly becoming specialties in their own right, but it would be unfortunate if these were to be divorced entirely from clinical EEG work.

Contrary to former predictions in some quarters, the vast majority of electroencephalographers are still recording EEGs on paper and analysing them by eye. Consequently, almost all our illustrative examples have been recorded in this way. The use of bipolar derivations from electrode arrays based on the international 10–20 system is in keeping with customary practice in the United Kingdom, but should not be taken as an adverse reflection on the use of common reference methods and other electrode placements in appropriate circumstances. All scalp recordings have been made with pad or stick-on electrodes of chlorided silver. Unless otherwise stated, amplifier time constants of 0·3 second and high frequency attenuation of 30 per cent at 70 Hz have been used throughout.

We are indebted to numerous authors, editors and publishers for permission to make use of illustrations and tables from other sources, and to Dr. D. D. Barwick and Miss B. P. Longley for access to their EEG data in the Regional Neurological Centre, Newcastle General Hospital.

We are grateful to the staff of the Department of Photography in the Medical School, University of Newcastle upon Tyne, for their preparation of the prints and diagrams, and to Elizabeth Armstrong, Yvonne Chisholm, Dorothy Deason and Jane Glass for their secretarial help. Marian Osselton has eased the burden of reading proofs and compiling the index.

L.G.K.
J.W.O.

INTRODUCTION

The distinction of making the first observations of the electrical activity of the brain goes to Caton who, in 1875, reported that he had detected currents from electrodes placed on the skull or exposed brain in rabbits and monkeys. Notwithstanding extensive investigation of the function of the nervous system in the intervening years by electrophysiologists in several European countries (Brazier, 1961), it was not until half a century later that Hans Berger (1929) recorded the first human electroencephalogram (EEG) from electrodes on the scalp. Over the ensuing decade he recorded from a wide variety of patients, including many with psychiatric disorders, and evolved an elaborate theory regarding the psychophysiological significance of the EEG. His findings were published between 1929–38, principally as a series of papers in the *Archiv für Psychiatrie und Nervenkrankheiten* ; these are available in an English translation by Gloor (1969). Although Berger took many precautions to avoid contamination of his records by artefacts, his original publications were received with scepticism. It was not until some five years after they first began to appear that Adrian and Matthews, in 1934, obtained confirmation of his findings and by a demonstration to the Physiological Society, ensured their recognition.

The initial reluctance of physiologists to accept Berger's work was in part because of legitimate doubt about the reliability of his technique, which initially consisted of connecting a galvanometer directly between a pair of electrodes either inserted into or placed on the scalp, and in part because of the unfamiliar form of the brain potentials themselves. A galvanometer that is sufficiently sensitive for the indication of heart potentials of the order of a millivolt is not a satisfactory instrument for the examination of brain potentials which may be ten to a hundred times smaller. No electrical amplification was used and the optical system whereby he first recorded the oscillations of a mirror galvanometer on moving film might well have been susceptible to mechanical vibration. Thus some of Berger's early photographic records showed only the merest ripple of allegedly cerebral activity; and while the electrocardiogram and the action potentials of muscle and peripheral nerves were well enough known, the fluctuating rhythmicity and relatively smooth contour of brain potentials had little resemblance to them. Furthermore, the electrical activity of the former bore a distinct relationship to their physiological activity, whereas the rhythms from the brain appeared to be greatest during mental relaxation. These considerations contributed to the general view that Berger's records were artefactual.

The work of Adrian and Matthews (1934 a & b) carried out with the aid of a valve amplifier and pen recorder, left no doubt about the authenticity of Berger's findings which, by the end of 1934, had been repeated by Davis and Jasper in the United States of America. The potentialities of the new technique were then appreciated and workers in several centres began to apply it to the investigation of cerebral disorders. Berger's observation that epileptic seizures were accompanied by major electrical disturbances in the brain was confirmed and Walter (1936) was the first to demonstrate an association between the presence of focal slow waves in the EEG and a cerebral tumour.

Many of these pioneers are actively engaged in EEG work today and would testify that their discoveries have gone hand in hand with the great technological advances that have been made over the last 40 years. Displacement of the thermionic valve by the transistor, has so improved the performance and reduced the bulk of modern equipment that there remain few human conditions and situations in which attempts have not been made to monitor the electrical activity of the brain.

REFERENCES

Adrian, E. D. and Matthews, B. H. C. (1934a). 'The Interpretation of Potential Waves in the Cortex.' *J. Physiol.* **81,** 440
— — (1934b). 'Berger Rhythms: Potential Changes from Occipital Lobes in Man.' *Brain* **57,** 355
Berger, H. (1929). 'Uber das Elektrenkephalogramm des Menschen.' *Arch. Psychiat. NervKrankh.* **87,** 527
Brazier, M. A. B. (1961). *A History of the Electrical Activity of the Brain.* London and New York; Macmillan
Caton, R. (1875). 'The Electric Currents of the Brain.' *Br. med. J.* **2,** 278
Gloor, P. (1969). 'Hans Berger on the Electroencephalogram of Man'. *Electroenceph. clin. Neurophysiol.* Suppl. 28
Walter, W. G. (1936). 'The Location of Cerebral Tumours by Electroencephalography.' *Lancet* **2,** 305

CHAPTER 1

ANATOMY AND PHYSIOLOGY OF THE CEREBRAL CORTEX

In order to understand the origin of the electrical activity which can be recorded from the surface of the head it is necessary to study the structure and function of those cells in the cerebral cortex which are generating the activity. Therefore succeeding parts of this chapter deal with the gross anatomy of the brain, the morphology of typical cortical nerve cells and the different kinds of electrical activity developed by cortical cells. The architecture of the cerebral cortex is described and is followed by accounts of the dynamic interrelationships of cells and of the functional properties of large areas of cortex. Finally, consideration is given to two regions of the brain which are of particular relevance to EEG phenomena—the thalamus and the reticular formation. The various aspects of cortical structure and function are integrated in Chapter 2, which describes the neural mechanisms underlying the EEG.

GROSS ANATOMY OF THE BRAIN

The brain consists of two cerebral hemispheres, the cerebellum and the brainstem; the latter is sub-divided into the midbrain, pons and medulla *(Figure 1.1a)*. Occupying a large central region through-out the length of the brainstem is a diffuse complex of nerve cells and fibres termed the *reticular formation*. In a rostral direction the reticular formation merges with the *thalamus,* which is one of several large clusters of nerve cells *(nuclei)* lying at the base of each cerebral hemisphere *(Figure 1.1b)*. The large inner part of each hemisphere contains only the fibres of nerve cells and therefore appears white; the bodies of the cells are restricted to the outermost 1–4 mm where they form the cerebral cortex. The surfaces of the two hemispheres are indented by a number of fissures *(sulci)* of which the largest are the central (Rolandic) and lateral (Sylvian); the rounded areas of cortex lying between the fissures are termed *gyri*. The fissures have been used to subdivide the cerebral cortex on each side into four lobes—frontal, parietal, occipital and temporal *(Figure 1.1c)*. Running between the two cerebral hemispheres is a large band of nerve fibres termed the *corpus callosum* (CC in *figure* 1.1A).

MORPHOLOGY OF NEURONES

The central nervous system is made up of two types of cell—the nerve cell proper, or *neurone*, and the *glial* cell. The glial cells far outnumber the neurones and provide a structural framework within which the latter are held; they also form myelin coverings for the axons of some neurones. In addition, the close proximity of glial cells to neurones raises the possibility of important metabolic interrelationships. Although glial cells might conceivably contribute to very slow changes in cortical potentials, they do not discharge impulses or show any other evidence of excitability. In the next chapter it will be seen that the EEG can be adequately accounted for in terms of the known behaviour of neurones.

It has been estimated that there are in the region of $2 \cdot 6 \times 10^9$ neurones in the human brain (Pakkenberg, 1966) and that a slab of cortex with a surface area of 1 mm² contains approximately 50,000 (Thompson, 1899). The shapes and sizes of neurones vary enormously but all possess the same anatomical subdivisions *(Figure 1.2)*:

(1) The *soma*, or cell body, contains the nucleus, Golgi apparatus and Nissl substance (RNA). Apart from directing the metabolic activities of the whole neurone, the soma also receives information from other neurones through synapses on its surface.

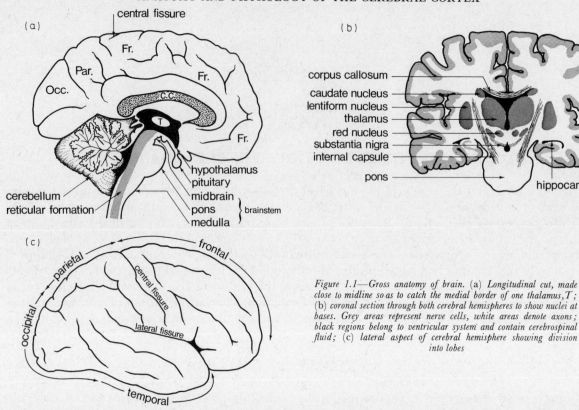

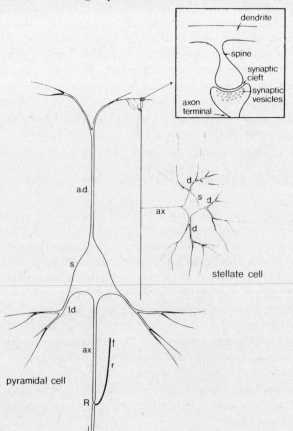

Figure 1.1—Gross anatomy of brain. (a) *Longitudinal cut, made close to midline so as to catch the medial border of one thalamus, T;* (b) *coronal section through both cerebral hemispheres to show nuclei at bases. Grey areas represent nerve cells, white areas denote axons; black regions belong to ventricular system and contain cerebrospinal fluid;* (c) *lateral aspect of cerebral hemisphere showing division into lobes*

(2) The *dendrites* are tapering structures arising from the soma which branch repeatedly; they are specialized for receiving inputs from other nerve cells through numerous synaptic connections.

Figure 1.2—Typical pyramidal and stellate (star) cells, in each case showing division into soma, dendrites and axon; inset shows diagrammatic electronmicrograph of a synapse (see text for dimensions). ax, axon; a.d., apical dendrite; d, dendrite; l.d., lateral dendrite; s, soma; r, recurrent axonal branch; R, node of Ranvier

2

(3) The *axon* is a process for sending impulses to other nerve cells. In some neurones the impulses are initiated at the junction of the axon and the soma—the axon hillock—and are then transmitted along the axon to other nerve cells. Some axons are surrounded by myelin sheaths derived from glial cells and this substantially increases the velocity of impulse propagation. When the axon nears its target cells it divides into many fine branches which form synapses on the soma, dendrites or axons of other cells.

(4) The *synapse* (*Figure 1.2*) is a specialized interface between two nerve cells where the respective membranes are separated by a narrow cleft, typically 200Å wide. The rounded swelling of the axon terminal contains various organelles including synaptic vesicles; these are spherical or ovoid structures some 500Å in diameter which are thought to contain the appropriate chemical transmitter substance.

ELECTRICAL ACTIVITY OF NEURONES

The advent of micro-electrode recording has made it possible to study the electrical behaviour of individual cortical neurones *in situ*; the most detailed information has been obtained by impaling the soma membrane with a micro-electrode and measuring the transmembrane potential with respect to a gross extracellular electrode. It has been found that all neurones possess an appreciable membrane potential at rest and that this can be modulated by excitatory or inhibitory synaptic inputs from other cells. The ionic basis of the membrane potential may now be considered.

RESTING MEMBRANE POTENTIAL

When a neurone is relatively quiescent, receiving minimal synaptic bombardment from other nerve cells, a potential difference exists across its membrane such that the inside of the cell is some 80 mV negative with respect to the outside. This 'resting potential' is a necessary consequence of the differences between concentrations of ions inside and outside the cell. These concentration differences result from two factors:

(1) The negatively charged ions (anions) inside the cell are mainly structural proteins and are not free to diffuse.

(2) The resting membrane is freely permeable to potassium ions (K^+) and chloride ions (Cl^-) but not to sodium ions (Na^+).

The internal anions exert an electrical force which attracts cations into the cell; however, only K^+ can diffuse freely across the membrane and hence their internal concentration is raised. Nevertheless the internal K^+ concentration is not quite sufficient to equalize the internal anions because K^+ tend to leave the cell by diffusing passively down their concentration gradient. The surplus of anions inside the cell is responsible for the internal negativity of the resting potential. Under equilibrium conditions the inward (electrically driven) flow of K^+ balances the outward (chemically driven) one; the potential across the membrane (E_m) is then the potassium 'equilibrium potential' (E_k) and its relationship to the potassium concentrations inside and outside the cell is given by the Nernst equation:

$$E_k = \frac{RT}{F} \log_e \frac{(K_i^+)}{(K_o^+)}$$

where R is the universal gas constant, T is the absolute temperature and F is the Faraday constant; (K_i) and (K_o) are the internal and external concentrations of potassium respectively.

On the outside of the cell Na^+ and Cl^- are the predominant cation and anion.

SYNAPTIC POTENTIALS

In the central nervous system the nerve cell membrane is never completely at rest since it is continually influenced by activity arising in other neurones, with which it has synaptic connections. These influences may be excitatory or inhibitory but, although the final effects on the cell are different, the preliminary stages in synaptic transmission are similar. The most likely sequence of events may be summarized in the following way:

(1) The arriving nerve impulses depolarize the axon terminal.

(2) This depolarization allows calcium ions (Ca^{++}) to enter the axon terminal.

(3) The calcium ions cause many, possibly several hundred, synaptic vesicles to empty their transmitter substance into the synaptic cleft. Each vesicle probably contains several thousand molecules of transmitter substance.

(4) The transmitter molecules rapidly diffuse across the cleft and combine with receptor molecules on the 'postsynaptic' membrane of the dendrite or soma.

The subsequent stages depend on the nature of the transmitter.

(5) If the transmitter is *inhibitory*, it increases the permeability of the membrane for K^+ (and Cl^-) and 'stabilizes' the membrane. If the membrane is already partially depolarized the inhibitory transmitter action temporarily restores it to the resting level; this induced change in membrane potential is termed an *inhibitory postsynaptic potential* (IPSP: *Figure 1.3*).

If the transmitter is *excitatory*, it causes the sodium permeability of the post-synaptic membrane to increase and the membrane potential falls (depolarizes). If the excitatory synapse is on the soma or is situated close to the soma on a dendrite, this depolarization is termed the *excitatory postsynaptic potential* (EPSP; *Figure 1.3*).

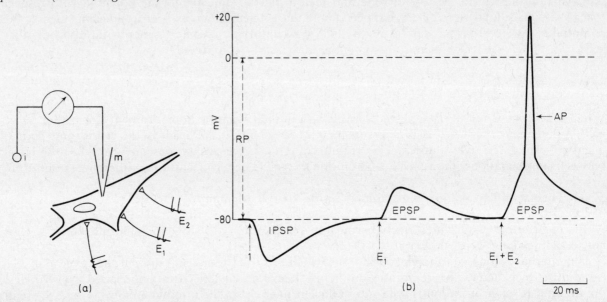

Figure 1.3—(a). *Technique for recording membrane potential from cortical neurone with intracellular micro-electrode* (m) *and extracellular indifferent electrode* (i). E_1 *and* E_2 *represent two groups of excitatory axons; I is an inhibitory group.* (b) *membrane potential of neurone at rest and following stimulation of inhibitory axons* (I), *one group of excitatory axons* (E_1), *and both groups of excitatory axons* ($E_1 + E_2$). RP, *resting potential; AP, action potential; IPSP, inhibitory postsynaptic potential; EPSP, excitatory postsynaptic potential (see text)*

(6) If the excitatory synapse is on a dendrite the depolarization may set up an impulse in the dendrite which propagates relatively slowly (for example, 0·3–0·5 m/s; Cragg and Hamlyn, 1955) towards the soma. The continued passage of the impulse will depend on the presence or absence of impulses in other parts of the dendritic tree. As the dendritic impulse approaches the soma it causes an increasingly large current flow across the membrane of the soma and axon hillock. It has recently been suggested (Diamond, Gray and Yasargil, 1969) that excitatory synaptic transmission will be particularly effective at synapses located on dendritic spines.

(7) If the depolarization of the soma or dendrite is sufficiently large, it causes an action potential to be set up in the axon hillock or soma of the neurone.

(8) The transmitter is hydrolysed by enzymes situated on the postsynaptic membrane and the reaction products enter the axon terminal for recombination.

The account of synaptic transmission given above probably applies to the majority of neurones in the CNS. However, recent experiments have raised the possibility that there may be some situations where synaptic transmission is not mediated by chemicals. Instead, sufficient 'electrotonic' current flows from the axon through the postsynaptic membrane to depolarize the latter. Finally, mention should be made of a second type of inhibition which, although widely present elsewhere in the brain and spinal cord, does not occur in the cerebral cortex and therefore need not be considered in detail. This inhibition takes place at synapses formed between two axon terminals and is termed *presynaptic*.

INITIATION OF ACTION POTENTIALS IN THE AXON HILLOCK

Although the somatic or dendritic membranes are depolarized, the membrane of the axon hillock possesses no synapses and therefore has a membrane potential which is initially at the resting level. The difference in potential between the various parts of the neurone causes current to flow outwards through the membrane of the axon hillock. This membrane has a certain resistance which is inversely related to the ease with which ions cross it (that is, to the membrane permeability). The effect of an outward flow of current across this membrane resistance is to reduce the transmembrane voltage, that is, to depolarize the axon hillock. This depolarization induces an increase in the sodium permeability of the membrane. The increased sodium permeability in turn causes further depolarization, thereby making the system regenerative. If the depolarization is sufficiently large, the sodium permeability increases until the inside of the cell becomes positive with respect to the outside. This reversal of membrane polarity constitutes the action potential (*Figure 1.3*); it lasts only a millisecond or so since the permeability of the membrane alters yet again, the sodium permeability declining and the potassium permeability increasing.

During the action potential a small change in the ionic composition of the neurone takes place. While the membrane sodium permeability is high, Na^+ will enter the cell under the influence of the Na^+ concentration gradient and the internal negativity. Correspondingly, during the ensuing phase of high potassium permeability, K^+ will leave the cell down their concentration gradient. The cell now pumps out the Na^+ in exchange for K^+; energy, derived from the hydrolysis of ATP, must be expended since work is done against the Na^+ and K^+ concentration gradients.

Once the action potential has been initiated in the axon hillock it flows backwards into the soma and, at the same time, starts to travel along the axon. In some cortical cells the action potential may be set up in the soma directly rather than in the axon hillock. The centrifugal conduction of the action potential in the axon depends on the passive outward flow of current across resting axonal membrane which takes place as the action potential approaches. The outward current depolarizes the membrane and induces the regenerative sodium permeability mechanism described above. If the axon is myelinated the flow of current through the membrane is restricted to the nodes of Ranvier; the action potential travels more rapidly than in a non-myelinated axon. In the largest axons of the dorsal spinocerebellar tract impulse velocities of 160 m/s have been recorded (Grundfest and Campbell, 1942); the maximal values in the other myelinated tracts are considerably lower than this, for example, 70 m/s for pyramidal axons in the cat spinal cord (Lance, 1954). If, as in many axons in the CNS, there is no myelin sheath, the conduction velocities are unlikely to exceed 1–2 m/s. Finally it is possible that, as in the retina, some cells with short axons transmit activity to their axon terminals by a passive flow of electrotonic current rather than by setting up impulses.

SYNAPTIC TRANSMITTER SUBSTANCES

Certain substances have now been provisionally identified as transmitters at synapses in the CNS. The evidence has come from observations on the distribution within the brain and spinal cord of either the suspected transmitter itself or of its synthesizing and hydrolyzing enzymes. In addition, the activities of single nerve cells have been studied following the application of the transmitter through a micropipette. Another approach has been to look for changes in spontaneous or evoked neuronal discharges after pharmacological blockade with the antagonist of the suspected transmitter. Lastly, in some situations it has been possible to collect the substance released from stimulated neurones. The following compounds are currently regarded as likely transmitters.

(1) Excitatory Transmitters

(a) *Acetylcholine (ACh)*. This substance has been conclusively identified as the transmitter released at synapses between motoneurones and Renshaw cells in the ventral horn of the spinal cord. It is probably involved in transmission through certain 'specific' thalamic nuclei (for example, VPM, VPL, VL, LG in *Figure 1.12*) and in the caudate nucleus. In the cortex ACh excites cells in layer V, particularly in the sensory areas and motor cortex. ACh is also released during EEG 'activation' induced by stimulation of the reticular formation (Kanai and Szerb, 1965).

(b) *L-glutamic and L-aspartic acid*. These amino-acids are distributed widely in the brain and spinal cord; they excite cells by a depolarizing action.

(2) Inhibitory Transmitters

There is good evidence that γ-amino-butyric acid (GABA) is an inhibitory transmitter in the nervous systems of invertebrates and it is likely that it has a similar role in the mammalian brain. The substance occurs in high concentrations in the brain and, when applied iontophoretically or topically, depresses neural activity. Recent intracellular recordings from cortical cells have shown that this inhibition is associated with hyperpolarization of the membrane, as in naturally occurring IPSPs. In the spinal cord evidence is accumulating that glycine acts as an inhibitory transmitter substance.

(3) Other Transmitters

Three monoamines are secreted by cells in the brainstem and are also thought to act as transmitters; they are dopamine, noradrenaline and 5-hydroxytryptamine. The influence of these substances on membrane excitability is less well understood than in the case of the transmitters considered above. Amongst other possible locations, dopamine has been found to occur in the substantia nigra, noradrenaline in the medullary reticular formation and 5-hydroxytryptamine in the raphe nuclei.

D.C. POTENTIALS

Under normal circumstances there is a steady (or d.c.) potential across the thickness of the cerebral cortex such that the surface is some 5–20 mV positive with respect to electrically indifferent areas (Bures, 1957). It is probable that this potential results mainly from a steady potential difference between the apical dendrites and somas of the pyramidal cells. Thus intracellular recordings from pyramidal cells, for example, during experimentally induced seizures, reveal 'slow changes' (that is, lasting several seconds) in transmembrane potential which are in phase with alterations in the transcortical d.c. potential (Sugaya, Goldring and O'Leary, 1964). It is possible that the glial cells also contribute to shifts in d.c. potential since they have been shown to undergo slow changes in membrane potential; these result from the extracellular accumulation of potassium ions released by discharging neurones (Orkand, Nicholls and Kuffler, 1966). Although individual glial cells are too small to act as effective dipoles, a series of glial cells orientated radially to the cortical surface might do so. Differing from the conditions in neurones, the areas of contact between glial cells are characterized by low electrical resistances which would allow appreciable current to flow from one cell to another. In addition to epilepsy, the d.c. cortical potential is reduced during anoxia, anaesthesia and the 'spreading depression' of Leão (1944). In this last condition, which results from any form of severe cortical damage, it has now been shown that there is a marked depolarization of neurones as the depression advances over the cortex (Collewijn and van Harreveld, 1966).

ARCHITECTURE OF THE CEREBRAL CORTEX

In the cerebral cortex the cell bodies are either conical, star or spindle shaped; accordingly the cells are classified as pyramidal, stellate and spindle respectively. Each *pyramidal cell* (*Figures 1.2 and 1.6*) possesses a long apical dendrite which usually reaches almost to the surface of the cortex; in comparison the lateral dendrites are relatively short. The synaptic connections are made either on the shafts of the dendrites or on protruding spines and a single cell may have several thousand synapses on its total area of membrane. Initially the axons run from the cell bodies perpendicular to the cortical surface; subsequently they may end in deeper parts of the cortex or they may turn back to innervate more superficial cells, or they may bifurcate to do both. Such axons are relatively short, a few millimetres at most, but others may leave the cortex altogether and the longest of these terminate in the lumbosacral cord.

The morphology of the *stellate cells* (*Figures 1·2 and 1·6*) is less consistent. They usually have small somata around which the dendrites branch repeatedly; most axons are short and terminate on neighbouring cells in the cortex.

The *spindle cells* have dendrites at each extremity of the spindle; the axons may leave the cortex, or less frequently, project superficially.

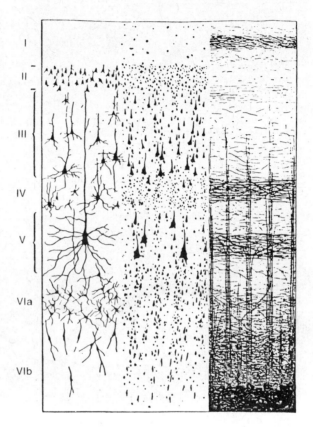

Figure 1.4—Diagram of structure of the cerebral cortex. Left: *from a Golgi preparation;* centre: *from a Nissl preparation;* right: *from a myelin sheath preparation.* I, *plexiform layer;* II, *external granular layer;* III, *pyramidal layer;* IV, *internal granular layer;* V, *ganglionic layer;* VI, *multiform layer*

(From Brodal (1969) by courtesy of the author and Oxford University Press, after Brodmann and Vogt)

The cells and fibres (axons and dendrites) of the cortex appear to be arranged in six layers (*Figure 1.4*).

(I) The most superficial, or *plexiform layer*, is characterized by abundant fibres running 'horizontally' (that is, parallel to the surface of the cortex) and contains very few cells.

(II) The *external granular layer* is composed of small cells, both pyramidal and stellate, which are packed tightly together.

(III) The *pyramidal layer* is made up of medium sized pyramidal cells.

(IV) The *internal granular layer*, like the outer granular layer, contains numerous small cells which are mainly stellate; there is also a dense band of horizontal fibres.

(V) The *ganglionic layer* is characterized by the largest pyramidal cells in the cortex.

(VI) The *multiform layer* is composed of spindle cells.

This six-layered pattern is a feature of the greater part of the cerebral cortex (neocortex) but is absent from a small area in the medial part of the hemisphere (allocortex). In this latter region, which includes the *hippocampus*, the cortical architecture appears less complex; for example, the pyramidal cell bodies are restricted to a single layer. The simplified structure of the hippocampus has been used to advantage in neurophysiological studies for it has allowed potentials recorded with micro-electrodes to be interpreted with some confidence.

Although the six-layered pattern is common to most areas of cortex a number of regional variations are evident. Thus in the motor cortex the pyramidal bodies in layer V are unusually large (*Betz cells*) while a prominent band of horizontally running fibres in layer IV distinguishes the striate cortex.

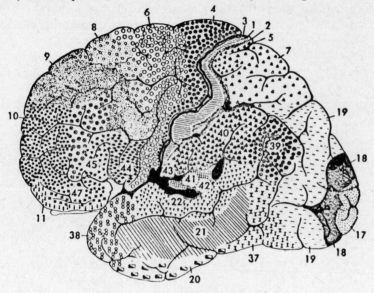

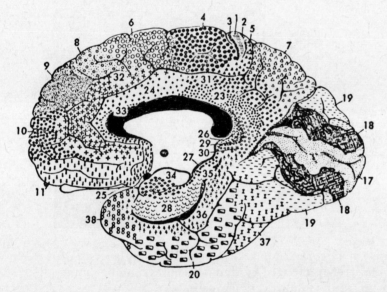

Figure 1.5—Brodmann's cytoarchitectural map of the human brain showing lateral and medial aspects of cerebral hemisphere (upper and lower figures respectively). The various areas have been assigned numbers and labelled with different symbols

(From Brodal (1969) by courtesy of the author and Oxford University Press, after Brodmann)

In the scheme proposed by Brodmann (1909) some 52 different cortical areas are identified (*Figure 1.5*). Although there have been arguments concerning the validity of such schemes recent neurophysiological experiments have demonstrated functional differences between some of the adjacent areas. Furthermore, the Brodmann scheme is now widely used as a topographical reference for anatomical and physiological studies and will be referred to subsequently.

COLUMNAR ORGANIZATION

In addition to the horizontal lamination described above, there is also evidence that the cells and fibres exhibit an intimate structural organization in columns (that is, in an axis perpendicular to the cortical surface). This organization is suggested by three features, namely:

(1) The cell bodies lie one above the other so as to form columns.

(2) The longest dendrite of each pyramidal cell, the apical dendrite, runs perpendicular to the cortical surface.

(3) The axons and recurrent branches of most pyramidal and stellate cells project in a vertical axis to deeper, or to more superficial, layers of the cortex. Incoming axons also run vertically before terminating.

CONNECTIONS OF CORTICAL CELLS

An account has now been given of the arrangements of cells within the cortex and of the potentials which the cells generate; the present section describes the probable sequence of neural activity in the cortex following different types of input. These inputs may be derived from other areas of cortex or from subcortical structures. So far as the former are concerned, axons are received from the corresponding region of the opposite hemisphere via the corpus callosum (callosal fibres) and from other cortical areas in the same hemisphere (association fibres). Of the subcortical structures the thalamus is especially important since it passes on to the cortex information received by way of all the sensory pathways, with the exception of the olfactory path. It also handles important inputs from other subcortical structures including the reticular formation, cerebellum and basal ganglia. The thalamus itself will be considered more fully later but, from a cortical standpoint, it is convenient to recognize two groups of thalamic nuclei:

(1) *Specific nuclei*, each of which projects to a relatively circumscribed region of cortex of the ipsilateral hemisphere.

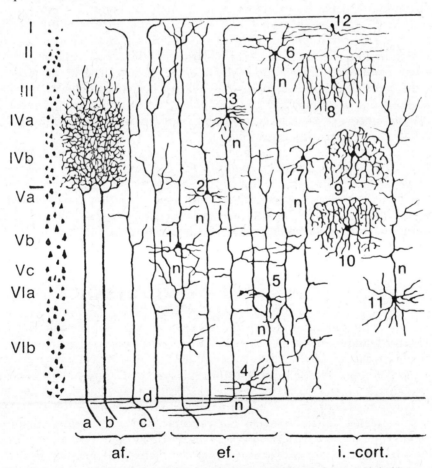

Figure 1.6—A very simplified diagram of different types of neurones in the cerebral cortex, with dendrites, axons and collateral axonal branches af, afferent axons from specific thalamic nuclei; (a,b), non-specific thalamic nuclei (c) and association areas (d); ef, neurones sending their axons out of cortex; cell 1 projects to subcortical structures, cells 2–5 to association areas; note that cell 4 is a spindle cell and remainder are pyramidal; i-cort, cells, mostly stellate, whose axons terminate within cortex.

(From Brodal (1969) by courtesy of the author and Oxford University Press, after Lorente de Nó)

(2) *Nonspecific nuclei*, each of which ultimately projects to an extensive area of the ipsilateral cortex and sometimes of the contralateral cortex as well.

The projections from the specific and non-specific thalamic nuclei differ in another way for, whereas the nonspecific axons are distributed to all layers of the cortex, the specific axons end exclusively in layer IV (*Figure 1.6*). Although the specific thalamic input is directed mainly to cells in layer IV it is also able to influence directly cells lying more deeply; this excitatory influence is executed through synapses on apical dendrites which extend through layer IV on their way to the cortical surface. In contrast to the thalamic inputs the majority of commissural and association axons terminate in layers II and III.

Once an input has gained access to the cortex, the information contained within the message of nerve impulses is processed by the cortical neurones. The business of processing is transacted in a vertical axis, that is between cells lying in columns perpendicular to the surface of the cortex. Within the columns certain directions of synaptic transmission are evident. Whereas cells in layer IV can influence those in all other layers, the projection of cells in layers II and III is largely restricted to layers V and VI. The cells in layers V and VI are 'output' cells responsible for sending processed information away from the columns of cells; however, they also modulate the activity of superficial cells through recurrent branches of their axons. Among the cells activated by these recurrent branches are neurones which feed inhibition back on to the output cells and in the hippocampus they have been identified as *basket cells*; each basket cell has been estimated to influence approximately 400 pyramidal cells.

The output from the cortical columns is sent to other cortical areas as well as to subcortical nuclei. By analogy with the input, commissural axons pass through the commissures to the corresponding area of the opposite hemisphere, while association axons carry information to other regions within the same hemisphere. Behavioural studies of various species in which the corpus callosum has been sectioned suggest that in 'lower' animals (for example, the cat) the corpus callosum is used to replicate permanently in one hemisphere information which has been acquired in the other. In primates, including man, this wasteful duplication does not occur; instead, whenever the need arises, the corpus callosum allows one hemisphere to gain temporary access to information stored in the other (Sperry, 1964). Of the subcortical structures the thalamus receives a very large input from the cortex; in general each thalamic nucleus which projects to the cortex receives fibres from the same cortical area. Other fibres are sent to the basal ganglia (caudate nucleus, putamen, globus pallidus, subthalamic nucleus and substantia nigra), cerebellum (via the pontine nuclei), red nucleus, reticular formation and optic tectum. The cortical fibres proceeding to the spinal cord form an important anatomical landmark on the ventral aspect of the brain stem since they are collected into two large bundles abutting the midline. These bundles are the *medullary pyramids* and the cortical cells from which the fibres originate are accordingly referred to as pyramid tract (PT) cells. In man there are about one million fibres in each pyramid.

REGIONAL CORTICAL NEUROPHYSIOLOGY

Now that cortical functioning has been described at a cellular level, the organized activities of whole cortical areas may be considered. Largely on the basis of neurophysiological studies three types of cortical area have been distinguished. These functional subdivisions of the cortex are not absolute; thus somatic evoked potentials can be recorded from 'motor' cortex and movements may be elicited by stimulation of somatic 'sensory' cortex. These observations are not altogether surprising since during natural behaviour, as opposed to experimental situations, the motor and sensory functions of the nervous system are closely interwoven. For example, the perception of shape and texture is achieved by carefully running the tips of the fingers over the object in question. Nevertheless, although the functioning of one area of cortex is probably never completely independent from that of all other areas, some regions are particularly concerned with one type of activity. It is upon these differences in emphasis that the following scheme for subdividing the cortex into areas depends.

(1) *Motor areas* are those in which relatively weak electrical stimulation produces movements of the body; in the human brain there are at least two, and possibly three, such areas in each hemisphere.

(2) *Sensory receiving areas* (somatic, auditory, visual, olfactory and gustatory). These are regions of

cortex from which the largest and earliest evoked potentials can be recorded following stimulation of the appropriate sensory pathway. Some of the sensory modalities project to more than one cortical area; accordingly primary, secondary and even tertiary receiving areas are recognized.

(3) *Association areas*. These areas are not concerned with the immediate reception of sensory data or with programming movements. Consequently they are regarded as dealing with the 'higher' domains of mental activity such as the integration of incoming sensory information from various sources and the checking of this new information against that previously acquired. In addition some parts of the association cortex are involved with the complex cerebral activities necessary for speech while others are closely associated with emotional responses. It is probable that 'consciousness' normally results from the collective properties of all the cortical areas as well as of subcortical structures.

MOTOR AREAS

The primary motor area occupies the precentral gyrus (Brodmann area 4 and part of 6) together with the floor and posterior wall of the central sulcus; it also extends on to the medial aspect of the hemisphere (*Figure 1.7*). The nature and magnitude of the movements evoked by stimulation within

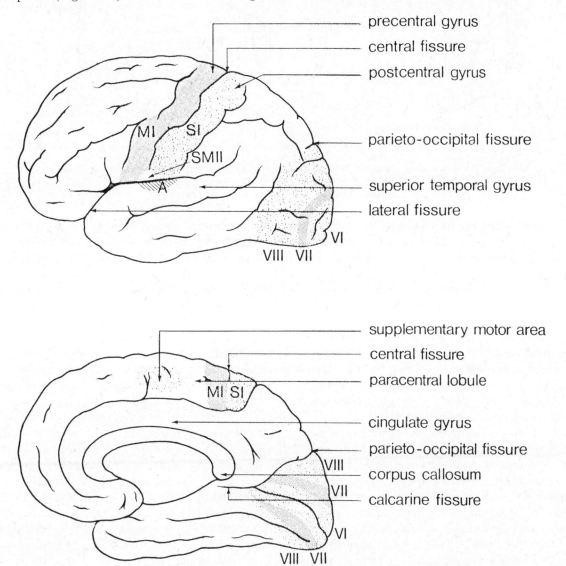

Figure 1.7—Lateral and medial aspects of cerebral hemisphere to show motor and sensory areas. S, somatosensory; A, auditory; V, visual; M, motor; primary, secondary and tertiary areas indicated by roman numerals. Remainder of hemisphere comprises association areas

11

this area depend to a large extent on such factors as the type and level of anaesthesia, the form of electrical stimulation, and the initial position of the limbs. Nevertheless, when relatively weak stimuli are employed sufficient to cause slight contractions only, it is found that movements on the opposite side of the body are represented in an orderly sequence within the motor area (*Figure 1.8*). This representation is inverted; thus the leg occupies the paracentral lobule on the medial aspect of the

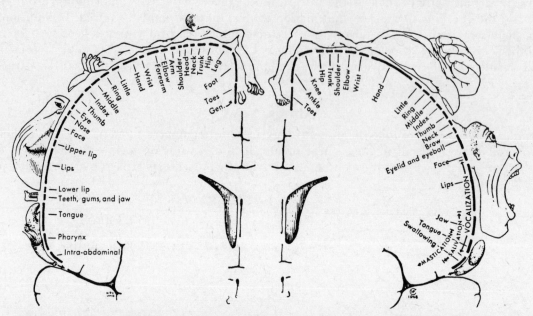

Figure 1.8—Diagram showing (left) the projection of the contralateral body surface on to the primary somatic sensory area in man (postcentral gyrus). On the right is the corresponding representation of movements in the primary motor cortex (precentral gyrus). The maps are based on the responses of unanaesthetized patients to electrical stimulation of the exposed cortex. Note the different extents of cortex allotted to various parts of body and the inverted representations.

(From Penfield and Rasmussen (1950) by courtesy of the authors and Macmillan)

hemisphere while the foci for the face and mouth reach the lateral fissure (Penfield and Rasmussen, 1950). The regions devoted to the mouth and to the fingers are particularly large and presumably reflect the importance and complexity of speech and manual skills within the spectrum of daily activities.

The main outflow of axons from the motor area to motoneurones is through the pyramidal tract (PT). In the cat the PT axons end on interneurones in the spinal grey matter and influence the motoneurones indirectly. In primates and presumably in man the PT axons may terminate directly on a-motoneurones, particularly those of flexor muscles. The PT cells are not functionally homogeneous, for only those with fast-conducting axons actively engage in the preparation for voluntary movement (Evarts, 1965); in contrast, those with slowly conducting axons are tonically active and cease firing when movement is anticipated. The PT cells are organized in colonies; thus each a-motoneurone in the cord and brain stem can be excited by a certain number (*colony*) of cortical cells and the colonies for different motoneurones overlap (Landgren, Phillips and Porter, 1962). Even repetitive stimulation of PT axons does not produce sufficiently large excitatory postsynaptic potentials (EPSP) to cause motoneurones to discharge. This finding implies that the PT cells normally act in conjunction with other descending pathways (reticulospinal, rubrospinal, vestibulospinal and tectospinal); of these the cortico-rubro-spinal projection appears to be especially important in man (Brodal, 1969). In addition it is now known that during voluntary contraction stretch reflexes are active and, by driving the a-motoneurones, may have an extremely important role in the final control of movement. It is therefore relevant that stimulation of the motor cortex has been shown to activate γ-motoneurones (Mortimer and Akert, 1961); by causing the intrafusal muscle fibres to contract, the γ-motoneurones are able to adjust the sensitivity of muscle spindles to stretch. Although the primary area is the largest and most important one, two other motor areas are also known. The *supplementary motor area* is situated on the medial aspect of the frontal lobe anterior to the primary area; the face is represented anteriorly and the leg posteriorly. The *secondary motor area* lies within the lateral fissure where it is co-extensive with the secondary somatic sensory area; the details of its somatotopic organization have not yet been elucidated in man.

The exact role of the cortical motor areas in the genesis of movement is far from clear. It is a common clinical observation that a patient who has suffered an infarction of the motor areas following thrombosis of the middle cerebral artery during the night may be perplexed to find, on waking, that he is unable to move his arm to switch off the alarm clock. It appears that the very first phase in the institution of movement, the formulation of the 'desire' to move, has not been impaired by the cortical lesion. It is probable that the 'desire' is conceived by subcortical structures. Thus Parkinson's disease, in which the primary lesion is thought to involve the substantia nigra, is characterized by a marked poverty of willed movement which is dramatically overcome by administration of L-dopa (the precursor of the brain transmitter substance, L-dopamine). Of the other subcortical nuclei closely connected with the early stages of movement the lateroventral (VL) nucleus of the thalamus is likely to be especially important in view of its strong projection to the motor cortex. Recent micro-electrode studies in man have demonstrated that some VL cells have a generalized alerting role and fire when movement of any part of the body is attempted while other cells may only be concerned with flexion or extension of a single joint (Crowell *et al.*, 1968). If the motor cortex is not involved with the 'desire' to move, the extensive topographical representation of movements render it well equipped to undertake the detailed 'programming' of motoneurones. This programming activity is probably continued and elaborated within the spinal cord since within its grey matter lie systems of interneurones to ensure that contraction of one group of muscles is associated with relaxation of others. This integrative potentiality of the human brain stem and spinal cord has been well documented in studies of an anencephalic child, aged several months, who was possessed of a considerable repertoire of reflex movements (Gamper, 1926).

Somatic Sensory Areas

The largest somatic sensory receiving area is the *primary area* (SI, *Figure 1.7*) situated in the postcentral gyrus (Brodmann areas 3, 1 and 2). In man it has been studied both by stimulation of exposed cortex in conscious patients (Penfield and Rasmussen, 1950) and by recording evoked potentials either directly from the cortical surface or through the scalp. The feelings evoked by stimulation are those of tingling, numbness, tickling and pressure, though not pain; with threshold stimuli patients are able to localize sensations to small sharply defined regions on the opposite side of the body. The main pathway to SI is from the dorsal column and trigeminal nuclei via the VPL and VPM thalamic nuclei respectively (*see* page 18). The primary area resembles the adjacent primary motor area in three major respects. Firstly, it is concerned with events on the opposite side of the body; secondly, the body has inverted representation and thirdly, the representation is distorted due to the large areas of cortex devoted to sensations from the hand and face. This emphasis on the hand and face is not a new neural development imposed by the cortex but simply reflects the large numbers of neurones at all levels in the somatosensory pathways (that is, receptors, cord, brainstem and thalamus) which are concerned with these particularly important areas.

The information arriving at SI comes predominantly from receptors which are sensitive to mechanical displacements and are situated in the skin and deep tissues. Very little mixing of the outputs from the different types of receptor takes place as the information is passed through the various sensory nuclei on its way to the cortex (*Figure 1.9*). On the other hand the neurones within these nuclei are subjected to inhibitory influences from populations of interneurones (that is, cells with short axons). This inhibition is of the *surround* type. It reduces the number of neural elements required to carry information onwards by restricting impulse activity to the neural channels excited most strongly by the peripheral stimulus. In this way contrast between the centrally stimulated and surrounding regions of skin is enhanced within the sensory message (*Figure 1.10*). It appears that inhibition of the surround type is a general property of sensory systems, since it has also been demonstrated in the visual and auditory pathways (*see Figure 1.11*). In the somatic sensory system it is well developed in the dorsal column and the trigeminal nuclei and to a lesser extent in SI but is largely absent from the thalamus.

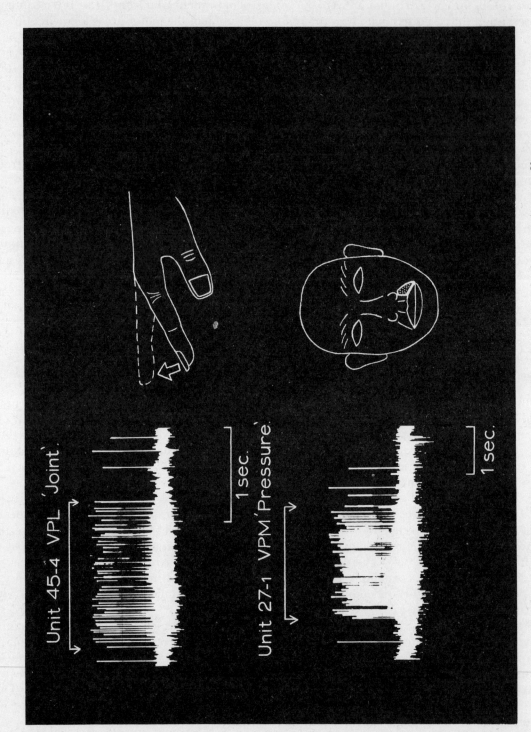

Figure 1.9 — Two thalamic somatosensory neurones investigated in patients undergoing stereotaxic surgery. Upper: 'joint' unit in VPL which discharges briskly when the metacarpophalangeal joint of the contralateral index finger is extended. Lower: cutaneous unit in VPM which responds to pressure above upper lip. In each case the appropriate stimulus is maintained during that portion of the trace indicated by arrows

(From McComas, Wilson and Hankinson, unpublished observations)

Within the SI area each vertical column of cells receives information from a certain type of receptor within a restricted 'receptive field' on the body surface (Powell and Mountcastle, 1959). Since the receptive fields of neighbouring columns overlap, stimulation of a single point on the skin will activate

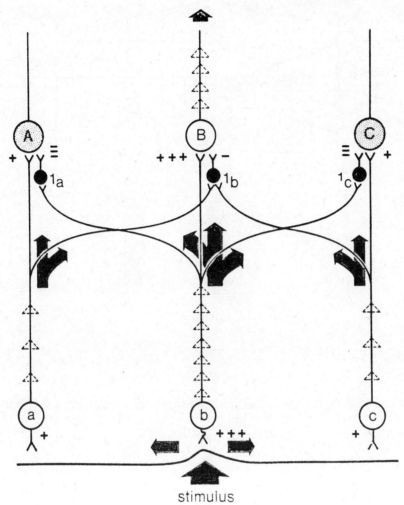

stimulus

Figure 1.10—Surround inhibition in the somatic sensory system. At the bottom of the figure the skin has been indented by a tactile stimulus, causing maximal excitation in the neighbouring mechanoreceptor (b). The impulses, indicated by broken-line triangles, travel centrally and cause strong postsynaptic excitation of the second-order neurone B. Through the axonal branches of (b) the inhibitory interneurones 1_a and 1_c will also be strongly excited and will put powerful inhibition on to the second-order neurones A and C. However, A and C will only receive weak excitation from their corresponding mechanoreceptors (a and c) which are some distance from the stimulus. Hence the combination of weak excitation and strong inhibition prevents A and C from firing. The net result is that whereas 3 mechanoreceptor axons were originally excited by the stimulus, only 1 second-order axon (B) conveys the message onwards; the spatial contrast in the sensory message has been enhanced

several columns of cortical cells. While the columns in area 3 receive information from superficial cutaneous receptors, those in area 2 are excited only by deep receptors (such as those in joints and fascia).

The *secondary somatic area* (SII), lies within the lateral fissure. Although much smaller than SI it receives information from cutaneous receptors on both sides of the body.

Among the outputs from SI and SII is a powerful projection through the pyramidal tract to the various subcortical somatosensory nuclei (dorsal horn, dorsal column and trigeminal nuclei, VPM and VPL of thalamus) where the descending axons form excitatory connections with inhibitory interneurones. It is possible that this pathway enables the cortex to improve the spatial contrast of

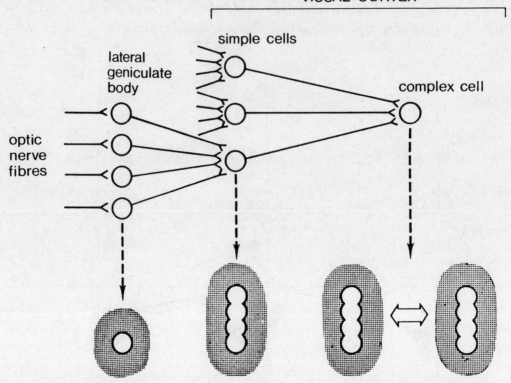

Figure 1.11—Retinal receptive fields of neurones at different levels in the visual pathway. The fields are shown at the bottom of the figure; light falling on the central (white) areas of the retina causes excitation of cells and light falling on the surrounding (shaded) areas causes inhibition. Note how the fields become progressively more complex by changing from a circular to a linear pattern (see text); this is due to convergence of one group of cells upon another, as indicated at top of figure

incoming somatic messages by accentuating surround inhibition. On the other hand overwhelming inhibition might serve to suppress somatic information entirely in favour of rival claims for cortical attention from other sensory modalities (Hernández-Peón, 1959).

VISUAL AREAS

The contralateral visual field is represented in triplicate within the occipital lobe (*see Figure 1.7*). The *primary visual area* (VI) is also known as the *striate cortex* on account of the prominent band of horizontally running fibres in layer IV. It corresponds to Brodmann's area 17 and is situated around the calcarine fissure on the medial aspect of the hemisphere. The central (macular) area of the contralateral visual field is projected posteriorly and lies at the pole of the occipital lobe. The *second* and *third visual areas* (VII and VIII; areas 18 and 19 respectively) are referred to as the *prestriate cortex* and surround area 17 in concentric fashion; they include large areas of the lateral aspect of the occipital lobe and VIII encroaches on to the temporoparietal cortex. All three visual areas receive fibres from the lateral geniculate (LG) body, which itself takes the bulk of the retinal output; in addition VI projects to VII which in turn activates VIII. It has been estimated that each LG axon has the opportunity to establish synaptic connections with 5000 cortical cells (Sholl, 1956). Stimulation of any of the visual areas in conscious patients usually gives rise to simple sensations such as flashes, spots and stars of light which are sometimes coloured (Penfield and Rasmussen, 1950). More complex sensations, for example those of people or objects, have been reported during excitation of prestriate cortex (Foerster, 1929).

The evoked potentials generated in the three visual areas by pulses of light are easily recorded in man through the scalp and are described in a later chapter. Recordings from single cells in cats and monkeys have led to an understanding of the way in which visual information is sequentially analysed within the cortex (Hubel and Wiesel, 1962). For each of the cells studied a map was made of the areas within the visual field in which illumination caused excitation or inhibition of the cell. These studies have shown that whereas LG cells are concerned with circular areas of light and shade, cells in VI are activated maximally by linear patterns—bars of light or shade, and edges (*Figure 1.11*). Moreover, each cortical cell responds best to a certain critical orientation of the linear stimulus within the visual field. The critical orientation is the same for all cells in a cortical column—further evidence of the importance of vertical connections between cells. Within columns, three functional types of cells can be differentiated. *Simple cells* are those which are only excited when the linear pattern occupies a relatively small area of the visual field. In contrast, *complex cells* are activated by similar patterns occupying any position within a larger area of the visual field. A third type of neurone, the *hypercomplex cell*, has even more elaborate stimulus requirements. The simple, complex and hypercomplex cells are thought to reflect successive integrative stages in visual processing as information is passed from VI to VII and thence to VIII.

The preoccupation of the cortical cells with straight borders between light and shade has been made use of in human evoked-potential studies. In these experiments a chequer-board pattern of alternate light and dark squares is presented. Reversal of the pattern, so that light squares become dark and vice versa, causes appreciable evoked potentials even though the total light energy falling on the retina remains the same.

Outside the three visual areas lies another cortical region which is concerned with visual processing at an even higher level; this is the inferior convexity of the temporal lobe. Ablation studies in monkeys (Klüver and Bucy, 1937) have shown that this region is required for the correct interpretation of visual information in regard to previous experience; without this area the significance of information received by the visual areas is lost.

AUDITORY AREAS

The primary auditory area (AI) is situated in a small region of the superior temporal gyrus (Brodmann area 41) which is buried in the lateral fissure (*see Figure 1.7*). In patients, electrical stimulation of this area produces simple sensations such as clicks, ringing, humming and buzzing (Penfield and Rasmussen, 1950). Potentials evoked by auditory stimuli can be detected on the scalp but their amplitudes are small, possibly due to the deep location of AI. Within the primary area, different frequencies of sound are represented in an orderly sequence. Thus individual cortical cells respond maximally to a certain frequency which is similar for all the cells in a vertical column. Some cells are concerned with the more complex sounds, such as rising and falling notes (Whitfield and Evans, 1965).

From studies on animals it appears that the primary area is only one of several cortical regions receiving auditory information from the medial geniculate bodies. Little is known about these secondary areas in man although they apparently include the frontal and parietal operculum (Celesia *et al.*, 1968).

ASSOCIATION AREAS

The association areas are those regions of cortex remaining after subtraction of the sensory and motor areas. They include the frontal lobe anterior to the motor areas (misleadingly called the 'prefrontal' cortex), most of the temporal lobe and the large area of parietal lobe behind the postcentral gyrus (*see Figure 1.7*). These areas are difficult to investigate since, unlike the regions considered so far, their responses to various kinds of peripheral input and the sensations evoked by direct cortical stimulation are complex and very susceptible to the conditions of the experiment, particularly the choice of anaesthetic. Only with anaesthetics such as chloralose or in unanaesthetized brains can evoked potentials be recorded from these areas; the responses are characterized by relatively long latencies and variability. Another quality of the responses is their lack of specificity; thus a single cell in an association area may be excited by a flash of light, a click or a tap on the skin. It is clear that these cells are equipped to integrate information received from the various sensory pathways. Some of this information will be received from the sensory receiving areas through association fibres but there is also another very important input from the non-specific thalamic nuclei.

17

Apart from integrating the continuous flow of information from the various sensory receptors, these areas are required to interpret these new data in the light of previous experience. One region especially concerned with the interpretation of visual data has already been mentioned; this is the inferior convexity of the temporal lobe. This lobe appears to be particularly important for memory since Penfield and Rasmussen (1950) found that electrical stimulation of the superior temporal gyrus conjured up scenes or incidents from the past. Ablation experiments in animals together with surgical and pathological studies in patients suggest that, within the temporal lobe, the hippocampus plays an important role in the initial 'laying-down' process of memory.

The interpretive properties of the parietal lobe are evident from the various agnostic syndromes associated with discrete injuries to this part of the brain. In these syndromes there may be a lack of awareness of part of the body even though the sensory areas are still informed. Sometimes there may be an inability to consider an object in terms of its structure or to use numbers. If the dominant cerebral hemisphere is involved, various disturbances of speech appear. Thus a lesion in the parietotemporal cortex may prevent the understanding of speech, either spoken or written. Damage to part of the frontal lobe (*Broca's area*) causes another type of speech impairment in which words conceived normally cannot be expressed correctly, even though there is no weakness of speech muscles. Other parts of the frontal lobe, particularly the cingulate gyrus and orbital cortex, seem to be especially concerned with mood and behaviour, as evidenced by the effects of prefrontal leucotomy.

THE THALAMUS

The importance of the thalamus in relation to cortical function has already been stressed and several thalamic nuclei have been mentioned. These nuclei were all 'specific' since they projected to relatively small areas of the ipsilateral cerebral hemisphere; they comprised the following:

Medial geniculate body (MGB) projecting to auditory area I.
Lateral geniculate body (LGB) to visual areas I, II and III.
Medial posteroventral nucleus (V.PM), to the somatic regions in SI and SII representing the face.
Lateral posteroventral nucleus (VPL), to the somatic areas representing the trunk and limbs.
Lateroventral nucleus (VL), to the primary motor area (MI).
Because these nuclei have prominent fibre pathways leading to them and discrete outflows to the

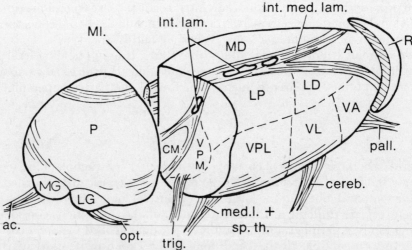

Figure 1.12—Diagram of a three-dimensional reconstruction of the right human thalamus seen from the dorsolateral aspect. The posterior part is separated from the rest by a cut to display some features of the internal structure. Only the rostral tip of the reticular nucleus is included. The main afferent inputs to some of the major nuclei are indicated. The abbreviations for the thalamic nuclei are those derived from the Latin nomenclature, as follows: A, anterior; CM, centromedian; Int. lam, intralaminar; LD and LP, dorsolateral and posterolateral; LG and MG, lateral and medial geniculate bodies; MD, dorsomedial; Ml, midline; P, pulvinar; R, reticular; VA, anterior ventral; VL, lateroventral; VPL and VPM, lateral and medial posteroventral. Abbreviations for fibres; ac, accoustic; opt, optic; trig, trigeminal; med 1, medial lemniscus; sp.th, spinothalamic; pall, pallidal; cereb, cerebellar

(From Brodal (1969) by courtesy of the author and Oxford University Press)

18

cortex, they have been the easiest to investigate and consequently most is known about them. Three less understood nuclei may be added to the 'specific' list to complement the account of cortical neurophysiology given above. These are the *pulvinar*, which projects to the temporoparietal cortex and is possibly concerned with speech mechanisms, the *dorsomedial nucleus* (MD), which sends fibres to the orbital cortex of the frontal lobe, and the *posterolateral nucleus* (LP), which supplies the parietal association area.

In contrast to these specific nuclei, stimulation of the *non-specific nuclei* activates large areas of the ipsilateral cortex and sometimes the contralateral cortex as well. The largest of these nuclei in man is the *centromedian* (CM) and others include the *parafascicular nucleus* (Pf), the *nuclei of the midline* and *anterior ventral nucleus* (VA). The pathways linking the non-specific nuclei to the cerebral cortex are not known since only VA appears to have direct connections. It is possible that the other non-specific nuclei make synaptic relays in VA or else use some other route, as yet unknown.

As knowledge of the thalamus increases, a more detailed and satisfactory functional classification of the nuclei should be possible. For example, it now appears that the *reticular nucleus* (R) feeds inhibition back on the various specific nuclei which it covers, and therefore cannot be categorized as specific or non-specific.

The positions of the different nuclei within the thalamus are shown in *Figure 1.12;* in general the non-specific nuclei lie medially and centrally and are surrounded by the specific nuclei.

THE RETICULAR FORMATION

The reticular formation is a large complex of nerve cells and fibres which occupies the central region of the entire brain stem (that is, midbrain, pons and medulla). Within the diffuse entanglements of cells and fibres certain features of structural organization are evident. For example, whereas the neurones with large cell bodies are situated in the medial two-thirds of the reticular formation, the smaller cells lie laterally; in some areas the cells are clustered together to form recognizable nuclei. The *axons* of the reticular cells run considerable distances in the long axis of the brain stem. Most of the rostrally situated cells project caudally while the caudal cells send axons rostrally; many axons bifurcate and run in both directions. Throughout the brain stem the axons give off branches to innervate the various cranial nerve nuclei. Ascending axons terminate in the 'non-specific' thalamic nuclei, the hypothalamus, the caudate and lentiform nuclei. Descending axons run in the ventral and lateral columns of the cord before ending on interneurones in the anterior horns.

In contrast to the axons, the *dendrites* of the reticular cells are arrayed in planes perpendicular to the long axis of the brain stem. They receive information concerning all the different modalities of sensation through the following connections:

Spinoreticular tract (from the skin and deep tissues of limbs and trunk).

Nucleus of spinal trigeminal tract (from tissues of the face).

Cochlear nuclei (hearing).

Vestibular nuclei (balance).

Superior colliculi and optic tectum (vision).

Fornix: it is possible that the fornix conveys information about smell.

In addition, the reticular cells accept inputs from the sensory and motor areas of the cortex as well as from the globus pallidus and hypothalamus.

The varied input connections to the reticular formation enable some cells to respond to widely differing forms of stimulation—clicks, flashes of light or pressure on the skin; presumably such cells perform an integrative function. Conversely, the extensive connections of individual reticular axons would permit the reticular cells to co-ordinate neural activity in large areas of brain. Among the specific functions of reticular neurones is the control of cortical excitability, which will be dealt with in the next chapter. Other reticular neurones are involved in the regulation of the cardiovascular and respiratory systems, and in the control of muscle tone and movement. Possibly because of the complex polysynaptic pathways within its structure, the reticular formation is particularly sensitive to anaesthetics and other metabolic agents.

REFERENCES

General reviews

Brodal, A. (1969). *Neurological Anatomy in Relation to Clinical Medicine.* 2nd ed. London; Oxford University Press

Curtis, D. R. (1969). 'Central Synaptic Transmitters'. In *Basic Mechanisms of the Epilepsies*, pp. 105–129. Ed. by H. H. Jasper, A. A. Ward Jr. and A. Pope. London; Churchill

Eccles, J. C. (1964). *The Physiology of Synapses.* Berlin; Springer

Katz, B. (1966). *Nerve, Muscle and Synapse.* New York; McGraw-Hill

Lorente de No, R. (1949). 'Cerebral Cortex: Architecture, Intracortical Connections, Motor Projections'. In *Physiology of the Nervous System* (Fulton), 3rd ed. pp. 288–312. New York; Oxford University Press

Mountcastle, V. B. (1968). *Medical Physiology*, 12th ed., Volume 2, ch. 59, 60, 62, 65, 68. St. Louis; Mosby

Penfield, W. and Rasmussen, T. (1950). *The Cerebral Cortex of Man.* New York; Macmillan

Original papers

Brodmann, K. (1909). *Vergleichende Lokalısatıonslehre der Grosshirnrinde.* Leipzig; Barth

Bures, J. (1957). 'The Ontogenetic Development of Steady Potential Differences in the Cerebral Cortex in Animals'. *Electroenceph. clin. Neurophysiol.* **9,** 121

Celesia, G. G., Broughton, R. J., Rasmussen, T. and Branch, C. (1968). 'Auditory Evoked Responses from the Exposed Human Cortex'. *Electroenceph. clin. Neurophysiol.* **24,** 458

Collewijn, H. and van Harreveld, A. (1966). 'Membrane Potential of Cerebral Cortical Cells during Spreading Depression and Asphyxia'. *Exp. Neurol.* **15,** 425

Cragg, B. G. and Hamlyn, L. H. (1955). 'Action Potentials of the Pyramidal Neurones in the Hippocampus of the Rabbit'. *J. Physiol.* **129,** 608

Crowell, R. M., Perret, E., Siegfried, J. and Villoz, J. P. (1968). ' "Movement Units" and "Tremor Phasic Units" in the Human Thalamus'. *Brain Res.* **11,** 481

Diamond, J., Gray, E. G. and Yasargil, G. M. (1969). 'The Function of Dendrite Spines: an Hypothesis'. *J. Physiol.* **202,** 116P

Evarts, E. V. (1965). 'Relation of Discharge Frequency to Conduction Velocity in Pyramidal Tract Neurons'. *J. Neurophysiol.* **28,** 216

Foerster, O. (1929). 'Beiträge zur Pathophysiologie der Sehbahn und der Sehsphäre'. *J. Psychol. Neurol., Lpz.* **39,** 463

Gamper, E. (1962). *Z. Neurol. Psychiat.* **102,** 154; **104,** 49. Cited by Jung and R. Hassler in *Handbook of Neurophysiology* **3,** ch 35. Ed. by J. Field. Washington; American Physiological Society

Grundfest, H. and Campbell, B. (1942). 'Origin, Conduction and Termination of Impulses in the Dorsal Spino-cerebellar Tract of Cats'. *J. Neurophysiol.* **5,** 275

Hernández-Peón, R. (1959). 'Reticular Mechanisms of Sensory Control'. In *Sensory Communication*, pp. 497–520. Ed. W. A. Rosenblith. Cambridge, Mass; M.I.T. Press

Hubel, D. H. and Wiesel, T. N. (1962). 'Receptive Fields, Binocular Interaction and Functional Architecture in the Cat's Visual Cortex'. *J. Physiol.* **160,** 106

Kanai, T. and Szerb, J. C. (1965). 'Mesencephalic Reticular Activating System and Cortical Acetylcholine Output'. *Nature, Lond.* **205,** 80

Klüver, H. and Bucy, P. C. (1937). 'Psychic Blindness and Other Symptoms Following Bilateral Temporal Lobectomy in Monkeys'. *Am. J. Physiol.* **118,** 352

Lance, J. W. (1954). 'Pyramidal Tract in Spinal Cord of Cat'. *J. Neurophysiol.* **17,** 253

Landgren, S., Phillips, C. G. and Porter, R. (1962). 'Cortical Fields of Origin of the Monosynaptic Pyramidal Pathways to some Alpha Motoneurones of the Baboon's Hand and Forearm'. *J. Physiol.* **161,** 112

Leão, A. A. P. (1944). 'Spreading Depression of Activity in the Cerebral Cortex'. *J. Neurophysiol.* **7,** 359

Mortimer, E. M. and Akert, K. (1961). 'Cortical Control and Representation of Fusimotor Neurons'. *Am. J. Phys. Med.* **40,** 228

Orkand, R. K., Nicholls, J. G. and Kuffler, S. W. (1966). 'The effect of Nerve Impulses on the Membrane Potentials of Glial Cells in the Central Nervous System of Amphibia'. *J. Neurophysiol.* **29,** 788

Pakkenberg, H. (1966). 'The Number of Nerve Cells in the Cerebral Cortex of Man'. *J. comp. Neurol.* **128,** 17

Powell, T. P. S. and Mountcastle, V. B. (1959). 'Some Aspects of the Functional Organisation of the Cortex of the Postcentral Gyrus of the Monkey: a Correlation of Findings Obtained in a Single Unit Analysis with Architecture'. *Bull. Johns Hopkins Hosp.* **105,** 133

Sholl, D. A. (1956). *The Organisation of the Cerebral Cortex.* London; Methuen

Sperry, R. W. (1964). 'The Great Cerebral Commissure'. *Scient. Am.* **210,** 42

Sugayo, E., Goldring, S. and O'Leary, J. L. (1964). 'Intracellular Potentials Associated with Direct Cortical Response and Seizure Discharge in the Cat'. *Electroenceph. clin. Neurophysiol.* **17,** 661

Thompson, H. B. (1899). 'The Total Number of Functional Cells in the Cerebral Cortex of Man'. *J. comp. Neurol.* **9,** 113

Whitfield, I. C. and Evans, E. F. (1965). 'Responses of Auditory Cortical Neurons to Changing Frequency'. *J. Neurophysiol.* **28,** 655

CHAPTER 2

THE NEURAL BASIS OF THE EEG

NEUROPHYSIOLOGICAL MECHANISMS

Many mechanisms have been proposed to account for the repetitive slow potentials that can be recorded from the surface of the brain or from the scalp. An adequate explanation depends on knowledge of the following:

(1) The identities of the cells generating the electrical potentials.

(2) The type of electrical potential involved.

(3) The neural network determining the frequency and variation in amplitude of the potentials.

(4) The neural mechanisms responsible for modifying the potentials when the excitability of the brain is altered.

Since Berger's original description of the EEG it has generally been assumed that the EEG results from the electrical activity of cells in the cerebral cortex, although this is questioned by Lippold (1970). It has long been known that certain areas of the brainstem and thalamus exercise powerful influences on cortical activity but it was only with the advent of intracellular recording using micro-electrodes that the changes in cell membrane potential responsible for the EEG could be studied adequately. Although it is true that most of the experimental observations have been made on anaesthetized animals, it is probable that barbiturate spindles are produced by neural mechanisms similar to those responsible for the *alpha* rhythm. At the present time there is good agreement about the nature of these neural mechanisms though many important details require clarification. Before the pertinent experimental observations are cited, the neurophysiological basis of the EEG may be summarized conveniently in the following manner.

(1) The repetitive waves which can be recorded from the surface of the brain or from the scalp are summated synaptic potentials generated by the pyramidal cells in the cerebral cortex.

(2) The synaptic potentials are the responses of the cortical cells to rhythmic discharges from thalamic nuclei.

(3) The frequencies and sizes of the thalamic discharges (and hence of the cortical potentials) are determined by the special arrangements of excitatory and inhibitory interconnections among thalamic cells.

(4) During 'activation', inputs from the reticular formation abolish the rhythmic discharges in the thalamic nuclei and cause the cortical potentials to become desynchronized.

CELLS GENERATING EEG POTENTIALS

The three types of cell found in the cerebral cortex have already been described and classed as stellate, spindle or pyramidal. A consideration of the respective cell structures and of cortical architecture indicates that of the stellate, spindle and pyramidal cells, only the pyramidal cells are likely to contribute to slow waves recorded over the surface of the cortex. Thus, since EEG recording electrodes are large and distant from the cell potential generators, they will only detect the summed activities of large numbers of adjacent dipoles disposed in the same axis. The pyramidal cells are the only ones uniformly orientated (perpendicular to the cortical surface) and with dendrites long enough to form effective dipoles. Dusser de Barenne and McCulloch (1938) showed that the deeper pyramidal cells were especially important since slow wave activity persisted even if superficial layers of the cortex were destroyed by heat. Finally, direct evidence of pyramidal cell involvement has been obtained from intracellular recordings of characteristic synaptic potentials.

Electrical Activity Responsible for Cortical Slow Waves

In the next section it will be seen that EEG potentials result from the flow of current in the extracellular fluid surrounding nerve cells. It has already been shown that the nerve cell membranes exhibit several types of activity.

(1) Propagating dendritic potentials.

(2) Non-propagating somatic and dendritic postsynaptic potentials (excitatory and inhibitory).

(3) Action potentials of axon hillock and soma.

(4) Action potentials of axon.

It is unlikely that activity in *axons or fine dendrites* can contribute substantially to surface waves. The reason in both cases is that the narrow diameters of the structures impose considerable internal resistance to the flow of ionic current; hence the potentials developed extracellularly are small. Compelling evidence that axons are relatively unimportant in the genesis of the EEG was obtained by Bartley and Bishop (1933). In experiments on rabbits the vagus nerve was excised and laid in a groove cut on the surface of the cerebral cortex. Maximal stimulation of the nerve evoked propagated action potentials which were barely detectable by large electrodes on the surface of the cortex.

In contrast to the axons and fine dendrites, the extracellular potential developed during the soma (and axon hillock) action potential is relatively large. However, the duration of the soma action potential 'spike' is brief (for example, 0·3 ms) and perfectly synchronous firing amongst adjacent cells is unlikely; consequently there is little chance of the extracellular potentials summing effectively at the surface of the cortex. Furthermore, in animal experiments it is still possible to record spontaneous cortical waves when the anaesthetic dose is large enough to prevent the initiation of action potentials in cortical cells (Li and Jasper, 1953). For these reasons it is unlikely that soma action potentials make an important contribution to surface waves. All the available evidence suggests that these waves result from excitatory or inhibitory postsynaptic potentials developed by the soma and larger dendrites. The low internal resistances of these structures ensure that the extracellular potentials will be correspondingly large and the slow time courses of the postsynaptic potentials permit summation with those of other cells. It is also possible that propagating dendritic potentials will contribute to the surface waves,

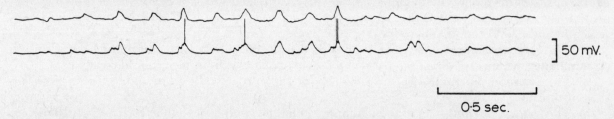

]50 mV.

0·5 sec.

Figure 2.1—Simultaneous recording from cortical surface (upper trace) and underlying cortical neurone (lower trace; intracellular recording)

(Modified from Creutzfeldt, Watanabe and Lux, (1966) *Electroenceph. clin. Neurophysiol.* **20**, 24, by courtesy of the authors and Elsevier)

especially when the larger dendrites are invaded. In conclusion, intracellular recordings strongly favour postsynaptic potentials as being responsible for surface waves. It has been found in many cortical neurones that repetitive postsynaptic potentials exhibit a close time relationship with potentials recorded on the surface of the overlying cortex (*Figure 2.1; see* also Jasper and Stefanis, 1965; Creutzfeldt, Watanabe and Lux, 1966).

Location of the EEG Pacemaker

The question next arises as to whether the repetitive postsynaptic potentials in the pyramidal cells are evoked by discharges from other cortical cells or from a subcortical pacemaker. One experimental approach has been to study the electrical activity in a slab of feline cortex which has been neurally isolated by cutting fibre connections to all other regions of the brain. Such unanaesthetized slabs remain viable since they receive an adequate blood supply through pial vessels and they can still respond to direct electrical stimulation. Unfortunately, conflicting observations have been made on such slabs for whereas Burns (1951) recorded no spontaneous potentials whatsoever, other workers have reported the occurrence of background activity, including spindles (Kristiansen and Courtois,

1949; Andersen and Andersson, 1968). From this last work it would appear that the cortex does contain neural networks which can generate spontaneous rhythms. On the other hand, two observations suggest that the cortical networks are normally driven by an external pacemaker. Firstly, it has already been seen that spontaneous waves can still be recorded when cortical impulse activity, and therefore intracortical driving, has been abolished by anaesthesia. Secondly, if the thalamus is removed on one side by suction it is found that spontaneous spindles are abolished for several hours in the ipsilateral hemisphere (Kristiansen and Courtois, 1949).

These last observations strongly suggest that some other part of the brain is normally responsible for driving the slow wave activity in the cortex. Bremer (1935) showed by a simple but very meaningful experiment that the site of the pacemaker lay above the brain stem. He found that if the midbrain of a cat was completely transected, the spontaneous electrical activity that could be recorded from the unanaesthetized cerebrum (cerveau isolé) was dominated by slow waves. Soon afterwards, Dempsey and Morison reported a highly original series of investigations in which the non-specific thalamic nuclei were identified as the probable pacemaker region for the EEG. In their initial study (Dempsey,

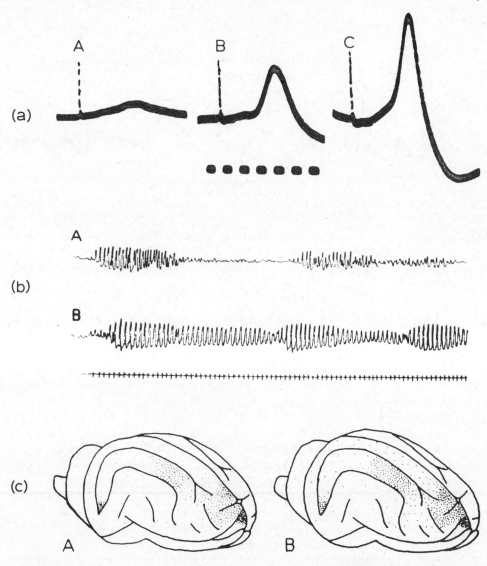

Figure 2.2—(a) *Recruiting responses in cat association cortex following successive stimuli at 8 per second* (A, B, C) *to non-specific thalamic nuclei. Time trace: 10 ms intervals. Nembutal anaesthesia;* (b) *similarity of spontaneous 8–12 Hz barbiturate spindle* (A) *and recruiting responses in same area of cat cortex* (B). *Notice waxing and waning of potentials in both records;* (c) *map of cat cortex showing distribution of recruiting response* (A) *and of spontaneous 8–12 Hz rhythms* (B)

(Figures (a) and (c) are from Morison and Dempsey (1942) *Am. J. Physiol.* **135,** 288, 289; Figure (b) is from Dempsey and Morison (1942). *Am. J. Physiol.* **135,** 297, by courtesy of the American Physiological Society)

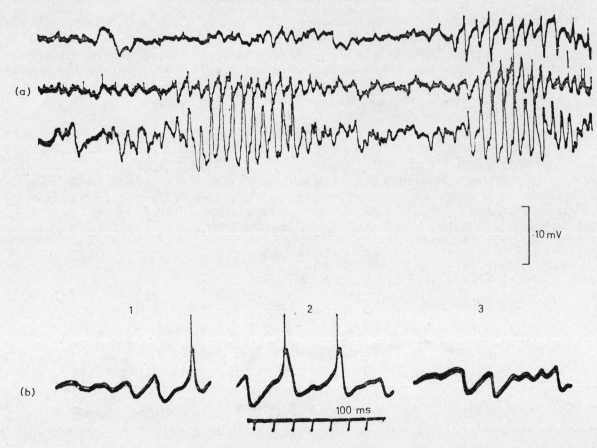

Figure 2.3—(a) Correlation between spindle activity in the thalamus and cortex. The top two traces are from medial and lateral thalamic nuclei respectively while the lower trace is from cortical area to which the lateral thalamic nucleus projects. During the first spindle (left) there is good correspondence between discharges in lateral thalamic nucleus and cortex; the medial thalamic nucleus is silent. In the second spindle (right) both thalamic nuclei discharge suggesting that excitation may have spread within the thalamus from the lateral to the medial thalamic nuclei

Figure 2.3—(b) Intracellular recording from cat thalamic neurone during barbiturate spindle showing alternating excitatory and inhibitory postsynaptic potentials (upward and downward deflections of oscilloscope trace respectively). Records are taken at start (1), in middle (2), and at end of spindle (3)

(a) from Andersen, Andersson and Lømo (1967), J. Physiol. **192,** 289; (b) from Andersen and Sears (1964), J. Physiol. **173,** 469, by courtesy of the authors and Cambridge University Press

Morison and Morison, 1941) these workers stimulated the central end of the cut sciatic nerve in the cat and recorded an early response in the primary somatosensory (SI) cortical area followed by a secondary (non-specific) response which was widely distributed over both hemispheres. They then made lesions in various parts of the thalamus to delineate the neural pathway responsible for the secondary response and were able to establish that the 'specific' somatosensory thalamic nucleus (VPL) was not involved.

Subsequently Dempsey and Morison (1942 a, b; Morison and Dempsey, 1942) found that electrical stimulation of the non-specific thalamic nuclei evoked cortical potentials which had the same form and distribution as the secondary responses. The amplitude of these responses to successive stimuli fluctuated in a characteristic manner. While the first response was small, subsequent ones became progressively larger; accordingly Dempsey and Morison termed these potentials *recruiting responses* (*Figure 2.2a*). If the stimulation was continued the potentials declined in amplitude. This waxing and waning of responses strongly resembled the spontaneous EEG spindle activity that could be recorded in the same animal under barbiturate anaesthesia (*Figure 2.2b*). Furthermore the recruiting responses were largest in those regions of cortex displaying the most prominent EEG spindles, the association areas (*Figure 2.2c*). It was also noted that good recruiting responses could be obtained only when a spindle was about to begin. This last observation, together with the similarities in appearance and cortical distribution of the recruiting responses and EEG spindles, suggested that the two types of activity were using the same neural pathway, that is, the non-specific nuclei. Further suggestive evidence that these nuclei were involved in the genesis of EEG activity was that, like the cortex, they exhibited spontaneous runs of potentials which waxed and waned and could be time-locked to corresponding waves in cortical spindles (Morison, Finley and Lothrop, 1943; *see also Figure 2.3a*). More recently it has been shown by intracellular recording that the waves in these thalamic spindles are alternating excitatory and inhibitory postsynaptic potentials (Andersen and Sears, 1964; *Figure 2.3b*).

Andersen and Sears (1964) have suggested a neural circuit which would account for the frequency and for the waxing and waning of the thalamic waves *within* a thalamic nucleus (*Figure 2.4*). In this scheme a small number of the thalamic neurones projecting to the cortex (thalamocortical relay or TCR cells) develop EPSPs elicited by background synaptic bombardment from other sites. The impulses discharged by a cell such as E in the first column of *Figure 2.4* will activate an inhibitory inter-

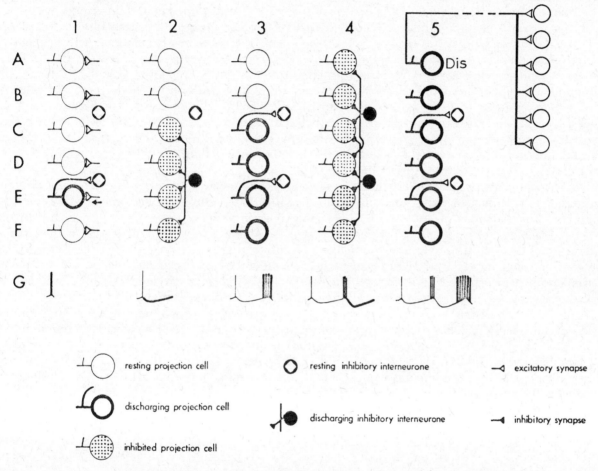

Figure 2.4—*Diagrammatic representation of the neural events during the initiation of a thalamic spindle; note the key role of the inhibitory interneurones in 'phasing' the discharges (see text). Notice also how distributor neurone (Dis) transmits spindle activity to other parts of thalamus*

(Modified from Andersen and Sears (1964) *J. Physiol.* **173,** 475, by courtesy of the authors and Cambridge University Press)

neurone. This interneurone then inhibits a relatively large number of TCR cells, including C, D and F (*Figure 2.4, column 2*) which had not developed a previous EPSP and impulse. All these TCR cells (namely C, D, E and F) now become silent during the large IPSP evoked by the inhibitory interneurone. As the IPSP declines, the same cells become hyperexcitable due to a fundamental biophysical property of nerve membranes (as in postanodal exaltation). Once more the TCR cells, now including the C, D and F fraction, respond to background excitation and develop EPSPs (*Figure 2.4, column 3*). The discharge of cell C activates an additional postsynaptic inhibitory neurone so that an even larger fraction of the TCR pool is now inhibited (cells A, B, C, D, E and F in column 4). Subsequently all these cells (A–F) discharge and the process continues; each time, the number of discharging thalamic cells increases. After a certain number of cycles the thalamic activity declines, possibly because the discharges of the TCR cells begin to lose synchronicity. The length of each cycle in the spindle will be the combined durations of an EPSP and an IPSP (approximately 100 ms). This periodicity corresponds to a frequency of 10 Hz, which is within the *alpha* range (8–13 Hz). Andersen (1966) has recently shown that a computer model of the thalamus, embodying recurrent axonal branches to postsynaptic inhibitory interneurones, can generate synchronized activity which waxes and wanes. Andersen and Andersson (1968) suggest that the synchronization of spindle activity between different thalamic nuclei is brought about by *distributor cells*; these cells have very long axons which extend from one nucleus to another (Dis, *Figure 2.4*).

The impulses set up in the thalamic cells during an EPSP will trigger EPSPs in the cortical cells to which they are linked. A large thalamic discharge will excite a correspondingly large number of cortical neurones and elicit a good sized surface wave. It has already been seen that the axons from the non-specific thalmic nuclei terminate in all layers of the cortex. An arrangement of this kind would cause the apical dendrites of pyramidal cells to depolarize throughout their entire length and would account for the negativity recorded at the cortical surface during the recruiting responses and EEG spindles. If the EPSPs evoked in the deep pyramidal cells are large, they will initiate action potentials and these, in turn, will activate cortical inhibitory interneurones through collateral axonal branches. The inhibitory interneurones will then feed postsynaptic inhibition back on to the deep cortical cells. As the IPSP dies away it will be succeeded by an EPSP evoked by the next thalamic discharge and the cycle is repeated. When the cortical pyramidal cells discharge during each phase of the spindle they will influence, amongst other cells, the thalamic pacemaker neurones. Nevertheless, the returning cortical volleys are not essential for thalamic rhythmicity since thalamic cells still fire repetitively after the cortex has been ablated (Adrian 1941, 1951).

The routes taken by the non-specific thalamic axons to the cortex are largely unknown, for only the anterior ventral nucleus (VA) has so far been shown to have a direct projection. It is possible that impulses from the remaining non-specific nuclei may relay in VA or in some other subcortical structure before reaching the cortex. A polysynaptic path of this kind would account for the rather longer latencies of the recruiting responses compared with those of the 'specific' responses. One subcortical region that may be involved in EEG phenomena is the anterior hypothalamus since low frequency stimulation here produces slow cortical waves together with other physiological manifestations of sleep (Hess, 1944, 1954). A second possibility is that the non-specific thalamic nuclei influence the specific nuclei, which in turn exert control over the cortical areas to which they project. Thus, stimulation of non-specific thalamic nuclei evokes alternating EPSPs and IPSPs in specific thalamic nuclei (Purpura and Cohen, 1962). The importance of the specific nuclei as the link between the non-specific thalamic nuclei and the cortex is particularly stressed by Andersen and Andersson (1968). In addition, these workers have experimental evidence that, on occasion, a specific nucleus may develop an autonomous rhythm which is then imparted to the cortex and to the remainder of the thalamus. According to Andersen and Andersson any part of the thalamus, specific or non-specific, has the capacity to act as a pacemaker (faculative pacemaker theory; *Figure 2.3*).

Normally, *alpha* or *beta* spindles can be recorded from the surface of the brain only during relaxation with the eyes closed or during drowsiness or barbiturate anaesthesia. If the relaxed subject opens his eyes or undertakes mental activity the *alpha* rhythm is replaced by fast irregular activity of small amplitude, that is, the recorded potentials have become desynchronized. A similar change occurs if strong sensory stimulation is given to a drowsy or lightly anaesthetised animal. In each of these situations the transition is associated with physiological evidence of awakening of the person or animal and since the cerebral cortex has presumably become more excitable, the phenomenon is termed 'activation' of the EEG. Because of their relationship to 'consciousness' the neural mechanisms involved in activation have been the subject of intensive study. One of the earliest and most important investigations was that of Bremer (1935). He observed that if the rostral brain stem of a cat was transected, the EEG activity of the isolated cerebral hemispheres (cerveau isolé) was characterized by repetitive slow waves. However, if the transection was made at the junction of the spinal cord and medulla (encéphale isolé) the cortical activity was desynchronized. Clearly some structure in the brainstem was necessary for activation of the cortex. Soon afterwards, Magoun and his colleagues (Lindsley *et al.*, 1950) identified the activating region with the *reticular formation*. They showed that, in an otherwise intact cat, a lesion in the reticular formation caused the animal to become somnolent and to develop rhythmic cortical activity (*Figure 2.5a*). In distinction to this finding, a lesion made outside the reticular formation, so as to interrupt the important lemniscal somatosensory pathways, did not have this retarding effect on the animal's behaviour nor did it cause synchronization of the EEG. In a

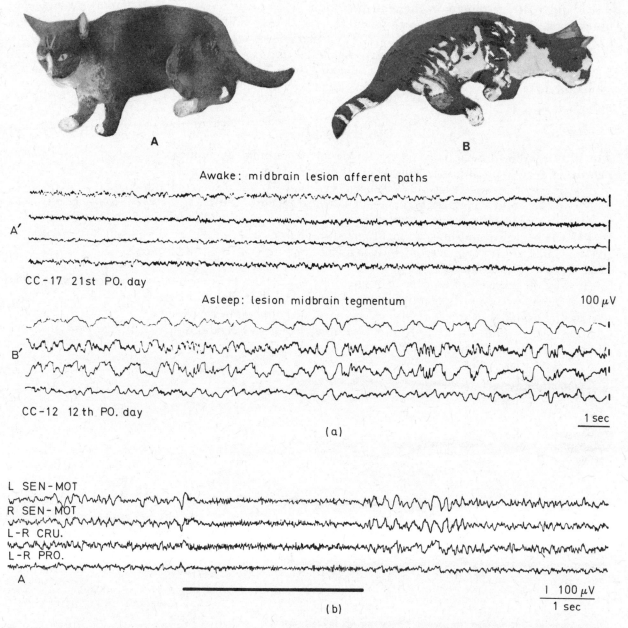

Figure 2.5—(a) *Animal with interruption of sensory paths in the midbrain, sparing central tegmentum, standing awake* (A), *with strip of characteristic waking EEG* (A′). *Animal with lesion in mesencephalic tegmentum lying asleep* (B), *with characteristic strip of sleeping EEG* (B′). *In A the reticular formation is intact but in B it will have been interrupted*

(From Lindsley, Schreiner, Knowles and Magoun (1950), *Electroenceph. clin. Neurophysiol.* **2**, 496, courtesy of the authors and Elsevier)

(b) *Effect of stimulation of medullary reticular formation on EEG activity in cat anaesthetized with chloralose (encéphale isolé preparation, see text). The period of stimulation is shown by the heavy line underneath record; it can be seen that the large slow waves in the EEG are replaced by low voltage fast activity*

(Modified from Moruzzi and Magoun (1949) *Electroenceph. clin. Neurophysiol.* **1**, 456, by courtesy of the authors and Elsevier)

different type of experiment Moruzzi and Magoun (1949) found that stimulation of the reticular formation produced activation of the EEG under light barbiturate anaesthesia (*Figure 2.5b*). These crucial experiments have been confirmed and it appears that the activating region is situated in the mesencephalic part of the reticular formation; in contrast, stimulation of the bulbar or lower pontine regions produces synchronization of the EEG. Since the reticular formation receives inputs from all the sensory pathways, almost any form of powerful stimulation will activate the EEG.

The pathway taken by the reticular axons involved in activation is not altogether clear although many apparently terminate in the non-specific thalamic nuclei. Within the thalamus the reticular fibres evoke excitatory postsynaptic potentials and block inhibitory ones (Purpura *et al.*, 1966). Consequently there is desynchronization of the thalamocortical relay cells and hence of the cortex itself. Other reticular fibres run to the hypothalamus and it is therefore of considerable interest that lesions of the *posterior hypothalamus* are associated with hypersomnia (von Economo, 1929) while stimulation of this area produces activation (French, Amerongen and Magoun, 1952).

ROLE OF EEG RHYTHMS

Are EEG rhythms functionally important or merely 'idling' phenomena of thalamic and cortical neurones? Several possible functions deserve consideration.

Level of consciousness.—It has already been seen that sleep is associated with repetitive slow wave activity at the cortical surface. It is possible that this synchronization of the EEG simply results from loss of adequate sensory stimulation during the unconscious period. On the other hand it is conceivable that slowly repeated and highly synchronized discharges and inhibitory periods in large masses of thalamic and cortical cells actively induce unconsciousness.

Modulation of evoked cortical potentials.—The cortical activity evoked by sensory stimulation is markedly affected by the presence or absence of on-going EEG activity. This interaction is reflected both in the form of the surface-evoked potential and in the discharges of individual neurones (Bindman, Lippold and Redfearn, 1964). Rather surprisingly it has proved difficult to demonstrate behavioural correlates with the *alpha* rhythm. Thus Walsh (1952) was unable to show a relationship between *alpha* rhythm and the reaction time to a visual stimulus, although later work has indicated the presence of a slight effect

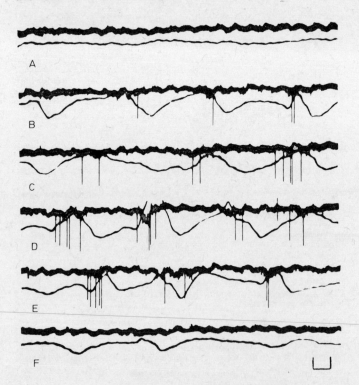

Figure 2.6—Correlation between spontaneous spindle waves and spike discharges of pyramidal tract. A: Simultaneous records from pyramidal decussation (upper) and motor cortex (lower) during inter-spindle period. B: Beginning of spindle waves and pyramidal spikes. C, D, E: During spindle. F: End of spindle, beginning of interspindle period. Horizontal bar = 50 ms, vertical bars = 50 μV (waves)

(From Whitlock, Arduini and Moruzzi (1953), *J. Neurophysiol.* **16**, 418, by courtesy of the authors and the American Physiological Society)

(Lansing, 1957; Callaway, 1962). Again, it has not been possible to demonstrate any correlation between visual pattern recognition and the *alpha* rhythm (MacKay, 1953).

Memory.—Andersen and Andersson (1968) suggest that spontaneous spindles, initiated in the thalamus and imparted to the cortex, are essential for learning processes. These authors envisage that the repeated activation of cortical neurones in each spindle renders more permanent any changes which occur at cortical synapses during the acquisition of recent sensory data. As a corollary, the thalamic spindle generators could also act as a 'readout system' by selectively activating areas of cortex in which the appropriate information is stored.

Descending influences.—In 1939 Adrian and Moruzzi noted that there was a discharge of impulses down the pyramidal tracts during each cycle of a barbiturate spindle in anaesthetized cats; an example of this corticofugal activity is given in *Figure 2.6*. Although the destination of these pyramidal tract impulses is not known, it is conceivable that during natural sleep they are involved in the suppression of sensory or motor activity in the spinal cord and brain stem (Morrison and Pompeiano, 1965 a, b).

DEVELOPMENT OF EXTRACELLULAR POTENTIALS

In *Figure 2.7* a pyramidal cell has been represented in terms of its two largest structural features—the soma, S, and the apical dendrite, D. At rest, the membrane of the entire cell is uniformly polarized, the inside being some 80 mV negative with respect to the outside (*Figure 2.7a*). Let us now suppose that

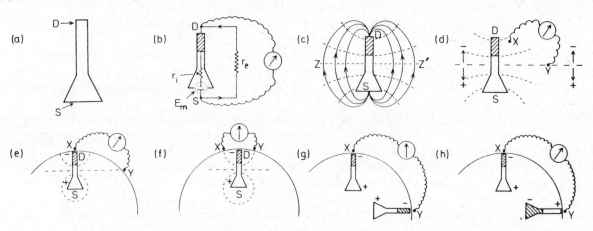

Figure 2.7—a–h, genesis of potentials around a pyramidal cell in which the apical dendrite is depolarized. See text for explanation of figure

an excitatory input causes the extremity of the apical dendrite to depolarize completely, that is, the membrane potential becomes zero. The pyramidal cell will now behave as a *dipole*—an elongated structure with a potential difference across its ends. Since both the cell protoplasm and the extracellular fluid contain diffusible ions, current will flow between the normally polarized soma ('source') and the depolarized apical dendrite ('sink') (*Figure 2.7b*). By Ohm's law, the magnitude of this synaptic current (I) will be directly proportional to the membrane potential at S (E_m) and inversely proportional to the sum of the internal (protoplasmic) resistance r_i and the external (extracellular fluid) resistance r_e; the membrane resistances are small in comparison and can be ignored.

That is,
$$I = E_m/(r_i + r_e)$$

The distribution of potentials between S and D will also depend on the internal and external resistances.

Thus the potential E_{SD} (measured with two extracellular electrodes) $= E_m \times r_e/(r_i + r_e)$.*

The current between S and D will travel widely within the volume of fluid surrounding the cell and can be represented diagrammatically in *Figure 2.7c* (continuous lines). Since the shortest extracellular path has the least resistance, the current density will be greatest in the immediate vicinity of the cell.

---

*Note if r_i is large, as in a fine dendritic branch, then E_{SD} will be small; therefore activity in very fine dendrites contributes little to the EEG. Notice also that these simple equations do not take into account the capacitance of the neural membrane. The effect of the capacitance is that the extracellular current, and therefore the extracellular potential, will be somewhat briefer than postsynaptic potentials recorded with an intracellular electrode in the soma (Rall, 1960; Holmes and Short, 1970).

At any point within the volume of fluid around the cell there will be a potential intermediate between those at S and D. In *Figure 2.7c*, points at the same potential have been joined by contours (interrupted lines); it can be seen that these transect the current paths at right angles. The equipotential line Z–Z' is of particular significance since any point lying upon it will be at a potential midway between those of S and D. Furthermore it is evident that this contour is the only one to extend to infinity; therefore a reference electrode Y placed at a considerable distance from the cell will lie on this contour. Imagine that an 'active' electrode X is now brought close to the cell. If X is moved above Z–Z' so as to lie nearer to D than to S, it will be negative with respect to Y (*Figure 2.7d*). Conversely if X lies closer to S than to D it will become positive in relation to Y. On the head the freedom of electrode movement is limited so that unless a cell lies in a sulcus, it will have an axis perpendicular to the surface of the head. Consequently a scalp electrode can only move close to D; it will always be some distance from S. The largest potential between X and the indifferent electrode Y will be recorded when X lies directly over D (*Figure 2.7e*).

If X is found to be negative with respect to Y it indicates either: (1) a depolarization of the apical dendrite by EPSPs or propagated dendritic potentials, or (2) a hyperpolarization (IPSP) of the soma. It will be appreciated that, although the cell membrane potentials are different in (1) and (2), in both instances the dendrite is negative relative to the soma and therefore the ionic current and extracellular potential gradient will be in the same direction.

If X is positive with respect to Y it indicates either (1) a hyperpolarization (IPSP) of the apical dendrite or (2) a depolarization (EPSP) of the soma.

Electrical activity in the proximal part of the apical dendrite will not be considered separately since it will induce similar surface potentials as activity in the adjoining soma. Strictly the term 'apical dendrite' as used in this and the following sections, denotes only that region of the dendrite near to the cortical surface.

It is obvious from what has already been said that the positions of the electrodes are critical if electrophysiological activity is to be correctly interpreted. Therefore it is important to recognize two recording conditions in which activity will not be detected. The first is when X is offset in relation to D while Y is brought closer so that it lies on the same equipotential contour as X (*Figure 2.7f*). In the second situation, X is placed optimally over D but simultaneous activity occurs in another dipole situated under Y (*Figure 2.7g*). In each case, X and Y are at the same potential and no evidence of activity will be recorded. If, in this latter situation, the polarity of one of the dipoles reverses then the potentials at X and Y, instead of cancelling each other, will summate (*Figure 2.7h*).

Finally, it should be noted that the relatively large surface electrodes used in electroencephalography will average potentials projected to the surface of the scalp from many underlying dipoles. Consequently, a change in recorded potential indicates the creation of a large number of similarly orientated dipoles. In physiological terms, it means that a large cluster of pyramidal cells has become simultaneously excited or inhibited.

INTERPRETATION OF SURFACE POTENTIALS

In *Figure 2.8* the structure of the cortex has been simplified to show only three types of neurones. Thus S and D represent the soma and apical dendrite of a pyramidal cell, while E and I are star cells which have excitatory and inhibitory projections respectively on to the pyramidal cell. Two types of input fibre are also shown—specific thalamic (sp) and non-specific thalamic (non-sp). It will be remembered that the main termination of specific axons is in layer IV while non-specific axons are distributed to all layers. The assumption is made in *Figure 2.8a* that, amongst its other connections, each type of fibre will make excitatory connections with accessible apical dendrites or somata of pyramidal cells within its cortical layer of termination. It is also assumed that the inhibitory cell (I) will fire only when it receives inputs from several pyramidal cells, that is, during relatively massive cortical discharges. Finally, it has been shown in the preceding section that a surface negativity will be produced under two circumstances; first, during an excitatory depolarization (EPSP or impulse) in the apical dendrite and secondly, during an inhibitory hyperpolarization (IPSP) of the soma. In contrast, an EPSP confined to the soma (and proximal dendritic regions) will produce a surface

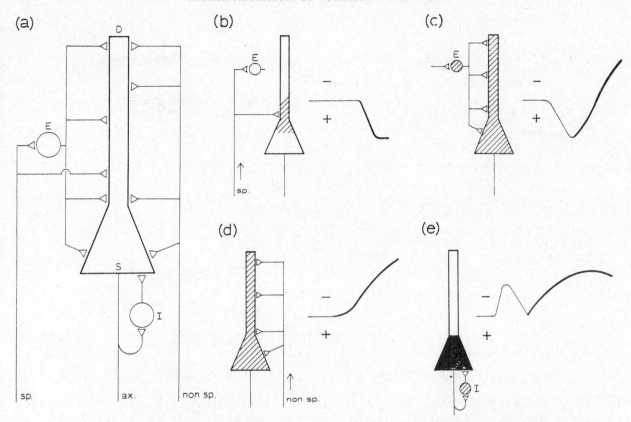

Figure 2.8—Greatly simplified diagram to show how different inputs to cortex cause evoked responses in pyramidal cells and hence characteristic potentials at cortical surface. In (a) S and D indicate soma and dendrite of pyramidal cell; soma lies in layer V of cortex. E is excitatory stellate interneurone in layer IV; I is postsynaptic inhibitory interneurone activated by recurrent branch from pyramidal cell axon (ax); sp and non sp are axons from specific and non-specific thalamic nuclei respectively. In b–e, depolarization (EPSP) of membrane shown by hatched lines, hyperpolarization (IPSP) by filled area. Potentials at surface of cortex are shown at side of each figure, heavy lines denoting the wave under consideration. See text for explanation

positivity. It is now possible to consider the genesis of the cortical potentials evoked by impulses arriving via specific and non-specific thalamocortical fibres.

(1) *Specific thalamic inputs* affect the pyramidal cell in two ways. Initially they cause a monosynaptic EPSP of the proximal dendritic region, thereby yielding a positive wave at the cortical surface (*Figure 2.8b*). They also activate excitatory star cells in layer IV which in turn induce widespread excitatory depolarization of the pyramidal cell, including the apical dendrite; this causes a surface negative wave to follow the initially positive one (*Figure 2.8c*). Although this sequence characterizes evoked activity in the primary somatosensory and motor areas, the situation in the visual cortex is somewhat different. Thus, Creutzfeldt *et al.* (1969) have shown that the initial large surface positive wave is associated with an IPSP which is presumably well developed in the apical dendrite.

(2) *Non-specific thalamic inputs* depolarize the pyramidal cell throughout its length; the depolarization of the apical dendrite is especially marked and causes a surface negativity (*Figures 2.8d, 2.9*). This mechanism will operate following any type of non-specific activity, whether during naturally occurring *EEG spindles* or experimentally-induced *recruiting responses*; the *non-specific response* and *K complex* (page 65) have a similar basis. Creutzfeldt, Watanabe and Lux (1966) have shown that each surface 'positive' wave during a cortical spindle simply reflects the delay before the next EPSP and that it may be enhanced by an IPSP, which is presumably well developed in the apical dendrite. To summarize, each negative wave in an EEG spindle results from excitation of pyramidal cells; each 'positive' wave signals the pause before the next excitation, with or without inhibition (*Figure 2.9*).

There is evidence to suggest that the spike and wave discharges characteristic of centrencephalic epilepsy may also employ the non-specific pathway. Thus Jasper and Drooglever-Fortuyn (1947) were able to evoke typical cortical spike and wave activity by low frequency (3 per second) stimulation of non-specific thalamic nuclei. Pollen (1964) has shown that the slow negative wave following the

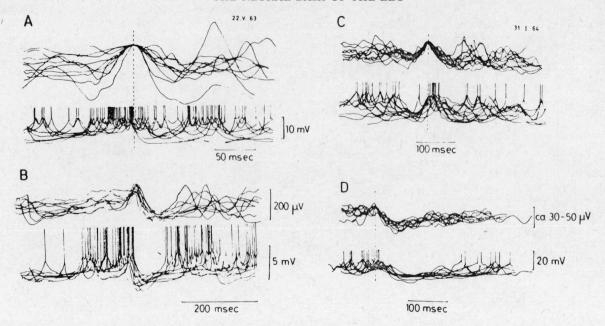

Figure 2.9—*Superimposed line drawings of two types of surface EEG waves (upper trace of each pair) and the simultaneous activity in an underlying cortical neurone (lower trace in each pair). Same cell in A and B, another cell in C and D. In A and C negative EEG waves have been superimposed and are seen to correspond to excitation (EPSPs and discharges) in cellular record. In B and D the surface negative wave is followed by a positivity which is associated with an IPSP in the cellular record*

(From Creutzfeldt, Watanabe and Lux (1966), *Electroenceph. clin. Neurophysiol.* **20**, 26, by courtesy of the authors and Elsevier Publishing Company)

initial negative spike is due to an IPSP; the IPSP is apparently restricted to the pyramidal cell soma and is probably achieved through the inhibitory feedback loop shown in *Figure 2.8d*.

(3) *Focal epileptic discharges.* Several methods have been employed to induce epileptic discharges in exposed mammalian cortex; they include intensive electrical stimulation, freezing, and the application of substances such as strychnine, alumina, cobalt and penicillin (Ajmone-Marsan, 1969; Prince, 1969). Within a varying period of time (for example, a few minutes with strychnine) spikes can be recorded from the surface of the treated cortex. Simultaneous intracellular recording from neurones reveals that these spikes are associated with massive depolarization of the cell soma (*paroxysmal depolarization shifts* or PDSs). Since the spikes usually have an initial negative polarity it is probable

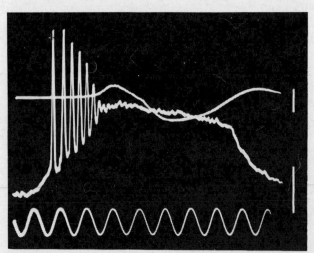

Figure 2.10—*Typical example of paroxysmal depolarization shift (PDS). Upper trace is from cortical surface, underneath is intracellular recording (Calibrations 1 mV and 10 mV respectively, positivity upwards; time trace 100 Hz)*

(From Matsumoto and Ajmone Marsan (1964), *Exp. Neurol.* **9**, 292, by courtesy of the authors and Academic Press)

that the depolarization extends up the apical dendrite and is well developed near the cortical surface. Although they are very much larger than excitatory postsynaptic potentials the PDSs are also thought to be synaptically mediated since they can be evoked by thalamic or cortical stimulation. During the paroxysmal depolarization, action potentials are fired; however, excessive depolarization inactivates the regenerative sodium conductance mechanism and causes the cell to cease discharging (*Figure 2.10*). Sometimes PDSs occur in rapid succession (tonic phase) and summate to produce a steady depolarization lasting a minute or more. During this phase the EEG is flat and the inactivation of the regenerative sodium conductance mechanism prevents firing. As the cell membranes repolarize, intermittent PDSs reappear and are associated with impulse generation (clonic phase). Since the membrane properties of 'epileptic' neurones appear normal when tested between PDSs, it is evident that the nature of the synaptic bombardment responsible for the PDS is a fundamental problem in epilepsy.

(4) *Contingent negative variation* (CNV; page 208). This wave was originally described by Walter and his colleagues in 1964. In their experiments a subject was presented with a warning stimulus and then a second stimulus to which a response was required. Following the first stimulus a slow negative potential built up which could be recorded best over the frontal and vertex areas. Recently McSherry (1971) has investigated the neural mechanism of this response in monkeys using intracortical electrodes. He found that the CNV had a patchy distribution throughout the frontal lobe, being largest in the premotor cortex. McSherry also noted that the surface negativity was sometimes associated with a deep cortical positivity. The CNV was interpreted as resulting from excitatory depolarizations (EPSPs) in the apical dendrites of pyramidal cells with inhibitory hyperpolarizations (IPSPs) of the corresponding somas.

REFERENCES

General reviews

Amassian, V. E. (1961). 'Microelectrode Studies of the Cerebral Cortex'. *Int. Rev. Neurobiol.* **3,** 67

Andersen, P. and Andersson, S. A. (1968). *The Physiological Basis of the Alpha Rhythm.* New York; Appleton-Century-Crofts

Bremer, F. (1958). 'Cerebral and Cerebellar Potentials'. *Physiol. Rev.* **38,** 357

Creutzfeldt, O. D. (1969). 'Neuronal Mechanisms Underlying the EEG'. In *Basic Mechanisms of the Epilepsies*, pp. 397–410. Ed. by H. H. Jasper, A. A. Ward Jr. and A. Pope. London; Churchill

— Lux, H. D. and Watanabe, S. (1966). 'Electrophysiology of Cortical Nerve Cells'. In *The Thalamus*, pp. 209–230. Ed. by D. P. Purpura, and M. Yahr. New York; Columbia University Press

Purpura, D. P. (1959). 'Nature of Electrocortical Potentials and Synaptic Organizations in Cerebral and Cerebellar Cortex'. *Int. Rev. Neurobiol.* **1,** 47

Original papers

Adrian, E. D. (1941). 'Afferent Discharges to the Cerebral Cortex from Peripheral Sense Organs'. *J. Physiol.* **100,** 159

— (1951). 'Rhythmic Discharges from the Thalamus'. *J. Physiol.* **113,** 9 *P*

— and Moruzzi, G. (1939). 'Impulses in the Pyramidal Tract'. *J. Physiol.* **97,** 153

Ajmone-Marsan, C. (1969). 'Acute Effects of Topical Epileptogenic Agents'. In *Basic Mechanisms of the Epilepsies*, pp. 299–319. Ed. by H. H. Jasper, A. A. Ward Jr. and A. Pope. London; Churchill

Andersen, P. (1966). 'Rhythmic 10/sec Activity in the Thalamus'. In *The Thalamus*, pp. 143–151. Ed. by D. P. Purpura and M. D. Yahr. New York; Columbia University Press

— and Sears, T. A. (1964). 'The Role of Inhibition in the Phasing of Spontaneous Thalamocortical Discharge'. *J. Physiol.* **173,** 459

— Andersson, S. A. and Lømo, T. (1967). 'Some Factors Involved in the Thalamic Control of Spontaneous Barbiturate Spindles'. *J. Physiol.* **192,** 257

Bartley, S. H. and Bishop, G. H. (1933). 'Factors Determining the Form of the Electrical Response from the Optic Cortex of the Rabbit'. *Am. J. Physiol.* **103,** 173

Bindman, Lynn, J., Lippold, O. C. J. and Redfearn, J. W. T. (1964) 'Relation between the Size and Form of Potentials Evoked by Sensory Stimulation and the Background Electrical Activity in the Cerebral Cortex of the Rat'. *J. Physiol.* **171,** 1

Bremer, F. (1935). 'Cerveau Isolé et Physiologie du Sommeil'. *C. r. Séanc. Soc. Biol.* **118,** 1235

Burns, B. D. (1951). 'Some Properties of Isolated Cerebral Cortex in the Unanaesthetized Cat'. *J. Physiol.* **112,** 156

Callaway 3rd. E. (1962). 'Factors Influencing the Relationship Between Alpha Activity and Visual Reaction Time'. *Electroenceph. clin. Neurophysiol.* **14,** 674

Creutzfeldt, O. D., Watanabe, S. and Lux, H. D. (1966). 'Relations Between EEG Phenomena and Potentials of Single Cortical Cells. II. Spontaneous and Convulsoid Activity'. *Electroenceph. clin. Neurophysiol.* **20,** 19

— Rosina, A., Ito, H. and Probst, W. (1969). 'Visual Evoked Response of Single Cells and of the EEG in Primary Visual Area of the Cat'. *J. Neurophysiol.* **32,** 127

Dempsey, E. W. and Morison, R. S. (1942a). 'The Production of Rhythmically Recurrent Cortical Potentials After Localized Thalamic Stimulation'. *Am. J. Physiol.* **135,** 293

— — (1942b). 'The Interaction of Certain Spontaneous and Induced Cortical Potentials'. *Am. J. Physiol.* **135,** 301

— Morison, R. S. and Morison, B. R. (1941). 'Some Afferent Diencephalic Pathways Related to Cortical Potentials in the Cat'. *Am. J. Physiol.* **131,** 718

Dusser de Barenne, J. G. and McCulloch, W. S. (1938). 'The Direct Functional Interrelation of Sensory Cortex and Optic Thalamus'. *J. Neurophysiol.* **1,** 176

Economo, C. von (1929). *Die Encephalitis Lethargica, ihre Nachkrankheiten und ihre Behandlung.* Berlin; Urban und Schwarzenberg

French, J. D., Amerongen, F. K. von and Magoun, H. W. (1952). 'An Activating System in the Brainstem of Monkey'. *Archs Neurol. Psychiat., Chicago* **68,** 591

Hess, W. R. (1944). 'Des Schlafsyndrom als Folge diencephaler Reizung'. *Helv. physiol. pharmac. Acta* **2,** 305

— (1954). 'The Diencephalic Sleep Centre'. In *Brain Mechanism and Consciousness*. Ed. by J. F. Delafresnaye. Oxford; Blackwell

Holmes, O. and Short, A. D. (1970). 'Interaction of Cortical Evoked Potentials in the Rat'. *J. Physiol.* **209,** 433

Jasper, H. H. and Drooglever-Fortuyn, J. (1947). 'Experimental Studies on the Functional Anatomy of Petit Mal Epilepsy'. *Res. Publs. Ass. Res. nerv. ment. Dis.* **26,** 272

— and Stefanis, C. (1965). 'Intracellular Oscillatory Rhythms in Pyramidal Tract Neurones in the Cat'. *Electroenceph. clin. Neurophysiol.* **18,** 541

Kristiansen, K. and Courtois, G. (1949). 'Rhythmic Electrical Activity from Isolated Cerebral Cortex. *Electroenceph. clin. Neurophysiol.* **1,** 265

Lansing, R. W. (1957). 'Relation of Brain and Tremor Rhythms to Visual Reaction Time'. *Electroenceph. clin. Neurophysiol.* **9,** 497

Li, C-L and Jasper, H. H. (1953). 'Microelectrode Studies of the Electrical Activity of the Cerebral Cortex in the Cat'. *J. Physiol.* **121,** 117

— Cullen, C. and Jasper, H. H. (1956). 'Laminar Microelectrode Analysis of Cortical Unspecific Recruiting Responses and Spontaneous Rhythms'. *J. Neurophysiol.* **19,** 131

Lindsley, D. B., Schreiner, L. H., Knowles, W. B. and Magoun, H. W. (1950). 'Behavioural and EEG Changes Following Chronic Brain Stem Lesions in the Cat'. *Electroenceph. clin. Neurophysiol.* **2,** 483

Lippold, O. (1970). 'Origin of the Alpha Rhythm'. *Nature, Lond.* **226,** 616

MacKay, D. M. (1953). 'Some Experiments on the Perception of Patterns Modulated at the Alpha Frequency'. *Electroenceph. clin. Neurophysiol.* **5,** 559

McSherry, J. W. (1971). 'Intracortical Origin of the Contingent Negative Variation in the Rhesus Monkey'. Ph. D. Thesis. Houston; Baylor Coll. Med.

Matsumoto, H. and Ajmone-Marsan, C. (1964a). 'Cortical Cellular Phenomena in Experimental Epilepsy: Interictal Manifestations'. *Exp. Neurol.* **9,** 286

— — (1964b). 'Cortical Cellular Phenomena in Experimental Epilepsy: Ictal Manifestations'. *Exp. Neurol.* **9,** 305

Morison, R. S. and Dempsey, E. W. (1942). 'A Study of Thalamo-cortical Relations'. *Am. J. Physiol.* **135,** 281

— Finley, K. H. and Lothrop, Gladys N. (1943). 'Spontaneous Electrical Activity of the Thalamus and Other Forebrain Structures'. *J. Neurophysiol.* **6,** 243

Morison, A. R. and Pompeiano, O. (1965a). 'An Analysis of the Supraspinal Influences Acting on Motoneurons During Sleep in the Unrestrained Cat. Responses of the Alpha Motoneurons to Direct Electrical Stimulation During Sleep'. *Archs ital. Biol.* **103,** 497

— — (1965b). 'Pyramidal Discharge from Somatosensory Cortex and Cortical Control of Primary Afferents During Sleep'. *Archs ital. Biol.* **103,** 538

Moruzzi, G. and Magoun, H. W. (1949). 'Brain Stem Reticular Formation and Activation of the EEG'. *Electroenceph. clin. Neurophysiol.* **1,** 455

Pollen, D. A. (1964). 'Intracellular Studies of Cortical Neurons During Thalamic Induced Wave and Spike'. *Electroenceph. clin. Neurophysiol.* **17,** 398

Prince, D. A. (1969). 'Microelectrode Studies of Penicillin Foci'. In *Basic Mechanisms of the Epilepsies*. Ed. by H. H. Jasper, A. A. Ward Jr. and A. Pope. London; Churchill

Purpura, D. P. and Cohen, B. (1962). 'Intracellular Recording from Thalamic Neurons During Recruiting Responses'. *J. Neurophysiol.* **25,** 621

— Frigyesi, T. L., McMurtry, J. G. and Scarff, T. (1966). 'Synaptic Mechanisms in Thalamic Regulation of Cerebello-cortical Projection Activity'. In *The Thalamus*, pp. 153–170. Ed. by D. P. Purpura and M. D. Yahr. New York; Columbia University Press

Rall, W. (1960). 'Membrane Potential Transients and Membrane Time Constant of Motoneurones'. *Expl. Neurol.* **2,** 503

Walsh, E. G. (1952). 'Visual Reaction Time and the Alpha Rhythm: an Investigation of a Scanning Hypothesis'. *J. Physiol.* **118,** 500

Walter, W. G., Cooper, R., Aldridge, V. J., McCallum, W. C. and Winter, A. L. (1964). 'Contingent Negative Variation: an Electric Sign of Sensorimotor Association and Expectancy in the Human Brain'. *Nature, Lond.* **203,** 380

Whitlock, D. G., Arduini, A. and Moruzzi, G. (1953). 'Microelectrode Analysis of Pyramidal System During Transition from Sleep to Wakefulness'. *J. Neurophysiol.* **16,** 414

CHAPTER 3

TECHNOLOGY AND METHODOLOGY

APPARATUS

The essential components of an electrophysiological recording system comprise electrodes, amplifiers and a means of recording or displaying the electrical signals obtained. In addition, many laboratories use various kinds of stimulator and perhaps some form of computer to analyse the signals. This may be done *on-line*—as the investigation proceeds—or *off-line*—when the data are subsequently played back from magnetic tape. Such an analyser might be as simple as an *alpha* band filter or as complex as a large digital computer. Traditionally, EEG data are recorded on paper and analysed by eye. It is essential to master this basic technique before making use of more sophisticated methods.

ELECTRODES

The interface between the subject and the electrode should introduce the minimum possible resistance into the input circuit. Chlorided silver electrodes with electrode jelly or saline as the contact medium are the most satisfactory for general use. Electrodes are of two main types. *Stick-on* electrodes are attached either by means of a layer of collodion round the rim, or by covering with a gauze patch soaked in collodion which adheres to the surrounding scalp. *Pad* electrodes (Walter and Parr, 1963) are held in place by the bands of an elastic head cap; these are more easily displaced by movement and give rise to more frequent artefacts. Electrodes should be re-chlorided electrolytically whenever the surface shows signs of deterioration. The advantages of fast and slow chloriding methods are compared by Coles and Binnie (1968). When in regular use, electrodes should be kept in such a way that slow chloriding takes place continuously (Cooper, 1956). Over-chloriding, however, causes electrode resistance to increase (Geddes, Baker and Moore, 1969).

The reason for chloriding silver electrodes is to render them *reversible*. Small currents inevitably pass through a pair of electrodes when they are applied to the scalp and connected to the input stage of an EEG amplifier. This is because a circuit is thereby completed in which there are two sources of electromotive force (e.m.f.)—the fluctuating EEG potentials themselves and the relatively steady potential that arises at the interface between each electrode and the jelly or saline. The latter potential will, in general, be of the order of tens of millivolts and will be different for each electrode. Chloriding enables the electrode to present the same resistance to current flow in either direction, so that distortion of the EEG signal does not occur. Such an electrode is said to be reversible or non-polarizable (Cooper, 1962). A reversible electrode has a relatively stable potential with respect to the contact medium. It is this potential which gives rise to the effect known as *blocking* when a channel is switched from one pair of electrodes to another. The large change of steady potential at the amplifier input causes later stages to overload. The pen writer will deflect maximally in one direction and remain 'blocked' for an interval dependent on the time constant of the amplifier (Velate, 1962).

A number of other types of electrodes are used in some laboratories. Needles of platinum alloy or stainless steel are easy to insert into the scalp, but it is essential to use a fresh sterilized set for each patient. The impedance of a needle electrode is inversely proportional to the area of contact and is similar to that of a large resistor in parallel with a capacitor; thus there may be some attenuation of the signal at low frequencies (Zablow and Goldensohn, 1969). In contrast, a chlorided silver electrode presents a relatively low resistance which is constant at all frequencies within the EEG range. Solder-pellet electrodes embedded in bentonite paste (Taylor and Abraham, 1969) or attached to the scalp with paraffin wax (Kagawa, 1962) are also used, but are liable to be detached by traction on the lead. Cupped electrodes with flexible rims are very convenient for attachment to the skin of the face or neck by double-sided adhesive rings.

The contact resistance of a chlorided silver electrode when applied to the scalp should be less than 5,000 ohms. Values less than this can readily be obtained with the stick-on type. It is better to measure electrode resistance with a low frequency alternating current than with direct current. The latter may cause polarization if it is passed in one direction only and will give inconstant and very high readings with needle electrodes. To be realistic and to avoid damage to the electrode surface, only a small applied voltage should be used.

Margerison *et al.* (1967) give a comprehensive review of the construction, properties and maintenance of the different types of electrodes used in EEG work.

RECORDING EQUIPMENT

The first essential in an EEG laboratory is a multichannel recorder that will produce permanent records for immediate inspection. The majority of EEG machines have 16 channels. Although it is customary to operate all channels at the same sensitivity and with the same frequency characteristic, some of them may be required to record electrophysiological signals other than the EEG. Modern electrophysiological amplifiers use mainly transistors, but the input stage may have valves or field effect transistors, both of which give a high input resistance. This is important because the proportion of signal lost due to the finite resistance (r) of a pair of electrodes is approximately r/R, where R is the input resistance of the amplifier to which the electrodes are connected. For the usual types of EEG electrodes, R should be at least 1 megohm.

EEG amplifiers fall into three main classes: those in which the signal is amplified without any substantial change in its waveform; those in which the signal modulates the amplitude of a 'carrier', and those in which the signal is 'chopped' at the input by a vibrator. In the second and third types, the signal is reconstituted at the output of the amplifier by a process known as demodulation.

The first type of amplifier circuit uses a pair of matched transistors for each stage of amplification and is said to be *push-pull* in its operation. The signal to be amplified is connected to the input stage via leads that are conventionally named *black* and *white* or *Grid 1* and *Grid 2* in North America (*see* page 40). Balance between the two halves of a push-pull amplifier is maintained throughout all its stages, the intention being to minimize the amplification of any extraneous signal, such as mains (line) interference, which is *in phase* on both input leads and thus tends to cancel out. The desired signal, because it is applied between the two input leads, is essentially *out of phase*. The ratio between the gain of the amplifier as a whole for out-of-phase signals to that for in-phase signals is known as the *discrimination ratio*. It is commonly of the order of 10,000:1 for this type of amplifier. In carrier-modulated and chopper-type amplifiers, most if not all of the amplification takes place at the carrier or chopper frequency. Hence only the input circuit and frequency converter need be balanced to achieve a high discrimination ratio.

The maximum *gain* or *sensitivity* of an EEG amplifier has to be such that an input signal of 10 μV results in a pen deflection of at least 1 cm. The *noise*—random background activity—that is invariably present in the trace at maximum gain should not exceed the equivalent of 2 μV at the input. The range of signal voltages met with in EEG work varies from about 1000 μV down to zero. It is therefore essential to have calibrated gain controls (*attenuators*) whereby the degree of amplification can be adjusted and the pen deflections maintained within an appropriate range. There is regrettably no uniform practice in the choice of ratios by which stepped attenuators increase or decrease the gain. On some equipment the steps are marked in decibels (dB) above and below an arbitrary level designated 0 dB. The steps may be of 6, 5 or 3 dB corresponding to ratios of approximately 2·0, 1·8 and 1·4:1 respectively. If the gain is doubled, it is said to have changed by $+6$ dB; if it is halved, it has changed by -6 dB. In practice, the most convenient step is 3 dB which is equivalent to a ratio of $\sqrt{2}$:1. Absolute values of gain are expressed in μV/cm or μV/mm of pen deflection.

The important range of frequencies in clinical EEG work extends from 1 to 50 Hz (cycles per second), but the majority of EEG amplifiers are capable of giving an electrical output up to several kilocycles per second for the display of high frequency signals, such as the EMG, on a cathode ray oscilloscope. It is the pen writer which limits the maximum frequency that can be recorded. Nevertheless, it is essential to have high-frequency filters to attenuate muscle potential artefacts or mains interference

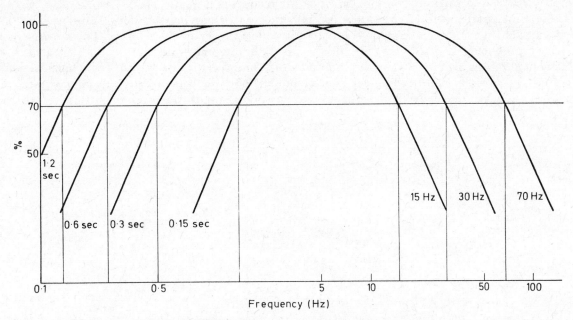

Figure 3.1—Idealized frequency response characteristic for recording system with different values of time constant and different degrees of high-frequency cut

when necessary. These filters modify the *frequency response characteristic* of the recording system in the manner shown in *Figure 3.1*. Each position of the filter control should be marked with the frequency at which the overall sensitivity of the system falls to 70 per cent of that in the centre of the passband.

Similarly, the low frequency response of the recording system can be modified by a control usually referred to as the *time constant*. The longer the time constant, the more faithfully will the recorder

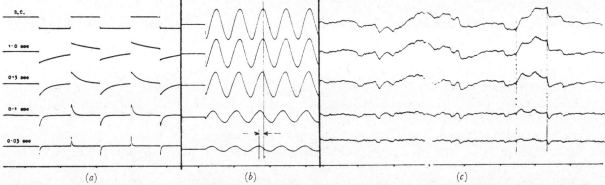

Figure 3.2—Effects of progressively shorter time constants on (a) calibration signal, (b) 1·5 Hz sine wave input and (c) EEG extract. Channel 1 directly coupled; channels 2–5 have time constants of 1·0, 0·3, 0·1 and 0·03 s respectively. In (b) note phase-shift of 130 ms (0·2 cycle or 72°) between channels 1 and 5

reproduce the low frequency components of an EEG signal. Typical values of time constant are 1·0, 0·3, 0·1 and 0·03 second. These correspond to a reduction of sensitivity to 70 per cent of that in the mid-passband at 0·15, 0·5, 1·5 and 5 Hz respectively (*Figure 3.1*). An amplifier that is capacitor (a.c.) coupled has a finite time constant, whereas one that is directly (d.c.) coupled throughout has, in effect, an infinitely long time constant and is capable of reproducing steady or very slowly changing potentials without distortion. The reproduction of sine and square wave inputs and of an EEG signal at different

37

time constants is shown in *Figure 3.2*. Note that progressive reduction of the time constant not only reduces the amplitude but also progressively shifts the *phase* of the sinusoidal output with respect to the input. This effect may become important when examining the time relationship between fast and slow waves in the EEG (Saunders and Jell, 1959). For instance, the waveform of a spike and wave complex depends on the time constant at which the recording is made (Weir, 1965).

The great majority of EEG machines use moving-iron or moving-coil pen recorders. The latter have a better high-frequency response but require more power to drive them. The pen tip moves in an arc producing a *curvilinear* trace. Because it is the angular deflection of the pen arm that is proportional to driving current, small amplitude and timing errors are introduced which are jointly known as *arc distortion*. Both types overshoot or undershoot when incorrectly *damped*, corresponding to an excessive or a deficient high-frequency response. The square wave responses of a pen recorder

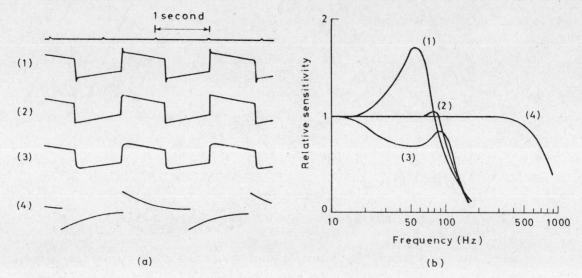

Figure 3.3—(a) *Response to a square-wave function.* (b) *Corresponding frequency response characteristics for a pen writer with damping controlled by electrical feedback:* (1) *very underdamped;* (2) *slightly underdamped;* (3) *overdamped;* (4) *equivalent responses for jet galvanometer*

with different degrees of damping are shown in *Figure 3.3a*; the corresponding frequency response characteristics are shown in *Figure 3.3b*. Damping depends on a number of factors but can be controlled electrically by feedback.

Pen recorders impose the principal limitation to the overall performance of an EEG machine, restricting the high-frequency response, limiting the amplitude of the maximum deflection and introducing arc distortion. These defects are largely overcome by high-pressure jet galvanometers which extend the high-frequency response by almost a factor of ten (*Figure 3.3b*). Their *rectilinear* write-out enables accurate timing measurements to be made between channels. The only disadvantage of these recorders is that they use a blue dye which has to be blotted by a porous roller and is rather more difficult to photograph than black ink.

A recommended specification for EEG recorders has been drawn up by the Committee on Apparatus of the International Federation of Societies for EEG and Clinical Neurophysiology (Knott, 1958).

OPERATIONAL TECHNIQUES

EEG recording is a dynamic procedure and the method adopted in an individual case will depend upon the information it is desired to obtain and upon whether special techniques or stimuli are to be employed. These, in turn, depend upon the clinical history and condition of the patient. Recording 'blind', that is, without prior knowledge of the clinical situation, is a procedure that should be reserved for comparative studies, either within a group of selected cases or in an individual case on different occasions, in which EEG features *per se* are to be related to clinical variables. Recording from patients in an intensive care unit, or in other hostile environments, may tax the performance of the apparatus and the skill of the technician to their limits. In these circumstances, only versatility and unorthodoxy of recording technique may yield the answer to the physician's query.

RECORDING PROCEDURE

The majority of initial EEG investigations follow a fairly standard pattern. When the patient has been put at ease, about a score of electrodes are applied symmetrically to the scalp. The International Federation has recommended a particular placement, known as the *10–20 system*, which is based on measurements from four landmarks on the skull (Jasper, 1958). A step-by-step account of how the measurements are made and descriptions of how different types of electrodes are applied are given by Cooper, Osselton and Shaw (1969). The 10–20 system has not received universal approval and a number of other systems are in use—for instance, those of Pampiglione (1956) and Hess (1966). Stick-on electrodes are coming into more general use because of their electrical stability and relative insensitivity to movement on the part of the patient. Where speed is important, pads or needles are still preferred by some technicians, although stick-on electrodes can be applied almost as quickly by someone who is experienced in their use.

The recording should preferably be carried out with the patient recumbent. Stick-on electrodes have an added advantage in that the head can rest on a soft pillow. With pad and needle electrodes, the back of the neck must be supported so that the posterior electrodes are not displaced by head movement. When the connections to the electrodes have been made, their contact resistances should be measured and if necessary reduced by means appropriate to the type of electrode in use. A calibration signal, usually 100 μV, is then recorded simultaneously on all channels and the gains adjusted until all channels give a deflection of 1 cm. An additional check of equalization can be made by recording with all channels connected to a single pair of electrodes, widely spaced on the head so that an adequate signal is obtained. These procedures should be carried out at a time constant of about 0·3 second, with no high-frequency attenuation and a paper speed of 30 mm/second.

All EEG machines have an electrode-switching unit with a *master selector*, whereby the technician can set up any pattern at will. These patterns of connection between the electrodes and the recording channels are known as *montages*. Different types of montages and their uses are discussed in a later section.

Once a recording has begun, it is usual to allow about 20 minutes for continuous stretches of record to be taken with the subject relaxed but awake, using a selection of the montages available and noting the effects of eye opening and closure with each. Minor adjustments to the electrodes may have to be made to eliminate artefacts, but the generally restful nature of the proceedings often induces drowsiness and sleep. Unless there is some specific reason to the contrary, sleep should not be discouraged: valuable information may thereby be acquired and the necessity for a further recording under sedation avoided. On the other hand, if a series of comparative recordings is to be carried out either on a single patient or upon a group, the conditions during recording must be the same on each occasion. Deliberate steps may have to be taken to maintain the patient in a constant state of alertness.

In most investigations, the use of a few standard montages is sufficient, but in some cases it will be necessary for additional montages to be used. The technician should be encouraged to make a running spatial analysis of the significant features of the record and to devise the most appropriate montages to display them. The record must at all times be carefully annotated with regard to changes in the patient's state and with particulars of the montage, control settings and stimuli employed.

The usual standard practice is to record at a paper speed of 30 mm/second and to adjust the master gain control so that the pen excursions fluctuate between 0·5 and 2 cm. If high voltage discharges are anticipated, the gain should be reduced to an extent that allows their waveform to be seen without distortion due to mechanical restriction of the pen deflections. When a record contains genuine low frequency components, as long a time constant as is practicable should be used and phase relations may be clarified by recording at 15 mm/second for part of the time. When it is desired to examine the waveform and phase relations of high-frequency components, no high-frequency attenuation should be introduced and the paper should be run at 60 mm/second. It may also be helpful to increase the gain and to reduce the relative amplitude of any slow components by shortening the time constants.

The record should end with a further set of calibration signals to check that the channels have remained equalized. Only then should the electrodes be removed from the patient's head.

POTENTIAL DISTRIBUTION

The distribution of potential changes over the surface of the head is complex and dynamic and the most that a clinical electroencephalographer can hope to do is to detect and locate their major components. A recording from scalp electrodes is but a sample of the activity near the surface of the brain; it is certainly attenuated and diffused and may be distorted by conduction through the cerebrospinal fluid, skull and scalp (Abraham and Marsan, 1958). Cooper *et al.* (1965) have shown that several square centimetres of cortex have to be involved in a synchronous electrical discharge for activity of comparable amplitude to be recorded from the overlying scalp. The ability to record in only two dimensions limits the accuracy with which the source of a particular EEG component can be located within the brain. In any case, there is no *a priori* reason to assume that each component must have a discrete source.

The cranium and its contents are far from being analogous to a container filled with a homogeneous conducting medium in which a number of generators are embedded. Nevertheless, whatever the current and voltage fluctuations may be within the brain as a whole, it is axiomatic that its net electrical charge and potential must at all times be zero. It is therefore permissible to regard certain discrete components of the EEG as being due to alternating dipole generators situated in particular parts of the brain (Shaw and Roth, 1955).

A dipole generator may be thought of as a source of electrical current, the length of which is small relative to the extent of the surrounding medium, and the poles of which are of equal potential but of opposite polarity. An alternating dipole is one in which the polarity is constantly reversing, perhaps many times per second. When such a dipole is embedded in a conducting medium, it gives rise to an alternating potential field which extends throughout the medium. Electrodes placed on the boundary of the medium will pick up voltages that fluctuate at the same frequency. Their magnitudes will be functions of the electrode spacing and of the orientation and distance of the dipole from the surface.

The only justification for using the dipole analogy is that *some* EEG phenomena give rise to a voltage distribution on the scalp as if they were originating from such a source (Brazier, 1951; Calvet *et al.*, 1964). One of the tasks of the electroencephalographer is to deduce the positions of these sources within the brain from an examination of the voltage distribution over the surface of the head.

MONTAGES

No specific recommendations have been laid down by the International Federation as to the montages that should be used for routine investigations, but the following general rules have been suggested (Jasper, 1958):

(1) Recording channels should be connected in sequence to rows of equidistant electrodes that lie along anteroposterior or transverse lines.

(2) The order of the channels, as read from top to bottom of the recording paper, should be such that those recording from the right side of the head come before those recording from the left.

(3) Channels recording anteriorly should come before those recording posteriorly.

When recording from anteroposterior rows, the second of these rules takes precedence over the third, whereas for transverse rows the order of precedence is reversed. The majority of examples in this book were recorded with montages that conform to these recommendations. A variant that is preferred by some workers for the comparison of the tracings from homologous areas is to allocate channels to right and left alternately, so that those recording from homologous areas are adjacent to each other on the paper.

The sense in which the recording pen reproduces the voltage fluctuations between a given pair of electrodes will depend upon the way in which the input leads of its amplifier are connected to them. Referring to these leads as *black* (Grid 1) and *white* (Grid 2), convention has it that, when the black lead becomes electro-negative with respect to the white, the recording pen makes an upward deflection. In diagrams of montages, black leads are drawn as full lines and white leads as broken lines, so that the relative polarity of a particular discharge can always be deduced. If an arrow between two electrodes is used to indicate the sense in which the channel is connected, it should point from *black* to *white*.

There are three basically different types of montages, commonly known as *bipolar, unipolar* (or monopolar) and *average reference* (or Goldman–Offner). The last named two types are also called *common reference* montages because they make use of a single electrode or reference potential which is common to all channels. There is a traditional preference for bipolar montages in European laboratories, but it should be appreciated that these different methods of *derivation* are complementary rather than mutually exclusive. A competent electroencephalographer should be familiar with the use of all three. A comprehensive review of these recording methods is made by Osselton (1966; 1969) and by Cooper, Osselton and Shaw (1969).

Bipolar Montages

A bipolar montage should be made up of sequential *linkages* of channels along anteroposterior or transverse rows of equispaced electrodes (Jasper, 1958), as shown in *Figure 3.4*. Each channel is con-

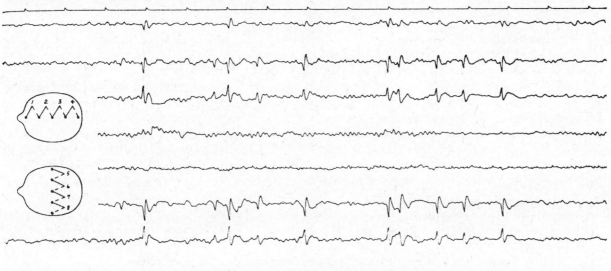

Figure 3.4—Demonstration of a focus of transient discharges at the vertex. Phase-reversals about vertex electrode common to two rows at right angles. Boy aged 9 years. Behaviour disorder. No history of epilepsy

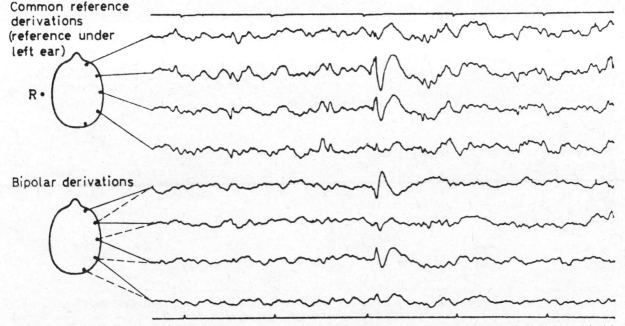

Figure 3.5—Simultaneous common reference and bipolar recordings of a sharp and slow wave complex the potential maximum of which is between the right anterior and mid-temporal electrodes

41

nected between a pair of 'active' electrodes on the scalp and records the potential difference between them. If a localized discharge occurs at or near one of the electrodes common to two channels, the latter will deflect in opposite directions, giving rise to a *phase-reversal*. In this particular example, the localized sharp waves occur at the vertex, giving rise to opposing deflections in channels 2 & 3 and 6 & 7. These pairs of channels are said to be *out of phase*: they demonstrate the presence of a *focus* at the vertex. The implication of such a finding is that the origin of the discharge lies perpendicularly below the site of the electrode. However, no indication is given as to its depth.

When a circumscribed discharge occurs midway between two electrodes, each will be affected equally by it; the electrodes are said to be *equipotential*. If these form part of a bipolar linkage, the channel connected between them will show no evidence of the discharge having occurred; the channel is said to be *isoelectric*. This circumstance is illustrated in channel 6 of *Figure 3.5* in which the anterior and midtemporal electrodes are almost equipotential with respect to the sharp and slow wave complex. A bipolar derivation, because it measures the potential difference between two electrodes, gives an indication of the *potential gradient* between them.

Unipolar Montages

Each channel in a unipolar montage records between one 'active' electrode on the scalp (via the *black* lead) and usually one relatively 'indifferent' electrode elsewhere. The latter is common to the *white* leads of all channels and is known as the *common reference*. At first sight, the advantages of having each channel register solely the voltage fluctuations under a single electrode on the scalp would seem to weigh heavily in favour of the unipolar method of recording. Unfortunately a major practical difficulty arises in the selection of a truly neutral reference. An electrode on the ear, the nose, the chin or the neck invariably picks up a certain amount of electrical activity from the nearest part of the brain and may be contaminated by a variety of non-cerebral potentials, all of which will be registered in all channels for which this electrode is the reference. Placing it away from the head and neck altogether immediately introduces a component of the electrocardiogram (ECG), the amplitude of which may be several times that of the EEG. A way of reducing this artefact has been described by Stephenson and Gibbs (1951), in which the reference is derived from one electrode over the right sternoclavicular junction and another over the seventh cervical vertebra. The ECG components, which are of opposite polarity under each electrode, are balanced out by variable resistors in series with them. However, the method is inconvenient for routine use and will not eliminate all trace of the ECG.

Some workers are prepared to tolerate a substantial common EEG signal in all channels and use a reference, such as the vertex, which is demonstrably 'hot'. In general, it is wiser to select a point as

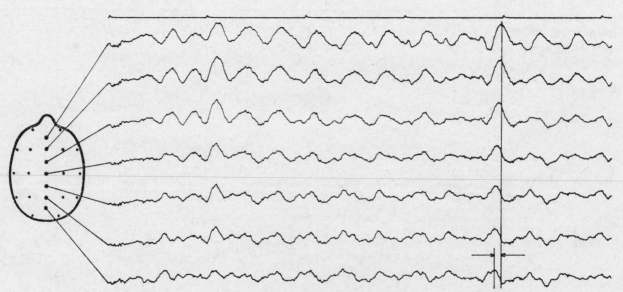

Figure 3.6—Progressive phase-shift from back to front of head equivalent to a total delay of 67 ms. Unipolar recording with chin reference. Recorded at 6 cm/s and with a time constant of 0–3 s in all channels

far as possible from the site of activity of greatest interest. The chin or a point on the neck about 5 cm below the external auditory meatus is often suitable (Sorel, 1969).

Some of the essential differences between unipolar and bipolar recordings are shown in *Figure 3.5*. When a discharge occurs synchronously at a number of electrodes, the unipolar derivations show deflections in the same sense. The amplitude of each deflection, assuming an indifferent reference, is proportional to the magnitude of the potential change that causes it. Hence measurements of the amount of any activity that is widespread, such as the *alpha* rhythm, should always be made with unipolar derivations. A bipolar derivation may well give an underestimate of amplitude because of cancellation of the common component at the electrodes from which the signal is derived. Furthermore, when small time differences exist between the occurrence of a widespread discharge at a number of electrodes, unipolar recording will demonstrate much more clearly what these differences are (*Figure 3.6*). If the activity in question is rhythmical, Cooper (1959) has shown that major ambiguities may arise with bipolar derivations.

Average Reference Montages

Each channel in an average reference montage records between an electrode on the scalp (via the *black* lead) and a common reference potential (via the *white* lead). The common reference potential is usually obtained by joining *all* the active electrodes on the scalp to a common point through high resistors of equal value. This point then assumes a potential which is the average of the potentials at the individual electrodes. The system was originally described by Offner (1950) and used by Goldman (1950), after whom it is sometimes known. If the potentials at the active electrodes were randomly related, then their average would tend towards zero the greater the number of electrodes employed. In practice, this is seldom the case with electrodes on the scalp. For instance, a widespread EEG feature, such as the *alpha* rhythm, or the electrical field accompanying an eye blink, may involve an appreciable number of electrodes simultaneously and will then contribute an appreciable potential to the average reference. This potential will affect all channels via their *white* leads, causing a reduction

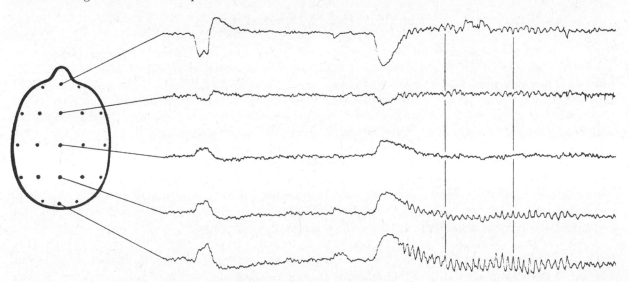

Figure 3.7—Common average reference recording showing inverted eye movement potentials posteriorly and phase-reversed alpha *rhythm anteriorly. Reference potential is derived from all 21 electrodes*

of amplitude due to cancellation in some and the appearance of an inverted signal in others (*Figure 3.7*). Average reference recording is therefore a difficult technique for the examination of activity that is spatially diffuse.

Notwithstanding these strictures, the technique is sometimes useful as an alternative to unipolar recording when no satisfactory site can be found for a reference electrode—perhaps due to pickup of the

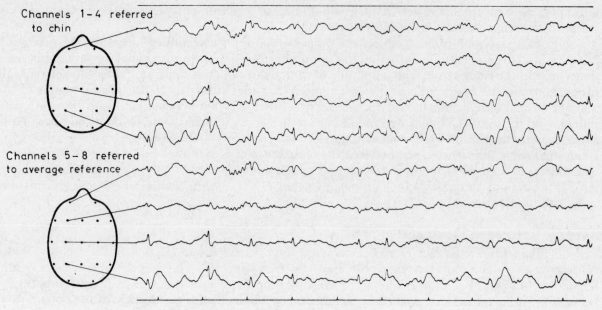

Figure 3.8—Unipolar and average reference derivations recorded at same sensitivity and time constant in all channels. Note equality of localized sharp waves in both sets of derivations, but partial cancellation of more diffuse slow activity in average reference derivations

ECG. A localized EEG feature extending to only two or three electrodes out of the full 10–20 placement, will hardly affect the average reference potential and the record will appear substantially the same as with an uncontaminated reference electrode (*Figure 3.8*).

DESCRIPTIVE TERMINOLOGY

The Terminology Committee of the International Federation has issued proposals (Storm van Leeuwen *et al*. 1966) as to the exact meaning that should be attached to a large number of terms used in EEG. The Committee also suggested that the features present in an EEG record should be classified into waves, activities, rhythms and complexes and that each feature should be described in terms of its frequency (or period), amplitude, phase relations, quantity, morphology, topography, reactivity and variability. The complexity of this classification emphasizes how difficult it is to describe in words what the eye can see. Some simplification is necessary when it comes to writing an EEG report.

The principal objective criteria by which a record is assessed are based upon the frequency, amplitude and shape of the waves of which it is composed, and upon their spatial and temporal distributions. Any one of these parameters might provide sufficient grounds for a record to be judged abnormal. Furthermore, few records are free from contamination by non-cerebral potentials of one sort or another and constant allowance must be made for these when a record is examined.

A cursory glance through a small selection of EEG records will show that they contain components of three basic kinds: those that are fairly continuous and very often rhythmical, those that are transient and those that comprise the background activity, upon which the two preceding kinds are superimposed, either singly or together. Whilst background activity may be broken down by analysis into a spectrum of many frequencies and may be of clinical significance, a statement of frequency can usefully be made only of regularly repetitive phenomena of which at least two complete cycles are present. Briefer discharges are better described in terms of their duration (period) and waveform.

As a matter of convenience, the EEG frequency spectrum is divided into bands that are designated as follows:

Delta:	less than 4 Hz
Theta:	from 4 Hz to less than 8 Hz
Alpha:	from 8 Hz to 13 Hz inclusive
Beta:	more than 13 Hz

Strictly speaking, these terms should be reserved for rhythmical discharges, but they are also used more loosely to describe irregular, non-rhythmical activity, the basic frequencies of which fall into a particular range. In general, they may be used irrespective of where the activity in question occurs. The only exception is the term *alpha rhythm* which refers to a particular phenomenon to be discussed later (*see* page 52). EEG records are sometimes described as 'fast' or 'slow'; these terms imply that their dominant frequency is respectively above or below the *alpha* range.

When stating the amplitude of a rhythm or other discharge, it is usual to refer to the peak-to-peak value in μV. In a given record one is more often concerned with the relative amplitudes either of one component with respect to another, or of one channel with respect to another. In serial studies, however, it may be necessary to know the actual magnitudes of particular components for the purpose of comparison from one occasion to the next. In this circumstance it is important to appreciate that a bipolar recording may give an inaccurate indication of absolute magnitude for reasons already discussed. Thus whenever it is desired to compare the amplitude or quantity (*abundance*) of a particular component in the EEGs of two or more subjects, it is preferable that an appropriate unipolar montage should be used.

Waveform is the most difficult descriptive feature to specify because it is a function of two variables: voltage and time. Hence the actual shape of an electrical phenomenon as recorded on moving paper

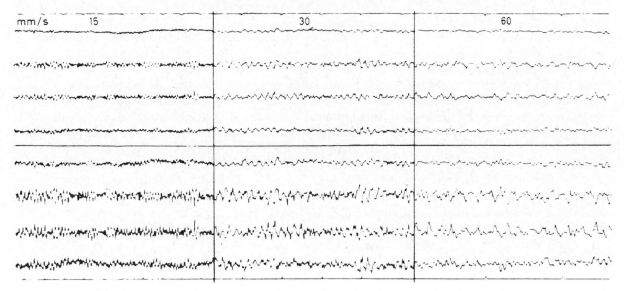

Figure 3.9—Effects of recording at paper speeds of 15, 30 and 60 mm/s and at sensitivities of 100 and 50 μV/cm from the same array of electrodes in the same subject over a short interval of time. The lower four channels portray the same avtivity as the upper four

depends upon both the sensitivity and the paper speed at which the recording is made. It also depends upon the overall frequency response of the recording system. What appears to be a spike at one sensitivity and speed will look much less dramatic at lower sensitivity or higher speed (*Figure 3.9*). The subjective quality of sharpness can only be specified in terms of rate of rise and subsequent rate of fall of voltage and of the overall duration of the discharge—parameters which it is both difficult and unnecessary to measure. What is important is the context in which such a transient occurs: the degree to which it stands out in amplitude and the extent to which it is qualitatively different from the activity amongst which it is seen. Its spatial distribution may also help to distinguish it from other components.

The activity recorded in each EEG trace is generally complex in waveform and essentially non-repetitive: it is impossible to predict what the next second will show. Nevertheless, over a short interval of time, it is often possible to break down the complex waveform into a small number of sinusoidal components. The opposite process is illustrated in *Figure 3.10* in which short samples of EEG activity have been simulated by the combination of only two sine waves. It does not, of course, follow that each component has a separate existence in the brain: only that the possibility of complex waveforms arising in this way should be considered when analysing an actual record. Sometimes it can be shown that

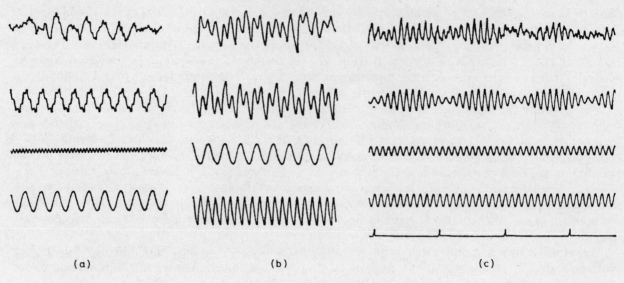

Figure 3.10—EEG waveforms simulated by the addition of two sine waves of (a) *high-frequency ratio,* (b) *medium-frequency ratio and* (c) *low-frequency ratio. In each example channel 1 shows the EEG waveform, channel 2 the simulated waveform and channels 3 and 4 its sine wave components*

there are indeed two components by demonstrating that each has a different spatial distribution or reactivity (Walter, 1963).

All EEG components fluctuate to a greater or lesser extent, either spontaneously or in response to stimuli, and considerable importance may attach to the way in which they do so, both during a particular recording and over longer periods of time. EEG maturation is a time process, extending over many years, in which delay may be of clinical significance. The general character of the EEG in normal subjects, recorded under the same conditions, is thought to remain stable for the greater part of adult life. In epilepsy, however, dramatic electrical discharges occur but may not be seen at all during a routine recording of half an hour's duration. It should always be remembered what a very small fraction of a patient's whole lifespan is sampled by such a recording. In cases of progressive organic disease of the brain, abnormalities which are intermittent in an initial recording may subsequently become more frequent or continuous. For these reasons, serial recordings over an interval of time dependent upon the clinical situation are always of greater value than a single examination, no matter how thorough.

EXTRACEREBRAL POTENTIALS

The ability to distinguish what is genuine cerebral electrical activity from what is spurious will sometimes tax the skill of the most experienced electroencephalographer, and there may be occasions when no rational explanation can be given as to why a particular discharge is thought to be an artefact. However, it is a mistake to regard all extracerebral potentials as an unmitigated evil: there are many circumstances in which they may be turned to good account if they provide information about the state of the subject while the recording is in progress. In certain experimental situations, deliberate steps may be taken to record physiological variables the intrusion of which, at other times, would be regarded as undesirable. Eye movements, pulse rate and respiration rate fall into this category. On the other hand, artefacts that arise from external sources of electrical interference, and those due to faults in the recording apparatus, are an embarrassment which every good technician will take immediate steps to eliminate.

ARTEFACTS FROM APPARATUS

It is not intended to discuss here the occasional electrical and mechanical faults which may occur in even the best designed recording equipment, except to say that those which develop progressively are more likely to be overlooked than those that are intermittent. Routine checking of amplifier noise and linearity of pen response may give advance warning of a fall-off in performance, but the majority of serious faults are unpredictable and must be dealt with as they arise.

Little difficulty should be experienced in recognizing the fuzziness or thickening of the trace due to interference from the alternating mains supply. This is at 50 Hz predominantly in Europe and

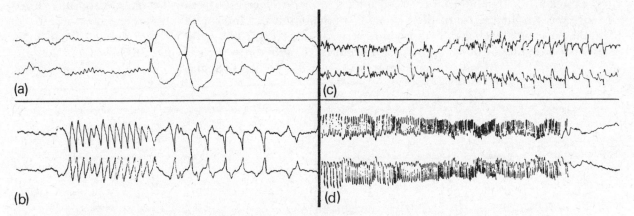

Figure 3.11—Artefacts arising at electrodes and in input leads: (a) *due to electrode movement;* (b) *due to imperfect electrode contact;* (c) *due to contamination of contact between electrode and clip;* (d) *due to contamination between input plug and socket.*

at 60 Hz in North America. It is colloquially known as *hum* or *ripple*. It may be detected to some extent in any building wired with alternating current mains and is particularly liable to be picked up from unscreened or unearthed (un-grounded) electrical apparatus in the EEG laboratory or in rooms adjacent to it. New EEG equipment should always be installed and tested *in situ* by the manufacturer's agent who will be able to advise what precautions should be taken. The discrimination ratio of modern EEG amplifiers is such that total screening of an EEG laboratory is unnecessary unless there is a potent source of interference, such as diathermy apparatus, nearby (Hospital Technical Memorandum No. 14, 1965). However, chopper amplifiers are prone to interference from certain kinds of hospital call systems (Dobbie, 1967) and special precautions may have to be taken with this type of EEG machine.

The area of contact between an electrode and the subject's scalp is probably the most critical link in the whole recording chain, and time spent in the preparation and proper application of electrodes will yield a generous return in terms of time saved on subsequent adjustment. Even so, an appreciable proportion of artefacts arise at this junction due to slight movements or alterations in pressure between the electrode surface and that of the scalp. These cause a momentary variation in contact impedance which, because of the minute currents that inevitably flow across the interface, are presented as voltage changes to the recording amplifier (*Figure 3.11a*). Variations in electrode potential ('pops') occasionally occur spontaneously, even in the absence of overt movements, and may then be mistaken for a rhythmical cerebral discharge (*Figure 3.11b*). Artefacts of a rather similar kind can also arise from faulty electrode leads, and from clips, plugs or sockets contaminated with saline or grease. These too can be either irregular or repetitive (*Figure 3.11c and d*). All such artefacts have a feature that greatly helps in their detection: they are strictly confined to the channel or channels connected to the component at fault and will give rise to mirror-image phase-reversals when these channels form part of a bipolar linkage.

Artefacts from Subject

The most prolific source of extracerebral potentials is the subject himself, whose muscles, eyes, heart and scalp can give rise to voltage changes, the magnitude of which may be many times that of the EEG. In so far as these provide information about the subject, they should not necessarily be eliminated or reduced. Muscular tension, for instance, is often a physical manifestation of anxiety which may in turn influence the character of the EEG. Similarly, eye blinks, heart rate and changes of skin resistance and potential may give a valuable indication of the degree of relaxation as the recording proceeds. Special techniques for recording these variables are discussed by Cooper, Osselton and Shaw (1969).

One of the temptations with artefacts of any kind is for the technician to reduce them by attenuation of the high or low frequency response of the recording amplifiers. This should be a last resort, not a first expedient, and should be reserved for excessive artefact that cannot be reduced by any other means. Indiscriminate use of these controls may complicate interpretation rather than simplify it. Muscle potentials are one of the commonest artefacts in EEG work (*Figure 3.12a*). Their high frequency attenuation may distort the waveform to something indistinguishable from *beta* activity (*Figure 3.12b*). In a tense subject, muscle activity is usually widespread, though maximal in the

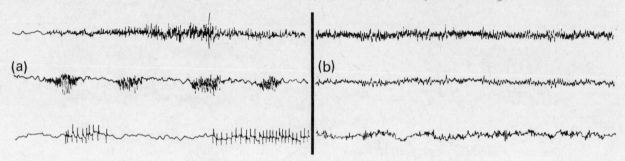

Figure 3.12—(a) *Examples of muscle activity recorded from scalp.* (b) *Upper trace: Unfiltered muscle activity. Centre trace: Identical activity with 30 per cent high-frequency cut at 24 Hz. Lower trace: Genuine* beta *activity*

temporal regions, but there are occasions when it may be picked up by a single electrode in the vicinity of a few active fibres. Its form is then likely to be that of the third example in *Figure 3.12a*, in which the individual spikes are probably single motor unit potentials. When these are picked up by only one electrode, phase-reversals will, of course, occur between the channels connected to it in a bipolar linkage.

Not infrequently, an electrode will inadvertantly be placed over or alongside an artery giving rise to a potential with a characteristic saw-toothed waveform in time with the pulse (*Figure 3.13a i*). This is caused by mechanical movement or by a change of contact pressure at the electrode due to pulsation in the vessel; it is much less likely to occur with stick-on electrodes than with pads. This artefact is not always obvious on casual inspection and may be mistaken for genuine low voltage slow activity (*Figure 3.13a ii*). It is more easily recognised by looking obliquely at the record in the direction of its travel. Once again, phase-reversals may be seen with bipolar linkages.

A further artefact due to cardiac activity is pick-up of the electrocardiogram. In the great majority of subjects, the head is fortunately equipotential with respect to the ECG field so that no trace of it is seen with bipolar montages; but there are some short-necked individuals in whom this is not the case. Repetitive sharp waves or less distinct complexes (*Figure 3.13a iii*) may then occur synchronously in a number of unrelated channels, as often in phase as out of phase with each other. In general, the situation is worse with unipolar montages, especially if a single reference electrode on the neck is used. Distances between the active electrodes and the reference are then much greater than the inter-electrode distances

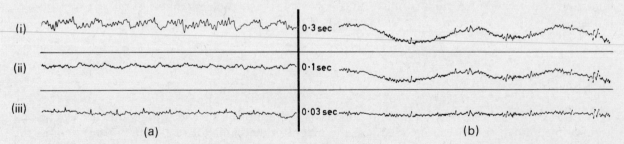

Figure 3.13—(a) *Artefacts due to cardiac activity. Upper traces due to pulsation; lower trace due to pick-up of ECG.* (b) *Effects of progressively reducing the time constant in three channels recording identical EEG signal and artefact due to perspiration*

of bipolar montages; pick-up is consequently enhanced and the deflections will be in phase in all channels. In these circumstances an average reference montage may be helpful. Occasionally, one or more complexes appear to be absent; this is more likely to be due to cancellation by a component of the EEG than to missed or premature beats. ECG artefact, unlike pulse artefact, cannot be eliminated by moving the electrodes, but it may be reduced by using transverse rather than anteroposterior bipolar linkages, depending on the orientation of the EEG field on the scalp.

A patient who is perspiring will cause very slow swings to appear in the record, usually in many channels simultaneously. These artefacts are due to changes in electrode contact resistance and in skin potential. They may be reduced by cooling the patient and, as a last resort, by reducing the time constants (*Figure 3.13b*).

There is a steady potential difference of the order of 100 mV between the aqueous and vitreous humours of the eye, the former being positive with respect to the latter. A movement of the eyeball consequently causes a potential field change that will be detected by electrodes in its vicinity. When the eyelids blink or are closed, the eyeball may make a momentary upward rotation. The potential change so produced is augmented by the effect of eyelid movement (Barry and Jones, 1965), an electrode on the forehead becoming electro-positive with respect to one situated more posteriorly. If an amplifying channel is connected between them with its *black* input lead anterior to the *white*, the

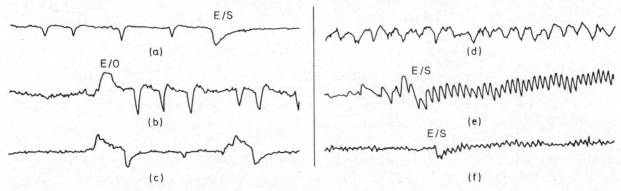

Figure 3.14—Eye movement potentials. (a), (b), (c), *due to blinking, eye opening and eye closure;* (d), (e), (f), *due to ocular tremor, nystagmus and eyelid flutter respectively*

recording pen will make a downward deflection (*Figure 3.14a*). Conversely, when the eyelids are opened an upward deflection will be produced (*Figure 3.14b*). Eye movements in a vertical plane should produce symmetrical deflections in anteriorly recording channels; these provide a useful check on electrode symmetry. A lateral movement of the eyes will produce potential changes of opposite polarity at the frontotemporal electrodes on each side (Nelligan, 1964). Random movements produce more varied artefacts. Those occurring during sleep (*see* page 210) and those associated with scanning a picture (*see* page 56) may have interesting EEG accompaniments. Apprehensive or inquisitive subjects may momentarily open their eyes when they are supposed to be closed and produce a combination of opening and closing artefacts (*Figure 3.14c*), while very anxious subjects or patients suffering from nystagmus may be unable to prevent an ocular tremor occurring when their eyelids are closed. A rhythmical discharge will then be picked up by frontal electrodes (*Figure 3.14d and e*) which it may subsequently be impossible to differentiate from genuine cerebral activity. A somewhat similar discharge can be produced during eyelid flutter (*Figure 3.14f*) which, according to Harlan, White and Bickford (1958), may occur in association with concentrated mental effort.

Kennedy *et al.* (1948) have described a rhythm which also occurs in association with mental effort but which they claim to be cerebral in origin. It is often of *alpha* frequency and is best recorded with a bipolar derivation between the anterior temporal electrodes on either side. They named it *kappa rhythm*. Further evidence in support of its cerebral origin was presented by Armington and Chapman (1959) and by Chapman, Armington and Bragdon (1962), but the possibility that it might be due to fine lateral eye movements was not convincingly eliminated.

It has not been possible to mention here more than a few of the commoner artefacts met with in practice, nor to discuss the ways in which they may be minimized. Although each has been considered separately, many of them can occur in combination, as in a restless subject who may move his head, talk and look around all at the same time. Such combinations, however, are so obviously extracerebral that they pose no problem in recognition. Clearly the best time to decide whether or not a doubtful discharge is genuine is during the recording itself and the responsibility to do so rests squarely on the technician. Scrupulous attention to electrode technique and consideration for the subject's physical and psychological comfort will do much to keep extraneous potentials to a minimum.

REFERENCES

Abraham, K. and Marsan, C. A. (1958). 'Patterns of Cortical Discharges and their Relation to Routine Scalp Electroencephalography'. *Electroenceph. clin. Neurophysiol.* **10,** 447

Armington, J. C. and Chapman, R. M. (1959). 'Temporal Potentials and Eye Movements'. *Electroenceph. clin. Neurophysiol.* **11,** 346

Barry, W. and Jones, G. M. (1965). 'Influence of Eyelid Movement upon Electro-oculographic Recording of Vertical Eye Movements'. *Aerospace Med.* **36,** 855

Brazier, M. A. B. (1951). 'A Study of the Electrical Fields at the Surface of the Head'. *Electroenceph. clin. Neurophysiol.* Suppl. 2, **38**; reprinted in *Am. J. EEG Technol.* (1967) **6,** 114

Calvet, J., Calvet, M. C. and Scherrer, J. (1964). 'Etude Stratigraphique Corticale de L'activité EEG Spontanée'. *Electroenceph. clin. Neurophysiol.* **17,** 109

Chapman, R. M., Armington, J. C. and Bragdon, H. R. A. (1962). 'A Quantitative Survey of Kappa and Alpha EEG Activity'. *Electroenceph. clin. Neurophysiol.* **14,** 858

Coles, P. A. and Binnie, C. D. (1968). 'An Alternative Method of Chloriding EEG Electrodes'. *Proc. electrophysiol. Technol. Ass.* **15,** 195

Cooper, R. (1956). 'Storage of Silver Chloride Electrodes'. *Electroenceph. clin. Neurophysiol.* **8,** 692
—   (1959). 'An Ambiguity of Bipolar Recording'. *Electroenceph. clin. Neurophysiol.* **11,** 819
—   (1962). 'Electrodes'. *Proc. electrophysiol. Technol. Ass.* **9** (**1**), 22; reprinted in *Am. J. EEG Technol.* (1963), **3,** 91
—   Osselton, J. W. and Shaw, J. C. (1969). *EEG Technology.* pp. 26, 75, 133. London: Butterworths
—   Winter, A. L., Crow, H. J. and Walter, W. G. (1965). 'Comparison of Subcortical, Cortical and Scalp Activity using Chronically Indwelling Electrodes in Man'. *Electroenceph. clin. Neurophysiol.* **14,** 191

Dobbie, A. K. (1967). 'A Special Interference Problem with Chopper-type Amplifiers'. *Wld. med. Electron.* **5,** 124

Geddes, L. A., Baker, L. E. and Moore, A. G. (1969). 'Optimum Electrolytic Chloriding of Silver Electrodes'. *Med. biol. Engng.* **7,** 49

Goldman, D. (1950). 'The Clinical use of the "Average" Reference Electrode in Monopolar Recording'. *Electroenceph. clin. Neurophysiol.* **2,** 209

Harlan, W. L., White, P. T. and Bickford, R. G. (1958). 'Electric Activity Produced by Eye Flutter Simulating Frontal Electroencephalographic Rhythms'. *Electroenceph. clin. Neurophysiol.* **10,** 164

Hess, R. (1966). *EEG Handbook.* p. 148. London; Sandoz

Hospital Technical Memorandum No. 14. (1965). 'Abatement of Electrical Interference'. London; H.M.S.O.

Jasper, H. H. (1958). 'Report of the Committee on Methods of Clinical Examination in Electroencephalography.' *Electroenceph. clin. Neurophysiol.* **10,** 370

Kagawa, N. (1962). 'Electroencephalography in Infants with Special Reference to the Newborn: Technique'. *Am. J. EEG Technol.* **2,** 99

Kennedy, J. L., Gottsdanker, R. M., Armington, J. C. and Gray, F. E. (1948). 'A New Electroencephalogram Associated with Thinking'. *Science* **108,** 527

Knott, J. R. (1958). 'Report of the Committee on Apparatus—recommendations to manufacturers.' *Electroenceph. clin. Neurophysiol.* **10,** 378

Margerison, J. H., St. John-Loe, P. and Binnie, C. D. (1967). 'Electroencephalography'. In *A Manual of Psychophysiological Methods.* Ed. by P. H. Venables and I. Martin, Amsterdam; North-Holland

Nelligan, D. P. (1964). 'Eye Movement Artefacts and Electrical Recording of Eye Position'. *Proc. electrophysiol Technol. Ass.* **11** (**2**), 25

Offner, F. F. (1950). 'The EEG as Potential Mapping: the Value of the Average Monopolar Reference'. *Electroenceph. clin. Neurophysiol.* **2,** 213

Osselton, J. W. (1966). 'Bipolar, Unipolar and Average Reference Recording Methods. I: Mainly Theoretical Considerations'. *Proc. electrophysiol. Technol. Ass.* **13,** 99; reprinted in *Am. J. EEG Technol.* (1966), **6,** 129
—   (1969). 'Bipolar, Unipolar and Average Reference Recording Methods. II: Mainly Practical Considerations'. *Am. J. EEG Technol.* **9,** 117; reprinted in *Proc. electrophysiol. Technol. Ass.* (1970), **17,** 45

Pampiglione, G. (1956). 'Some Anatomical Considerations upon Electrode Placement in Routine EEG'. *Proc. electrophysiol. Technol. Ass.* **7** (**1**), 20; reprinted *ibid* (1966), **13,** 166

Saunders, M. G. and Jell, R. M. (1959). 'Time Distortion in Electroencephalograph Amplifiers'. *Electroenceph. clin. Neurophysiol.* **11,** 814

Shaw, J. C. and Roth, M. (1955). 'Potential Distribution Analysis. II: A Theoretical Consideration of its Significance in Terms of Electrical Field Theory'. *Electroenceph. clin. Neurophysiol.* **7,** 285

Sorel, L. (1969). 'Les Montages Verticaux en Electroencéphalographie'. *Bull. Acad. r. Méd. Belg.* **9,** 587

Stephenson, W. A. and Gibbs, F. A. (1951). 'A Balanced Non-cephalic Reference Electrode'. *Electroenceph. clin. Neurophysiol.* **3,** 237

Storm, van Leeuwen *et al.* (1966). 'Proposal for an EEG Terminology by the Terminology Committee of the International Federation for Electroencephalography and Clinical Neurophysiology'. *Electroenceph. clin. Neurophysiol.* **20,** 306; reprinted in *Proc. electrophysiol. Technol. Ass.* (1966), **13,** 90

REFERENCES

Taylor, F. M. and Abraham, P. (1969). 'A Search for a Safe Bentonite Paste'. *Proc. electrophysiol. Technol. Ass.* **16,** 80

Velate, A. S. (1962). 'Amplifier Blocking—Part 1. The Mechanism, Effects and Possible External Causes'. *Proc. electrophysiol. Technol. Ass.* **8 (6),** 3

Walter, W. G. (1963). 'Technique—Interpretation'. In *Electroencephalography*. 2nd Edn., p. 82. Ed. by D. Hill and G. Parr. London; Macdonald

— and Parr, G. (1963). 'Recording Equipment and Technique'. In *Electroencephalography*. 2nd. Edn. p. 59. Ed. by D. Hill and G. Parr. London; Macdonald

Weir, B. (1965). 'The Morphology of the Spike-Wave Complex'. *Electroenceph. clin. Neurophysiol.* **19,** 284

Zablow, L. and Goldensohn, E. S. (1969). 'A Comparison between Scalp and Needle Electrodes for the EEG'. *Electroenceph. clin. Neurophysiol.* **26,** 530

CHAPTER 4

NORMAL FINDINGS

THE NORMAL ADULT EEG

The concept of the normal employed in the biological sciences is based upon examination of a sample of the population in question and the classification and measurement of its characteristics. The criteria of the normal EEG are established in a similar way, as indeed are the relationships between EEG findings and clinical conditions. The so-called normal EEG patterns now to be described are simply those that are most often found in people without demonstrable functional or structural cerebral abnormality. This stipulation in no way precludes their occurrence in patients who are manifestly ill; nor does it preclude the occurrence of statistically abnormal findings in people who in other respects satisfy the most stringent definition of normality.

Spontaneous Phenomena

Alpha Rhythm

One of the many things that Hans Berger discovered about the human EEG was that the majority of normal adult subjects had a dominant rhythm at about 10 Hz, but he was mistaken in believing it to be a product of the brain as a whole. Adrian and Matthews (1934) were the first to show that this *alpha rhythm*, as Berger named it, occurred predominantly in the posterior half of the brain, especially in the parieto-occipital regions, and that the anterior half of the brain was often relatively silent. They confirmed that the rhythm was most evident when the subject was relaxed with his eyelids closed and that it could be diminished or abolished by opening them. Afferent stimulation was also found to cause its reduction, but the effectiveness of a particular stimulus declined with repetition. Similarly, opening the eyes in total darkness caused only an initial reduction, the rhythm soon reappearing in the absence of a further stimulus, although it was once again reduced by a conscious effort to see. A comparable effect was observed during any form of mental concentration. Adrian and Matthews also showed that the two hemispheres produced *alpha* rhythms at apparently the same frequency and in approximately equal amounts, although the amplitudes did not always fluctuate together on the two sides.

Recent work, using highly specialized techniques, has shown that there is often more than one source of *alpha* activity in each cerebral hemisphere (Walter *et al.*, 1966). Perez-Borja *et al.* (1962), recording from multiple depth electrodes implanted in the occipital lobes, were able to demonstrate the existence of several rhythms in the range of 8–16 Hz. These were distributed widely throughout the occipital lobes and generally extended into adjacent temporal and parietal regions. They often fluctuated independently of each other and of the rhythms detected by electrodes on the scalp. Some were unaffected by visual stimuli. Although none of the subjects in whom these investigations were carried out was clinically normal, none was thought to have any structural anomaly of the occipital lobes.

The *alpha* rhythm is classically described as a bilateral posterior rhythm of substantially constant frequency in the range of 8–13 Hz which is diminished primarily by eye opening—this effect being described as *blocking* or *desynchronization*. The work of Perez-Borja *et al.* suggests that this is a misleading over-simplification. Nevertheless, in most clinical contexts, when recording from conventionally spaced scalp electrodes, it suffices to regard the *alpha* rhythm as monorhythmic, although its frequency may be observed to vary about the mean by ± 0.5 Hz in normal subjects under stable conditions. However, it may be as much as 2 Hz faster than the mean immediately after eye closure—the *squeak* phenomenon of Storm van Leeuwen and Bekkering (1958).

In the majority of adult subjects, the *alpha* rhythm has a mean frequency in the range of 9–10 Hz;

52

in some it is immediately above or below this range and in only a small number does it exceed 11 Hz. Conventional analysis usually reveals a spread of frequencies throughout the *alpha* range the proportions of which may change from epoch to epoch. The mean frequency in a given subject is more stable from one epoch to another if a constant level of alertness is maintained, for instance by the performance of a moderately difficult counting task. Margerison *et al.* (1964) have demonstrated a tendency for the abundance of activity in the low *alpha* frequency range to be reduced premenstrually. This would have the effect of slightly increasing the mean frequency.

When a large number of subjects is examined, it is found that their *alpha* rhythms are of higher mean voltage and of somewhat wider distribution over the right hemisphere. Since the *alpha* rhythm is best seen under conditions of relaxation, this finding may well be related to the fact that the majority of people are left hemisphere dominant. It raises the difficulty of deciding what degree of lateral asymmetry may be accepted as within normal limits. As has been discussed in Chapter 3 (*see* page 43), unipolar recording to a distant reference should always be employed if a true measure of amplitude is required. If the potential fields of the *alpha* rhythm over the two hemispheres are asymmetrically distributed, this fact alone is likely to give rise to an apparent amplitude asymmetry with a bipolar montage. In general, an overall difference in mean abundance of 2:3 is acceptable, so long as the greater is over the non-dominant hemisphere.

Toposcopic analysis by Cooper and Mundy-Castle (1960) of the phase relations of the *alpha* rhythm recorded with anteroposterior lines of scalp electrodes has provided evidence to suggest that its potential field may be either stationary or moving in a given individual at different moments. They found that in a group of normal subjects of about average intelligence the movement was generally anterior to posterior. They also found that exact synchrony between the hemispheres was rare. The latter finding has been confirmed by Liske *et al.* (1967) who found that there is often a small but consistent phase difference between the *alpha* rhythms over the two hemispheres in a given individual.

More importance attaches to relatively small differences in frequency between the two hemispheres. If there is a consistent difference of 1 Hz or more, then the side of lower frequency is likely to be involved in a pathological process.

Various hypotheses have been put forward as to the neurophysiological significance of the *alpha* rhythm, but the fact remains that a small minority of normal people, in their customary state of alertness, have little or none that can be demonstrated by conventional recording procedures and that they manifest no obvious handicap as a result of their deficit. Another small group have an *alpha* rhythm that persists even when the eyes are open, though its abundance in these circumstances is

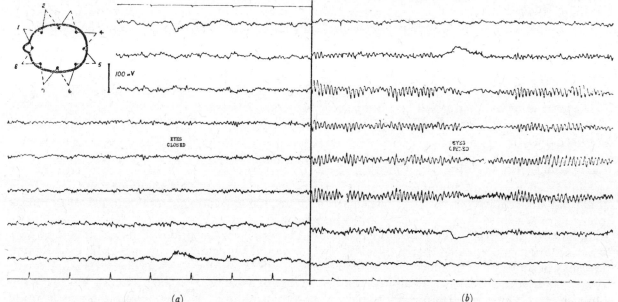

(a) (b)

Figure 4.1—(a) *M-type* alpha *subject. Normal man aged 27 years. EEG: Complete absence of* alpha *rhythm. Low voltage* beta *components not affected by eye closure.* (b) *P-type* alpha *subject. Normal man aged 18 years. EEG: Well sustained 11 Hz* alpha *rhythm suppressed for only about 1 second following eye opening*

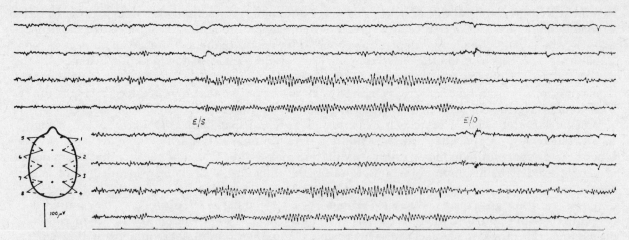

Figure 4.2—R-type alpha *subject. Normal woman aged 40 years. EEG: Well sustained 11 Hz* alpha *rhythm when eyes are closed (E/S). Persistent low voltage* beta *activity when eyes are open (E/O)*

usually reduced. The majority of people, as might be expected from the scatter of other human characteristics, occupy intermediate positions between these two extremes. These three *alpha* types are sometimes designated as M for *minus* or *minimal*, P for *persistent* and R for *responsive*; they are illustrated in *Figures 4.1 and 4.2.* It will be noted that the so-called persistent P-type *alpha* rhythm does in fact momentarily diminish as the eyes are opened. Complete unresponsiveness of the *alpha* rhythm to visual stimuli is a rare and unequivocally abnormal finding.

There have been numerous studies concerning the degree to which *alpha* abundance is affected by various kinds of peripheral stimulation or mental activity. There is general agreement that visual stimuli are the most effective in reducing *alpha* abundance and that the performance of mental arithmetic has a similar though less marked effect, depending on the degree of motivation (Glass, 1964). Kreitman and Shaw (1965) found that the performance of mental arithmetic, auditory tests and tactile tests respectively caused progressively smaller reductions in *alpha* abundance than visual tests. Indeed, the performance of tactile tests was more often accompanied by an enhancement of *alpha* abundance than a reduction.

There is good reason to suppose that the characteristics of the *alpha* rhythm and of other normal EEG features are genetically determined (Juel-Nielsen and Harvald, 1958; Vogel, 1965). Clarke and Harding (1969) compared the mean frequencies of the dominant posterior rhythms in an equal number of pairs of mono- and dizygotic twins. They found a greater degree of intra-pair similarity between the mean frequencies in the monozygotic twins, but only for the rhythms over the non-dominant hemisphere. However, a sophisticated computer comparison by Dumermuth (1968) revealed a much greater degree of similarity in the posterior EEG activities of pairs of mono- than of dizygotic twins.

The association between *alpha* types and personality structure is discussed on page 168. Relationships between mental ability and the EEG in normal subjects have been reported by Vogel, Broverman and Klaiber (1968).

Theta and Delta Activity

The presence of small amounts of activity at frequencies below the *alpha* range is not uncommon in normal adult subjects, even in the alert state, and it is difficult to define quantitatively the amount in excess of which such components should be regarded as abnormal. In general, the greater the abundance of the *alpha* rhythm, the more posterior slow activity is acceptable, but runs of *theta* activity of an amplitude approaching that of the *alpha* rhythm should be regarded with suspicion, even though they may occupy only a small fraction of the record. On the other hand, occasional *theta* components of this magnitude, either in the temporo-occipital regions or about the vertex, are acceptable in young adult subjects. Those in the former situation are likely to be reduced by eye opening and may be quite asymmetrical; those in the central regions are usually uninfluenced by eye opening but are enhanced during drowsiness.

Mundy-Castle (1951) detected *theta* activity to some extent in 64 per cent of a normal young adult group, but in only 24 per cent of a group of mentally normal old people. It was present in about one and a half times as many young women as young men; sometimes it was enhanced by embarrassment or during mental concentration. Picard *et al.* (1957) found the incidence of *theta* activity to be 36 per cent in a large group of potential air crew. These figures, of course, comprise those with both acceptable and excessive amounts of *theta* activity. Williams (1941), using the criteria given above, found the incidence of abnormal amounts of slow activity to be 5 per cent in a highly selected group of flying personnel as compared with 10 per cent in a group of other servicemen. It is generally accepted that between 10–15 per cent of the supposedly normal population at large have abnormal EEGs of a similar kind. These EEG patterns are discussed in greater detail on page 169.

On-going *delta* activity is abnormal in an alert adult subject under normal physiological conditions but allowance must be made for the various common artefacts which may occur in this frequency range in assessing the *delta* activity in a given record. However, Aird and Gastaut (1959) found occasional posterior waves in the 3–4 Hz range in 10 per cent of 500 normal subjects of 19–22 years of age. Picard *et al.* found an incidence of 7 per cent in their study.

Beta Activity

Beta activity is present to some extent in the EEGs of almost all normal adults. It can occur in a variety of locations in different subjects, but is seen most frequently in the precentral regions. When it occurs posteriorly it may well be masked by the *alpha* rhythm and becomes evident only when the eyes are open (*see Figure 4.2*). On the other hand, in the absence of an *alpha* rhythm in an M-type subject, opening the eyes may cause posterior *beta* rhythm to diminish. When it occurs anteriorly, it often behaves independently of the *alpha* rhythm and usually fluctuates asynchronously on either side. Mundy-Castle (1951) found that rhythmical *beta* activity, detectable on visual inspection, occurred in 53 per cent of his young adult group and in 62 per cent of his normal senile group and that its amount was inversely related to the amount of *alpha* rhythm. The seniles were found to have significantly less *alpha* and more *beta* activity than the young adult group—a finding that has been confirmed by Matousek *et al.*, (1967). As with low voltage *theta* components, *beta* components were demonstrated in about 60 per cent of young women and 40 per cent of young men. It must always be borne in mind when *beta* activity is seen that it may be related to the use or abuse of drugs (*see* page 192).

Mu Rhythm

Rhythmical fast activity is an extremely common finding in the frontal and precentral areas during electrocorticography, even in subjects who have had no general anaesthetic. Such activity in the

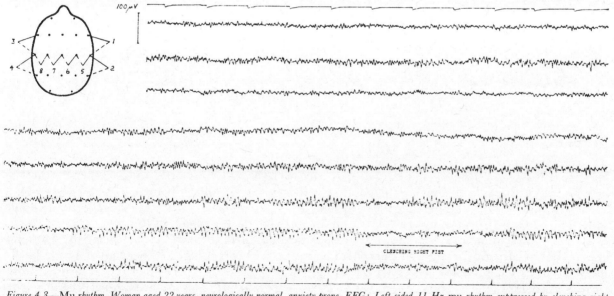

Figure 4.3—Mu *rhythm. Woman aged 22 years, neurologically normal, anxiety prone. EEG: Left-sided 11 Hz* mu *rhythm suppressed by clenching right fist. Less characteristic runs on right side.* Beta *activity at 20–22 Hz*

rolandic areas has been shown to be reduced during contralateral limb movements (Jasper, 1949); this effect is occasionally evident when recording from electrodes on the appropriate part of the scalp. A related and similarly responsive phenomenon is the *rhythme rolandique en arceau* of Gastaut, Terzian and Gastaut (1952). This takes the form of runs at 9 ± 2 Hz, the electro-positive half-cycles of which are rounded off and the electro-negative half-cycles pointed (*Figure 4.3*)—a waveform that could well be due to the presence of second or higher even-order harmonics. Because of its characteristic shape, this activity has variously been named *comb* or *wicket rhythm* and it is probably the same phenomenon as the *alphoid activity* described by Maddocks, Hodge and Rex (1951). It is now known as *mu rhythm*. When bilateral, it often occurs in independent runs on either side. It is not usually affected by visual stimuli or by intellectual effort. Chatrian, Petersen and Lazarte (1959) have shown that *mu* rhythm is reduced not only by overt movement of a contralateral limb but also sometimes when the subject formulates the intention of moving. The latter effect may be related to preliminary muscular tension in the limb in question. Gastaut estimates that *mu* rhythm can be seen in about 7 per cent of normal adults, its incidence declining in subjects over 30 years of age. Special electrode placements are sometimes necessary for its characteristic waveform to be revealed.

Evoked Phenomena

Lambda Waves

In general, all the phenomena described so far tend to be reduced by afferent stimulation of one sort or another and abnormal EEG components often respond in a similar way. In contrast, *lambda* waves are best seen when the subject is actively engaged in looking at something that arouses his interest. Characteristically, they consist of random electro-positive waves of up to 250 ms duration arising at the occiput but sometimes extending into the parietal regions. Their waveform is saw-toothed rather than spike-like and the initial electro-positive phase may be followed by a smaller one of opposite

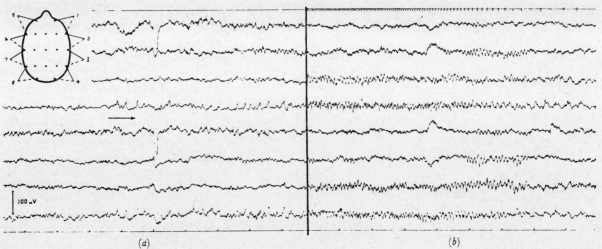

Figure 4.4—(a) Lambda *waves. Normal woman aged 23 years. EEG: Occipital* lambda *waves while subject examines picture presented at arrow. Eye movement artefacts in channels 1 and 5.* (b) *Response to photic stimulation in same subject. EEG: Bilateral posterior rhythm at flash frequencies of 2–23 per second*

polarity (*Figure 4.4a*). They were originally reported in 1949 by Evans (1953) and were subsequently described in greater detail by Gastaut (1951). Roth and Green (1953) point out that *lambda* waves are an essentially normal phenomenon that can be shown to occur in the great majority of adult subjects when a high recording sensitivity and an electrode in the region of the inion are employed. Scott *et al.* (1967) found that they occurred in 65 per cent of their normal controls during the scanning of a complex picture but in only 17·5 per cent of the group during reading; 17·5 per cent of their subjects showed spontaneous *lambda* waves whenever the eyes were open. Green (1957), recording from electrodes round the eyes, showed that each *lambda* wave was preceded by a small movement of the eyeball, the amplitude of which was often insufficient to give rise to a detectable artefact at the frontal electrodes of standard montages. Poor illumination diminished their incidence, even though the subject was still able to discern details of the picture.

There is a marked similarity between *lambda* waves and the responses to isolated photic stimuli. Both show the same distribution and have the same predominant polarity when the subject's eyes are open (*Figure 4.4b*). Subjects with clear *lambda* waves are very likely to show a marked response to rhythmic photic stimulation. It is significant that at low stimulation rates the latency of the major component of the photic response (70–90 ms) is approximately equal in the same individual to the interval between a *lambda* wave and the preceding eye movement. Sometimes a *lambda* wave follows a blink with substantially the same latency. Paradoxically, random waves of similar distribution and polarity, though of somewhat longer duration, are sometimes seen during light sleep (Roth, Shaw and Green, 1956). These observations have been confirmed by studies with implanted electrodes by Perez-Borja *et al.* (1962).

Vertex Waves

In a later section (*see* page 65), reference is made to a variety of discharges that may occur in the EEG in response to a sound or other stimulus during sleep. One of these—the electro-negative vertex wave (*V-wave*)—can sometimes be evoked by an auditory stimulus when the subject is fully awake (Roth, Shaw and Green, 1956). In these circumstances, the amplitude of the response may be relatively small in comparison with that of the spontaneous background activity and it may require a much louder evocative stimulus than would suffice if the subject were asleep. This led to the suspicion that the vertex wave might be an artefact, due either to an eye blink or to movement of the scalp, both of which comprise part of the more generalized startle reaction described by Landis and Hunt (1939). The first of these possibilities was investigated by Gastaut (1953), who demonstrated that the major component of the vertex wave was always electro-negative, whereas the electrical field change at the vertex accompanying an eye blink was always electro-positive. The second possibility has been discredited by Larsson (1960), who attached a strain gauge to the scalp at the vertex and was thus able to monitor any movements that occurred. Nevertheless, it is of interest that all three phenomena have latencies which fall into the range of 65 ± 25 ms. Auditory evoked responses are discussed in greater detail in Chapter 10.

Relatively high voltage—100 μV or more—vertex sharp waves occur in a very few fully alert subjects, usually children, in the absence of overt stimulus. It is doubtful if this can be regarded as a normal phenomenon but its significance is unknown. Usually there is a single focus at the midline (*see Figure 3.4*, page 41), but recording from a closely spaced transverse line of electrodes passing through the vertex will occasionally reveal bilateral foci that discharge synchronously. Gastaut (1953) reported *V-waves* in children between the ages of 7 and 15 years; most of these were cases of 'infantile encephalopathy'.

CHILDREN

Paediatric electroencephalography presents a number of special problems of a practical and theoretical nature. The difficulty of obtaining a satisfactory recording from an alert and possibly apprehensive child should not be underestimated, and constant allowance must be made in interpretation for the variety of artefacts that may occur. Stick-on electrodes should be used if the recording session is likely to be protracted, but a child's co-operation is better sustained if a number of brief recordings are made rather than a single long one. Often it is expedient to use fewer electrodes than the full number of the 10–20 system (Hellström *et al.* 1963). Familiarity with the procedure engenders confidence in the child and is probably the most important single factor in obtaining a technically successful record. When a child is known to be difficult and resists all approaches, recourse should be made to adequate sedation (*see* page 66) before attempting to apply the electrodes.

The interpretation of the EEG findings in children is often difficult because of the wide range of patterns that occur normally at any one age. Maturation of the EEG must bear some relationship to cerebral morphogenesis, but it is far from clear what this is. There are occasions when serial recordings show a trend opposite to that which might be expected from the clinical circumstances. The variability of the responses on different occasions to standard provocation techniques bears further witness to the fact that fluctuating states of cerebral excitability constitute a normal feature of childhood.

INFANCY—PATTERNS DURING ALERTNESS AND SLEEP

The EEG of a wakeful infant a few days old (*Figure 4.5a*) is of relatively low voltage, seldom exceeding 50 μV, and is composed of irregular and asynchronous *theta* and *delta* components. During drowsiness and sleep these increase in voltage and may have superimposed upon them discrete bursts of generalized *delta* activity of a few seconds' duration—a pattern named *tracé alternant* by Dreyfus-Brisac (1964)

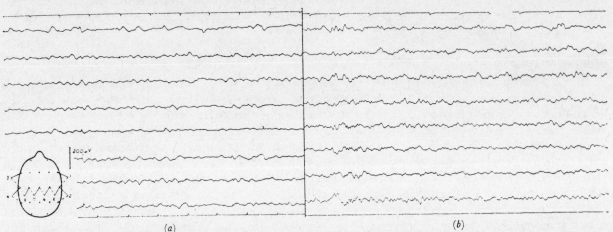

(a)   (b)

Figure 4.5—(a) *Normal infant, aged 10 days, awake. EEG: Irregular low voltage* theta *and* delta *components.* (b) *Normal infant, aged 6 weeks, awake. EEG: Moderate voltage* theta *and* delta *components with traces of activity at higher frequencies*

A sound stimulus is then likely to result in a period of generalized flattening, sometimes preceded by a burst of generalized slow waves analogous to the K-complex seen in later years (Ellingson, 1958).

As sleep deepens, two quite different states become apparent; these have been described as 'quiet' and 'active' (Parmelee *et al.*, 1968). Quiet sleep (*Figure 4.6a*) is characterized by regular heart and respiration rates, an absence of eye and limb movements, and the *tracé alternant* EEG pattern described

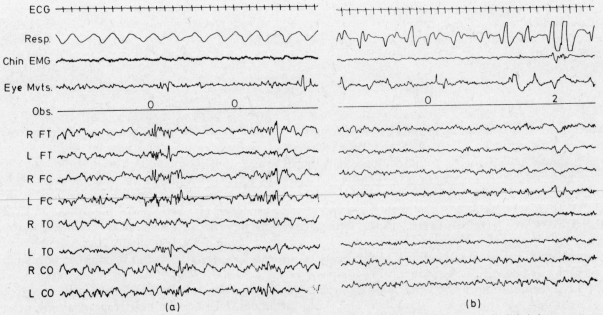

(a)   (b)

Figure 4.6—(a) *quiet,* (b) *active sleep in normal full-term newborn infant (see text).* Obs, *observation:* O, *no movement;* 2, *slight body movement*

(From Parmelee *et al.* (1968) in *Clinical Electroencephalography of Children.* Stockholm; Almqvist and Wiksell. Reproduced by courtesy of the authors and publishers)

above. Active sleep (*Figure 4.6b*) is characterized by irregular heart and respiration rates, frequent eye and limb movements, and a more constant polyrhythmic EEG pattern—a combination of features found in *paradoxical* sleep in adults (*see* page 212). Sleeping infants born and examined at term were found to spend approximately 50 per cent of the time in each of these sleep states. Episodes of quiet and active sleep occurred alternately with a cycle time of about 45 minutes. In contrast, premature infants spend a greater proportion of sleeping time in the active phase—up to 80 per cent when two months premature (Parmelee *et al.*, 1967). Nine months after conception, these infants also spent about half of their sleeping time in the active phase. Three months later the proportion had fallen to about 40 per cent in both the full-term and premature babies.

During the first few months of life there is a progressive and relatively rapid increase in the voltage of the low frequencies in the alert state and a tendency for these to become more rhythmical (*Figure 4.5b*). This is especially true of the *theta* components which at first tend to predominate in the central regions, subsequently becoming more generalized. Their amplitude is greatest at 6–9 months (up to 150 μV when the eyes are closed) and their dominant frequency, which is initially at 4 Hz, gradually increases with age. These *theta* components are often accentuated during crying—an effect that occurs also in older children. Rhythmical *delta* components in excess of 100 μV are seldom seen in the alert state, although they are common during drowsiness. The background is likely to consist of relatively low voltage random *theta* and *delta* components. *Beta* activity is uncommon in the alert state unless the infant has been given a hypnotic which induces this activity. A well documented survey of the EEG changes in normal alert infants during the first year of life is given by Hagne (1968).

OLDER CHILDREN—PATTERNS DURING ALERTNESS AND SLEEP

At about 18 months, intermittent low frequency *alpha* components may begin to appear and there may be quite a marked reduction in the amount of occipital activity on eye opening (Samson-Dollfus, Forthomme and Capron, 1964). The EEGs of children from about 2–12 years are usually polyrhythmic (*Figure 4.7a*), different components waxing and waning independently of each other. Not uncommonly

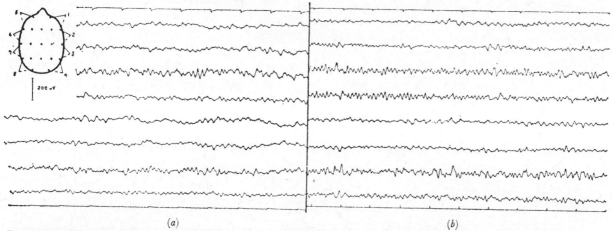

(a)   *(b)*

Figure 4.7—(a) *Normal child aged 3 years. Awake with eyes closed. EEG: Moderate voltage* theta *and* delta *components with ill-defined runs at 8 Hz.* (b) *Normal child aged 5 years. Awake with eyes closed. EEG: Moderate voltage* theta *components more marked on left side. Well-defined 8 Hz alpha rhythm more marked on right side*

these occur asymmetrically over the two hemispheres. There is a progressive tendency for all components to become more evident over the posterior part of the head. The *theta* rhythms usually predominate in the temporal or posterior temporal regions where they may be augmented during emotional stress. The *alpha* rhythm usually predominates rather more posteriorly and it becomes more obviously responsive to eye opening as the child matures. The amounts of *theta* and *alpha* activity are about the same at 5–6 years of age (*Figure 4.7b*). Thereafter, the faster rhythm gradually displaces the slower, although some *theta* activity may persist into adolescence. As the *alpha* rhythm develops with increasing age it becomes more clearly monorhythmic and distinct from the other components

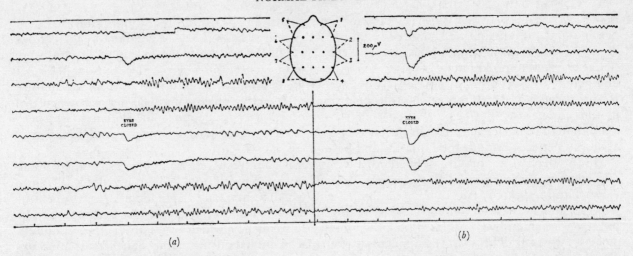

Figure 4.8—(a) *Normal child aged 7 years. EEG: 9 Hz* alpha *rhythm present only following eye closure.* Theta *components largely unaffected.* (b) *Normal child aged 10 years. EEG: 9–10 Hz* alpha *rhythm present only following eye closure. Low voltage* theta *components also more evident when eyes are closed*

while its dominant frequency increases in the majority of subjects to about 10 Hz (*Figure 4.8*). A quite marked asymmetry of *alpha* abundance, greater than the 2:3 ratio acceptable in an adult, may occur as a temporary feature in the maturation of a normal child's EEG. Churchill and Rodin (1968) have presented evidence to suggest that *alpha* asymmetry in children is related to head position at birth.

It cannot be emphasized too strongly that this outline of EEG maturation from infancy to adolescence is but an average picture and that many children will depart from it in any age group. For instance, those who are destined to have M-type records as adults may have little *alpha* activity at any age. *Theta* components, mixed with the *alpha* rhythm and quite often markedly asymmetrical, persist into adult life in 10–15 per cent of normal subjects. Patterns of this kind, that would be accepted as normal in children, are commonly described as 'immature'.

Corbin and Bickford (1955) carried out automatic frequency analyses on the EEGs of normal children between the ages of 1 and 10 years and demonstrated that, although there were wide differences in the findings at any one age, the EEG of an individual child had a relatively stable frequency composition in a standard environment. They showed further that, although there might be marked short-term asymmetries between homologous areas, the average analyses from them over a period of half a minute showed little difference, apart from a slight right-sided preponderance of the *alpha* rhythm in the majority of their subjects.

Drowsiness in children is sometimes associated with either or both of two strikingly rhythmical phenomena: (1) almost continuous and sometimes widespread sinusoidal 4–5 Hz activity and (2) bursts of higher voltage and frontally predominant 3–4 Hz activity of equally regular waveform

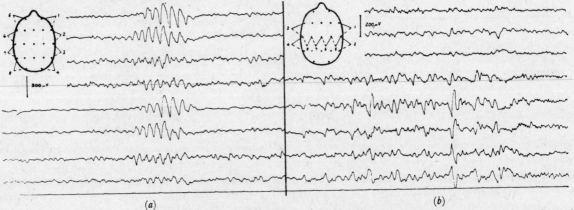

Figure 4.9—*Normal child aged 6 years.* (a) *During drowsiness. EEG: Bilateral burst of anteriorly predominant 4 Hz 'drowsy' waves.* (b) *During light sleep. EEG: Vertex sharp waves standing out from* theta *components in transversely recording channels*

(*Figure 4.9a*). The former is most frequently seen at 6–18 months, the latter at 3–10 years, but an individual child may show both kinds of discharge over a short interval of time (Kellaway and Fox, 1952). These patterns may recur when a child awakes from sleep, before full alertness is regained.

As sleep deepens, changes similar to those described for adults occur (*see* page 64), but voltages are generally higher and paroxysmal features more dramatic. Vertex sharp waves occur spontaneously in clusters during light sleep (*Figure 4.9b*) and bursts or more prolonged runs of high voltage *delta* activity occur in deep sleep (Monod, 1963). Sleep spindles and, less commonly, runs of *mu*-like rhythm predominate in the central regions, and sometimes occur independently on the two sides. K-complexes (*Figure 4.13*) are of higher voltage and longer duration than in an adult. Great restraint must be exercised in categorizing any of these phenomena as abnormal in the sleeping child.

There is no substitute for looking at large numbers of EEG records for an appreciation of the diversity of patterns that present during normal development in the child. The reader is therefore referred to the following atlases: Gibbs and Gibbs (1950); Laget and Salbreux (1967).

HYPERVENTILATION

Notwithstanding the universality of its use as a provocative procedure, it must be admitted that the value of hyperventilation has proved to be limited and its effects have been widely misinterpreted in the past. This is largely due to the dramatic nature of the response which may occur in young subjects. The technique consists of deep and regular respiration at a rate of about 20 per min for a period of 2–4 min, depending upon the perseverance of the subject and upon the EEG response obtained. In adults, this will cause an air exchange in the range of 20–50 litres per minute and a fall in plasma carbon dioxide in the range of 3–7 ml per cent (Morrice, 1956).

The characteristic hyperventilation response consists of a fluctuating crescendo of bilaterally synchronous and frontally predominant slow activity, initially of *theta* frequency, but slowing typically

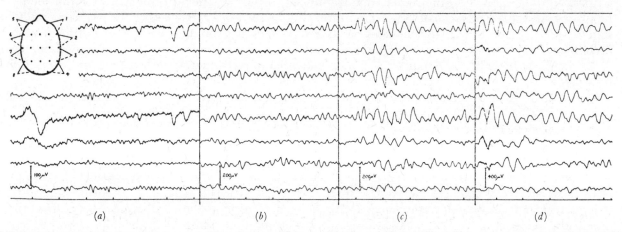

(a) (b) (c) (d)

Figure 4.10—Hyperventilation response in normal child aged 6 years. EEG: sampled before and after 0·5, 1·5, and 2·5 minutes hyperventilation. (a) Gain 50 μV/cm. Fluctuating 7–8 Hz components posteriorly of 40 μV peak. (b) Gain 100 μV/cm. 4–6 Hz components in all areas of 100 μV peak. (c) Gain 100 μV/cm. Predominantly 3 Hz runs anteriorly of 200 μV peak. (d) Gain 200 μV/cm. Continuous 2·5–3 Hz activity anteriorly of 500 μV peak

to 3 Hz (*Figure 4.10*). The final amplitude of this rhythmical discharge may reach 500 μV in normal children, although faintness or tetany may deter the subject from reaching this stage. Ingenious devices for encouraging children to overbreathe have been described by Lee (1965) and Gay and Muras (1969). Often the response is posteriorly rather than anteriorly predominant. In normal adults it is commonly much less marked, but there is a wide individual variation. Meyer and Gotoh (1960) have shown that the production of slow activity is related to hypocapnic constriction of cerebral vessels leading to a reduction of cerebral blood flow and consequent ischaemic anoxia.

The amount of slow activity evoked is increased in all subjects by quite mild degrees of hypoglycaemia, such as might exist three hours after a meal. It normally disappears within half a minute of the end of overbreathing. If it is prolonged, or continues to wax and wane, it should be ascertained that the subject is not continuing to overbreathe before accepting the response as abnormal. An additional check is provided by repeating the procedure 20 minutes after a glucose drink. Occasionally, the maximum effect is seen just after cessation of overbreathing when the subject is able to relax from his exertions. Apart from one that is prolonged, a response that is consistently asymmetrical is also abnormal at any age. Evoked discharges of epileptiform type are discussed on pages 80 and 93.

In view of the fact that few adults hyperventilate to the point at which *delta* activity is evoked, Prestwick *et al.* (1965) used a technique in which hyperventilation was immediately followed by hypoxia. Subjects hyperventilated with air through a face mask until a reduction in the end-tidal carbon dioxide concentration to about 50 per cent of the resting value was achieved. This was followed by breathing a 5 per cent oxygen–95 per cent nitrogen mixture, either until the appearance of *delta* rhythm in the EEG, which they defined as a positive end-point, or until an arterial oxygen saturation of 60 per cent was reached. The combined technique resulted in 80 per cent of their normal subjects reaching the end-point within 3 minutes, whereas only 5 per cent reached it with hyperventilation alone. The combined technique enabled a quantitative threshold to be determined which they found to increase with age, but to be relatively constant in a given subject from one occasion to another. However, the threshold was found to be lowered In two women during menstruation.

PHOTIC STIMULATION

Adrian and Matthews (1934) were the first to investigate the effects of rhythmical photic stimulation on the human EEG. Stimuli were derived from a constant light source in front of which a disc with cut-out sectors was rotated. Nowadays, an electronic stroboscope, using a gas discharge lamp as the light source, is the most convenient apparatus to use. Any model that will deliver blue-white flashes of 80,000 or more candles intensity over a range of 1–100 flashes per second is suitable but it is an advantage if a number of different intensities can be selected. The short duration of the flash precludes all possibility of damage to the retina. The translucent diffusing screen in front of the lamp should be placed a standard distance of 20–30 cm in front of the subject's eyes, so as to ensure an even illumination of the visual fields and the delivery of a supramaximal stimulus whether or not the eyelids are closed. The majority of stroboscopes allow an electrical pulse, synchronous with the discharge of the lamp, to be fed to an auxiliary stimulus marker mounted directly in line with the recording pens. However, registration of this pulse on the record is no guarantee that the subject received a stimulus. It is better to attach a small photocell to the forehead or nasion and to record the signals from this on one of the EEG channels

While an element of surprise sometimes plays a part in the nature of the EEG response obtained during photic stimulation, Jeavons (1969) emphasizes the danger of precipitating a clinical seizure and advocates the use of a standard procedure which is explained to the patient in advance. He recommends that stimulation should begin at 20 flashes per second, the frequency which he has found to be most effective in evoking paroxysmal discharges. The patient is requested to look at the centre of the screen and stimulation is commenced with the eyes open. If no abnormality has occurred within 5 seconds, the patient is asked to close his eyes while stimulation continues at the same flash rate for another 5 seconds. Other frequencies are selected in the range of 1–24 flashes per second and the procedure repeated in exactly the same way. Stimulation is stopped immediately when a paroxysmal discharge is evoked. Further testing for periods of 2 seconds over a wider range of frequencies can be performed to delimit the range over which the patient is photosensitive.

The normal primary response is occipital and is best seen with a montage that includes an electrode on the midline near the inion. At low frequencies of stimulation (*see Figure 4.4b*), or if isolated flashes are given, the major component of the response consists of an electro-positive wave that occurs with a latency of 70–90 ms (Cobb and Dawson, 1960). As the flash frequency is increased, these individual discharges merge to form a rhythm that tends to be sharp rather than sinusoidal in waveform, indicating the presence of higher order harmonics. When the eyes are open, the amplitude of this rhythm is likely to pass through a maximum in the 8–13 Hz range, though not necessarily at the frequency of the subject's *alpha* rhythm, thereafter declining as the frequency of stimulation is further increased. The terms *photic driving* or *photic following* are commonly used to describe a quasi-resonant response of this nature. Each implies a mode of causation which may not necessarily be true. To say simply that the response is at the flash frequency avoids all ambiguity. When the eyes are closed, the response in subjects who have a well-marked *alpha* rhythm is likely to be more complex as the evoked and spontaneous rhythms combine or temporarily displace each other. In those who have little *alpha* rhythm, there may be little difference between the responses with the eyes open and closed. There is a tendency for the responses to be of higher amplitude over the minor hemisphere.

When a marked occipital rhythm is evoked at the flash frequency, it is likely to extend into the parietal, temporal and even into the frontal areas. Its amplitude in these situations will be less and its waveform probably more complex, due to the presence of harmonic components. Subharmonics occur most often in the parieto-temporal regions and higher order harmonics most often anteriorly. Their amplitudes may well exceed those of the fundamentals in these situations, giving rise to the phenomena of frequency halving, doubling or trebling. Even when there is no obvious response in the occipital areas, averaging (*see* page 201) will reveal a small response at fundamental, harmonic or subharmonic frequencies of the flash rate (Werre and Smith, 1964).

The limitations of visual analysis and the restrictions imposed by insufficient recording channels are very evident when attempting to elucidate the detailed structure of widespread and complex responses to photic stimulation. Walter has always been a keen advocate of their clinical significance. He has developed toposcopic display equipment which provides a more comprehensive view and allows a more detailed study to be made of them (Walter, 1953). He has reported (Walter, 1950) that the nature of the response is influenced by such factors as the blood sugar level, mental activity, fatigue and the extent to which the subject 'abandons himself to the emotional tide' of the subjective sensations that accompany stimulation. Visual sensations of colour and pattern are frequently experienced, as well as kinaesthetic sensations of swaying or spinning. Autonomic and subjective emotional reactions occur less frequently in normals, but the latter are of special interest in that they may be accompanied by an evoked *theta* rhythm in the parieto-temporal regions, the frequency of which is usually, though not invariably, equal to or half that of the stimulus.

A considerable range of responses is obtained in normal children. Ellingson (1960) has shown that responses both to isolated and to rhythmical photic stimuli can be obtained in infants a few hours after birth, the average latency of the former decreasing from about 200 to 100 ms at 3 months. Walter (1951) reports that the responses in children up to the age of about 6 years are relatively small, but

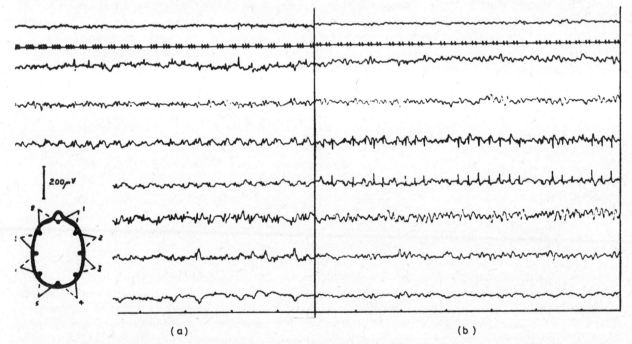

(a)   (b)

Figure 4.11—Responses to photic stimulation in normal children. (a) Boy aged 8 years. Groups of 20 per second flashes repeating at 3·5 per second. EEG: Traces of response at 20 Hz superimposed upon major occipital response at 3·5 Hz. (b) Boy aged 11 years. Pairs of flashes separated by 80 ms repeating at 4 per second. EEG: 4 per second occipital spike response. Sequence broken by occasional irregularity of stimulus timing

they can always be revealed by averaging techniques (*see* page 202). Subsequently rhythmical responses become much larger and may be particularly marked at low frequencies. This finding is in keeping with personal experience. Fundamental responses are often of highest voltage in the *theta* range with subharmonics occurring at *delta* frequencies. These are especially evident if pairs or repetitive groups of flashes are given (*Figure 4.11*), the response to the latter often comprising components at both the flash and group frequencies. Higher order harmonics are less common below the age of 10 years. The most striking response, seen in about 5 per cent of normal children, is the occurrence of paroxysmal slow activity, sometimes associated with sharp components and often posteriorly predominant.

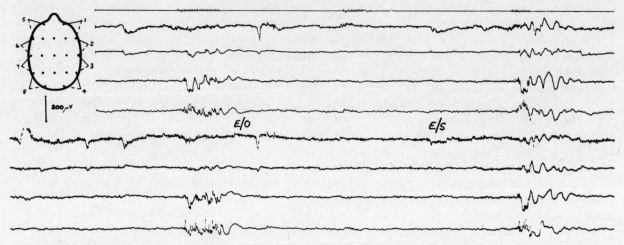

Figure 4.12—Paroxysmal responses to photic stimulation in normal girl aged 14 years. EEG: Bursts of posteriorly predominant polyspikes and slow waves on stimulation at 22 flashes per second only when eyes are closed

(*Figure 4.12*) (Petersén *et al.*, 1968). These discharges are seldom associated with objective changes and only a minority of the children experience unusual sensations. Photomyoclonic responses, similar to those described in adults (*see* page 80), occur much less often.

That subharmonic responses to photic stimulation are relatively frequent in young adults has been shown by Mundy-Castle (1953) who found their incidence to be 30 per cent as compared with 15 per cent in a group of normal seniles. Third harmonic responses occurred in 20 per cent and 52 per cent of the groups respectively. These differences he relates tentatively to the greater incidence and amplitude of spontaneous *theta* activity in young subjects and of spontaneous *beta* activity in seniles.

SLEEP

Few can have had the wide experience of Gibbs and his colleague (Gibbs and Gibbs, 1950) in observing the EEG phenomena of sleep, but all electroencephalographers are aware of the profound and sometimes striking changes that may occur during its various stages. When sleep is induced by drugs, these may modify the patterns that are obtained. Only the major changes that take place in spontaneous or drug induced sleep during conventional daytime recording will be dealt with here. Overnight sleep is discussed in Chapter 10.

Spontaneous Sleep

When an adult becomes drowsy, the first indication in the EEG is likely to be a reduction of any muscle potentials and movement artefacts that may be present and a slight augmentation of the amplitude and persistence of the *alpha* rhythm. The latter is then interrupted by periods of relatively low voltage activity during which slow lateral movements of the eyeballs often occur. These give rise to undulating low frequency deflections in anteriorly recording channels. The slightest stimulus during the episodes of low voltage EEG activity will cause immediate reappearance of the *alpha* rhythm—the reverse of the usual alerting effect in full consciousness and, for this reason, sometimes called the *paradoxical alpha response* (Goldie and Green, 1960). Periods of irregular low voltage activity and of higher voltage *alpha* rhythm may alternate spontaneously for a minute or two, the duration of the former progressively increasing until the latter no longer appears. At this stage the subject is lightly asleep.

In light sleep there is still an extreme sensitivity to sensory stimuli, but the response to a stimulus insufficient to produce arousal now takes the form of a sharp wave discharge phase-reversed about

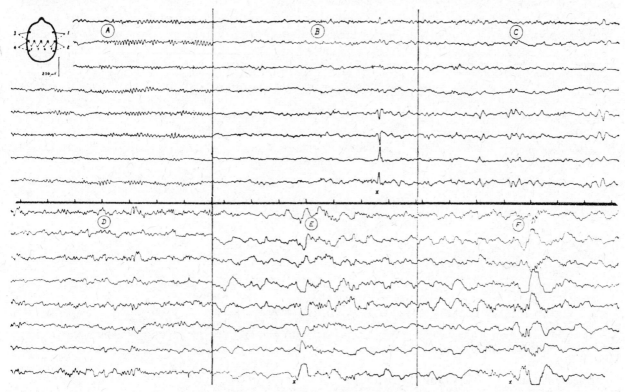

Figure 4.13—Progressive stages of drowsiness and sleep. Normal man aged 20 years. (a) Widespread alpha rhythm in early drowsiness. (b) Low voltage stage of drowsiness, showing vertex response to sound at X. (c) Theta dominant stage of light sleep. (d-f) Increasing random delta activity as sleep progressively deepens. Classical K-complex responses to sound stimulus at X

the vertex (*Figure 4.13b*). This predominantly electro-negative vertex wave probably involves the same mechanisms as are responsible for the similar discharge (*V-wave*) that can sometimes be elicited in the alert state. Particularly in sleeping children, it occurs frequently in the absence of an overt stimulus and is often of such high voltage and spike-like waveform that it is mistakenly regarded as epileptiform (*Figure 4.9b*).

These vertical sharp waves are essentially the same phenomenon as Gibbs' *biparietal humps* (Kiloh *et al.*, 1953) and may be regarded as rudimentary forms of the *K-complex* described by Davis *et al.* (1939). The K-complex is most readily evoked by an auditory stimulus and characteristically consists of a generalized burst of one or two high voltage slow waves (*Figure 4.13e–f*). Both these phenomena, like the paradoxical *alpha* response, are non-specific in the sense that they can be elicited by a stimulus in any modality.

Another phenomenon that may be seen at this stage of sleep is the occurrence of isolated or grouped, predominantly electro-positive waves in the occipital regions. These are similar in waveform, polarity and location to *lambda* waves (*see* page 56), but are usually of rather higher voltage and longer duration (Roth, Shaw and Green, 1956). They occur independently of vertex waves, but both may be seen at the same depth of sleep.

Following the stage of irregular low voltage activity there is a progressive increase of the *theta* and later of the *delta* components, while as sleep deepens the activity over the two hemispheres shows less and less synchrony; 12–14 Hz *sleep spindles* are then likely to appear. Typically these are of greatest amplitude in the anterior and central regions and, although often substantially synchronous and symmetrical, in children they sometimes wax and wane independently on either side (*Figure 4.14*).

At this depth of sleep (*Figure 4.13e*) the K-complex is more widespread, of higher voltage and longer duration and is composed of slower components than before. It may be accompanied or followed by a period of increased 12–14 Hz activity. It is difficult to measure the latency of the complex because of the ill-defined nature of the initial component and because of the variability of the waveform that is often seen in a given individual without apparent change in the depth of sleep. Davis *et al.* (1939) estimated that the average latency increased from the order of 100 ms in light sleep to 500 ms in very deep sleep. If a succession of identical stimuli was given at regular intervals of about 10 seconds, apparent adaptation occurred but seldom lasted for more than four or five stimuli; responses then

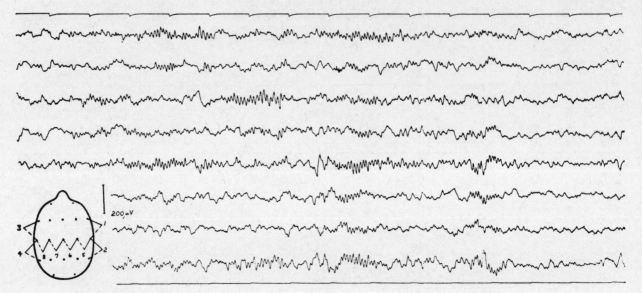

Figure 4.14—14 Hz spindles during natural sleep. Normal woman aged 17 years. Note independence of spindles on either side

reappeared. On the other hand, in pentothal-induced sleep, very little evidence of adaptation was found by Roth, Shaw and Green (1956), unless the interval between stimuli was reduced to about 2 seconds. It has been shown by Oswald, Taylor and Treisman (1960) that a significant stimulus, such as the sound of the subject's own name included in a tape recording of a succession of other names, evokes a more clear-cut response than do the others and may cause complete arousal. A similar observation has been made by Zung and Wilson (1966) during overnight sleep.

In very deep sleep, the EEG consists of generalized high voltage *delta* activity which may be asynchronous and as slow as 1 Hz. In adults, faster components will be intermixed with it, but in young children they may appear to be completely absent, because of masking by the very high voltage slow activity. In adults, this activity disappears almost immediately on arousal, being replaced by initially rather widespread *alpha* and *beta* and perhaps some *theta* activity, whereas in children rhythmical high voltage slow activity, similar to that seen in drowsiness, may persist until the child is fully awake (*see* page 60).

DRUG-INDUCED SLEEP

The induction of sleep by means of orally administered hypnotics is a routine procedure in most EEG laboratories. Of the barbiturates, quinalbarbitone sodium (Seconal) and pentobarbitone (Nembutal) are widely used. The initial dose of each of these drugs for an adult is 200 mg but on occasion this may have to be supplemented with a further 100 mg. In infants the initial dose is 50 mg. Occasionally, nausea, vomiting and ataxia occur as after-effects, whilst in children, especially those inclined to be hyperkinetic, barbiturates may produce restlessness; augmenting the dose then rarely aids sedation. In many laboratories non-barbiturate sedatives such as glutethimide 250–750 mg are preferred. Chlorpromazine too is used, especially in agitated patients, but the optimum dose may be difficult to estimate; often 100–200 mg is sufficient but much larger amounts may be required in some patients. Trimeprazine tartrate (2–3 mg/kg) or promazine (2 mg/kg) is more suitable for children.

The characteristic effect of barbiturates on the EEG—and one that is shared by many other hypnotics—is that they induce *beta* activity, often in the form of discrete runs or spindles and typically at a frequency of 18–24 Hz (Brazier and Finesinger, 1945). In higher dosage, persistent generalized *beta* activity may become the dominant feature. This activity usually has a fronto-central preponderance and, in normal subjects, is substantially symmetrical, although the runs may occur independently on either side. Consistent asymmetry is often of clinical significance. The intravenous injection of thiopentone sodium is the technique of choice for an examination of the distribution of this barbiturate fast activity (*see* page 93), but quinalbarbitone sodium by mouth may be almost as effective. Apart from the increased *beta* activity, the EEG changes following the exhibition of hypnotics (excepting intravenous barbiturates) are essentially the same as those seen in spontaneous sleep.

The intramuscular administration of a sedative for EEG purposes should be reserved for unco-operative patients in whom both oral and intravenous administration are impossible. Paraldehyde is the drug most frequently employed. An initial dose of 1 ml per year of age should be given up to the age of 5, increasing by 0·5 ml per year up to the age of 15 and remaining at 10 ml for all older subjects. The resulting sleep may be very deep and K-complexes may then be difficult to elicit. It is not uncommon for doses of this order to produce widespread activity at 12–16 Hz. A single or repeated intramuscular injection of 2 mg/kg promazine is a useful sedative for restless infants and young children.

The EEG changes that accompany narcosis induced by intravenous thiopentone sodium depend upon the dose and the rate at which it is given, upon the age of the subject and probably upon a factor of individual variability. Apart from special techniques, such as those referred to on pages 182 and 191, two rates of administration are commonly employed: 50 mg and 100 mg per minute. The slower rate is indicated for children and for adults in whom it is desired to induce only light sleep or in whom extra caution is advisable because of old age or infirmity. The faster rate is indicated for adults in good health and may need to be increased as the injection proceeds if the subject has a high tolerance and becomes restless. This is often the case with alcoholics.

The initial EEG change consists of the appearance of low voltage but widespread barbiturate fast activity and random *theta* components that progressively displace the *alpha* rhythm, followed by a

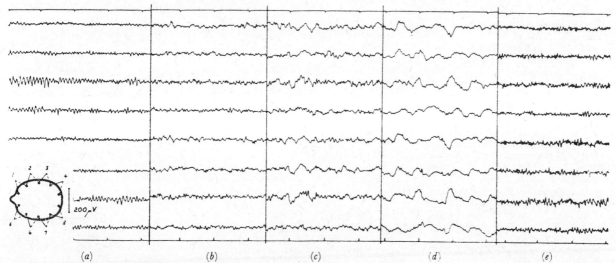

(a)   (b)   (c)   (d)   (e)

Figure 4.15—Progressive stages of thiopentone sodium narcosis. Neurologically normal subject with endogenous depression. Woman aged 35 years. (a) Beginning of injection. EEG: 10 Hz alpha dominant record. (b) 30 s later; total of 100 mg injected. EEG: Diffuse beta and random theta components. (c) 30 s later; total of 150 mg injected. EEG: Appearance of first delta components. (d) 30 s later; total of 200 mg injected. EEG: Generalized high voltage delta activity. (e) 30 s later; no further injection. EEG: Generalized moderate voltage beta activity

crescendo of generalized and bilaterally symmetrical *theta* and *delta* activity (*Figure 4.15*). Children and young adults show a much more dramatic build-up of slow activity at relatively low dosage levels than do older subjects, the amplitude of the delta activity often exceeding 200 μV shortly after consciousness is lost. In subjects over 40 years of age, such activity may only appear when the corneal reflex can no longer be obtained. If the injection is continued beyond this stage, the *delta* activity and faster components are interrupted by periods of relatively low voltage which become more prolonged as the level of anaesthesia deepens (Kiersey, Bickford and Faulconer, 1951). The alternating pattern of paroxysmal discharges occurring on a flat background is known as *suppression-burst* activity (*see Figure 8.9*). Although the occurence of respiratory embarrassment is rare, equipment for resuscitation should always be available. For this same reason, the investigation should not be carried out within 4 hours of a meal.

The injection should be discontinued when high voltage *delta* activity appears; the latter is then unlikely to persist for more than 30 seconds, giving way to moderate voltage generalized *beta* activity, with little or no activity of lower frequency. This state of light narcosis may last for 5–10 minutes, during which K-complexes are readily elicited (Roth, Shaw and Green, 1956), being terminated by arousal and the return of the *alpha* rhythm. Marked drowsiness will persist for some time and the subject, if undisturbed, may fall into a more natural sleep, with the reappearance of *theta* and *delta* components. *Beta* activity of gradually diminishing amplitude is likely to be evident during the whole of this period.

Methohexitone is claimed to have significant advantages over thiopentone for the controlled induction of sleep during EEG examination. In a comparative trial, Fenton and Scotton (1967) showed that recovery after an equivalent depth of narcosis occurred almost twice as quickly after methohexitone. The potency of methohexitone is about three times that of thiopentone and the drugs were therefore administered at rates of 10 and 30 mg per 15 seconds up to total doses of 1·76 and 5·28 mg per kg body weight respectively. The EEG changes were qualitatively similar with each drug, except that methohexitone produced rather less fast activity. Nevertheless, there was always sufficient for an adequate comparison between the two hemispheres to be made.

REFERENCES

Adrian, E. D. and Matthews, B. H. C. (1934). 'The Berger Rhythm: Potential Changes from the Occipital Lobes in Man'. *Brain* **57,** 355

Aird, R. B. and Gastaut, Y. (1959). 'Occipital and Posterior Electroencephalographic Rhythms'. *Electroenceph. clin. Neurophysiol.* **11,** 637

Brazier, M. A. B. and Finesinger, J. E. (1945). 'Action of Barbiturates on the Cerebral Cortex'. *Archs Neurol. Psychiat., Chicago* **53,** 51

Chatrian, G. E., Petersen, M. C. and Lazarte, J. A. (1959). 'The Blocking of the Rolandic Wicket Rhythm and Some Central Changes Related to Movement'. *Electroenceph. clin. Neurophysiol.* **11,** 497

Churchill, J. A. and Rodin, E. A. (1968). 'Asymmetry of Alpha Activity in Children'. *Devl. Med. Child Neurol.* **10,** 77

Clarke, L. G. and Harding, G. F. A. (1969). 'Comparisons of Mono and Dizygotic Twins with Respect to some Features of the Electroencephalogram'. *Proc. electrophysiol. Technol. Ass.* **16,** 94

Cobb, W. A. and Dawson, G. D. (1960). 'The Form and Latency in Man of the Occipital Potentials Evoked by Bright Flashes'. *J. Physiol.* **152,** 108

Cooper, R. and Mundy-Castle, A. C. (1960). 'Spatial and Temporal Characteristics of the Alpha Rhythm: a Toposcopic Analysis'. *Electroenceph. clin. Neurophysiol.* **12,** 153

Corbin, H. P. F. and Bickford, R. G. (1955). 'Studies of the Electroencephalogram of Normal Children: Comparison of Visual and Automatic Frequency Analyses'. *Electroenceph. clin. Neurophysiol.* **7,** 15

Davis, H., Davis, P. A., Loomis, A. L., Harvey, E. N. and Hobart, G. (1939). 'Electric Reactions of the Human Brain to Auditory Stimulation During Sleep'. *J. Neurophysiol.* **2,** 500

Dreyfus-Brisac, C. (1964). 'The Electroencephalogram of the Premature Infant and Full-term Newborn: Normal and Abnormal Development of Waking and Sleep Patterns'. In *Neurological and Electroencephalographic Correlative Studies in Infancy*, p. 186. Ed. by P. Kellaway and I. Petersén. New York and London; Grune and Stratton

Dumermuth, G. (1968). 'Variance Spectra of Electroencephalograms in Twins'. In *Clinical Electroencephalography of Children*, p. 119. Ed. by P. Kellaway and I, Petersén. Stockholm; Almqvist and Wiksell

Ellingson, R. J. (1958). 'Electroencephalograms of Normal, Full-term Newborns Immediately After Birth with Observations on Arousal and Visual Evoked Responses'. *Electroenceph. clin. Neurophysiol.* **10,** 31

— (1960). 'Cortical Electrical Responses to Visual Stimulation in the Human Infant'. *Electroenceph. clin. Neurophysiol.* **12,** 663

Evans, C. C. (1953). 'Spontaneous Excitation of the Visual Cortex and Association Areas—Lambda Waves'. *Electroenceph. clin. Neurophysiol.* **5,** 69

Fenton, G. W. and Scotton, L. (1967). 'The Use of Methohexitone in Sleep Electroencephalography'. *Electroenceph. clin. Neurophysiol.* **23,** 273

Gastaut, H., Terzian, H. and Gastaut, Y. (1952). 'Etude d'une activité électroencéphalographique méconnue: "le rhythme rolandique en arceau"'. *Marseille méd.* **89,** 296

Gastaut, Y. (1951). Un signe électroencéphalographique peu connu: les pointes occipitales survenant pendant l'ouverture des yeux'. *Revue neurol.* **84,** 640

— (1953). Les pointes négatives évoquées sur le vertex: leur signification psychophysiologique et pathologique'. *Revue neurol.* **89,** 382

68

REFERENCES

Gay, P. and Muras, J. S. (1969). 'A Device for Promoting Hyperventilation in Children'. *Proc. electrophysiol. Technol. Ass.* **16,** 270

Gibbs, F. A. and Gibbs, E. L. (1950). *Atlas of Electroencephalography*, Vol. I: *Methodology and Controls.* p. 90. Cambridge, Mass.; Addison-Wesley Press

Glass, A. (1964). 'Mental Arithmetic and Blocking of the Occipital Alpha Rhythm'. *Electroenceph. clin. Neurophysiol.* **16,** 595

Goldie, L. and Green, J. M. (1960). 'Paradoxical Blocking and Arousal in the Drowsy State'. *Nature, Lond.* **187,** 952

Green, J. (1957). 'Some Observations on Lambda Waves and Peripheral Stimulation'. *Electroenceph. clin. Neurophysiol.* **9,** 691

Hagne, I. (1968). 'Development of the Waking EEG in Normal Infants during the First Year of Life'. In *Clinical Electroencephalography of Children*, p. 97. Ed. by P. Kellaway and I. Petersén. Stockholm; Almqvist and Wiksell

Hellström, B., Karlsson, B. and Müssbichler, H. (1963). 'Electrode Placement in EEG in Infants and its Anatomical Relationship Studied Radiographically'. *Electroenceph. clin. Neurophysiol.* **17,** 115; reprinted in *Am. J. EEG Technol.* 1964, **4,** 71

Jasper, H. H. (1949). 'Electrocorticograms in Man'. *Electroenceph. clin. Neurophysiol.,* Suppl. **2,** 16

Jeavons, P. M. (1969). 'The Use of Photic Stimulation in Clinical Electroencephalography'. *Proc. electrophysiol. Technol. Ass.* **16,** 225

Juel-Neilsen, N. and Harvald, B. (1958). 'The Electroencephalogram in Uniovular Twins Brought up Apart'. *Acta Genet. Statist. med.* **8,** 57

Kellaway, P. and Fox, B. J. (1952). 'Electroencephalographic Diagnosis of Cerebral Pathology in Infants During Sleep. I: Rationale, Technique and the Characteristics of Normal Sleep in Infants'. *J. Pediat.* **41,** 262

Kiersey, D. K., Bickford, R. G. and Faulconer, A. (1951). 'Electroencephalographic Patterns Produced by Thiopental Sodium during Surgical Operations: Description and Classification'. *Br. J. Anaesth.* **23,** 141

Kiloh, L. G., Walton, J. N., Osselton, J. W. and Farrall, J. (1953). 'On the Significance of the Sharp Wave Occurring at the Vertex During the Early Stages of Sleep'. *Electroenceph. clin. Neurophysiol.* **5,** 621

Kreitman, N. and Shaw, J. C. (1965). 'Experimental Enhancement of Alpha Activity'. *Electroenceph. clin. Neurophysiol.* **18,** 147

Laget, P. and Salbreux, R. (1967). *Atlas d'Electroencéphalographie Infantile*, p. 652. Paris; Masson

Landis, C. and Hunt, W. (1939). *The Startle Pattern.* New York; Farrar and Rinehart

Larsson, L. E. (1960). 'Can the Non-specific EEG Response be an Artifact Caused by Scalp Movement?' *Electroenceph. clin. Neurophysiol.* **12,** 502

Lee, D. (1965). 'An Electronic Toy for Assisting Young Children to Hyperventilate'. *Proc. electrophysiol. Technol. Ass.* **12,** 161

Liske, E., Hughes, H. M. and Stowe, D. E. (1967). 'Cross-correlation of Human Alpha Activity: Normative Data'. *Electroenceph. clin. Neurophysiol.* **22,** 429

Maddocks, J. A., Hodge, R. S. and Rex, J. (1951). 'Observations on the Occurrence of Precentral Activity at Alpha Frequencies'. *Electroenceph. clin. Neurophysiol.* **3,** 370

Margerison, J. H., Anderson, W. McC. and Dawson, J. (1964). 'Plasma Sodium and the EEG During the Menstrual Cycle of Normal Human Females'. *Electroenceph. clin. Neurophysiol.* **17,** 540

Matoušek, M., Volavka, J., Roubíček, J. and Roth, Z. (1967). 'EEG Frequency Analysis Related to Age in Normal Adults'. *Electroenceph. clin. Neurophysiol.* **23,** 162

Meyer, J. S. and Gotoh, F. (1960). 'Metabolic and Electroencephalographic Effects of Hyperventilation'. *Archs Neurol.* **3,** 539

Monod, N. (1963). 'Les bouffées paroxystiques au cours du sommeil de l'enfant de 2 à 8 ans.' *Revue neurol.* **109,** 340

Morrice, J. K. W. (1956). 'Slow Wave Production in the EEG, With Reference to Hyperpnoea, Carbon Dioxide and Autonomic Balance'. *Electroenceph. clin. Neurophysiol.* **8,** 49

Mundy-Castle, A. C. (1951). 'Theta and Beta Rhythm in the Electroencephalograms of Normal Adults'. *Electroenceph. clin. Neurophysiol.* **3,** 477

— (1953). 'An Analysis of Central Responses to Photic Stimulation in Normal Adults'. *Electroenceph. clin. Neurophysiol.* **5,** 1

Oswald, I., Taylor, A. M. and Treisman, M. (1960). 'Discriminative Responses to Stimulation during Human Sleep'. *Brain* **83,** 440

Parmelee, A. H., Akiyama, Y., Schultz, M. A., Wenner, W. H., Schulte, F. J. and Stern, E. (1968). 'The Electroencephalogram in Active and Quiet Sleep in Infants'. In *Clinical Electroencephalography of Children*, p. 77. Ed. by P. Kellaway and I. Petersén. Stockholm; Almqvist and Wiksell

— Wenner, W. H., Akiyama, Y., Schultz, M. A. and Stern, E. (1967). 'Sleep States in Premature Infants'. *Devl. Med. Child Neurol.* **9,** 70

Perez-Borja, C., Chatrian, G. E., Tyce, F. A. and Rivers, M. H. (1962). 'Electrographic Patterns of the Occipital Lobe in Man: a Topographic Study Based on Use of Implanted Electrodes'. *Electroenceph. clin. Neurophysiol.* **14,** 171

Petersén, I., Eeg-Olofsson, O. and Selldén, U. (1968). 'Paroxysmal Activity in the EEG of Normal Children'. In *Clinical Electroencephalography of Children*, p. 167. Ed. by P. Kellaway and I. Petersén. Stockholm; Almqvist and Wiksell

Picard, P., Navarranne, P., Laboureur, P., Grousset, G. and Jest, C. (1957). 'Confrontations des Données de l'Electroencéphalogramme et de l'Examen Psychologique chez 309 Candidats Pilotes à l'Aéronautique'. *Electroenceph. clin. Neurophysiol.* Suppl. 6, 304

Prestwick, G., Reivich, M. and Hill, I. D. (1965). 'The EEG Effects of Combined Hyperventilation and Hypoxia in Normal Subjects'. *Electroenceph. clin. Neurophysiol.* **18,** 56

Roth, M. and Green, J. (1953). 'The Lambda Wave as a Normal Physiological Phenomenon in the Human EEG'. *Nature, Lond.* **172,** 864

— Shaw, J. and Green, J. (1956). 'The Form, Voltage Distribution and Physiological Significance of the K-complex'. *Electroenceph. clin. Neurophysiol.* **8,** 385

Samson-Dollfus, D., Forthomme, J. and Capron, E. (1964). 'EEG of the Human Infant during Sleep and Wakefulness during the First Year of Life: Normal Patterns and their Maturational Changes; Abnormal Patterns and their Prognostic Significance'. In *Neurological and Electroencephalographic Correlative Studies in Infancy*, p. 208. Ed. by P. Kellaway and I. Petersén. London; Grune and Stratton

Scott, D. F., Groethuysen, U. C. and Bickford, R. G. (1967). 'Lambda Responses in the Human Electroencephalogram'. *Neurology* **17,** 770

Storm van Leeuwen, W. and Bekkering, D. H. (1958). 'Some Results Obtained with the EEG-Spectrograph'. *Electroenceph. clin. Neurophysiol.* **10,** 563

Vogel, F. (1965). 'Genetic Aspects of the EEG'. *Electroenceph. clin. Neurophysiol.* **19,** 196

Vogel, W., Broverman, D. M. and Klaiber, E. L. (1968). 'EEG and Mental Abilities'. *Electroenceph. clin. Neurophysiol.* **24,** 166

Walter, D. O., Rhodes, J. M., Brown, D. and Adey, W. R. (1966). 'Comprehensive Spectral Analysis of Human EEG Generators in Posterior Cerebral Regions'. *Electroenceph. clin. Neurophysiol.* **20,** 224

Walter, W. G. (1950). 'The Functions of Electrical Rhythms in the Brain'. *J. ment. Sci.* **96,** 1

— (1951). 'The Effect of Physical Stimuli on the EEG'. *Electroenceph. clin. Neurophysiol.* Suppl. **2,** 60

— (1953). 'Toposcopy'. *Electroenceph. clin. Neurophysiol.* Suppl. **4,** 7

— and Shipton, J. (1957). 'La présentation et l'identification des composantes des rhythmes alpha'. *Electroenceph. clin. Neurophysiol.* Suppl. **6,** 177

Werre, P. F. and Smith, C. J. (1964). 'Variability of Responses Evoked by Flashes in Man'. *Electroenceph. clin. Neurophysiol.* **17,** 644

Williams, D. (1941). 'The Significance of an Abnormal Electroencephalogram'. *J. Neurol. Psychiat.* **4,** 257

Zung, W. W. K. and Wilson, W. P. (1966). 'Attention, Discrimination and Arousal during Sleep'. *Electroenceph. clin. Neurophysiol.* **20,** 623

CHAPTER 5

EPILEPSY

INTRODUCTION

Epilepsy is not easily defined. To say that epilepsy is a 'tendency to recurring epileptic seizures' (Penfield and Erickson, 1941) is mere tautology. To define it as 'paroxysmal cerebral dysrhythmia' (Gibbs, Gibbs and Lennox, 1937) is not only 'romantic' as Grey Walter has pointed out, but meaningless. Penfield later wrote that one could regard epilepsy 'physiologically, as a tendency to periodic involuntary neuronal explosions. For the patient it is a state of continuing dread (usually shared by his friends and family) interrupted by recurring attacks of involuntary behaviour.'

One important difficulty has arisen from the social implications of the diagnosis. In infancy, attacks of grand mal associated with fever are referred to as febrile convulsions; in tetany, attacks of grand mal are accepted as an integral part of the syndrome; and when fits occur after prolonged bouts of coughing, the use of the word epilepsy is vigorously contested by many clinicians, so that the condition has come to be known, most inappropriately, as laryngeal vertigo. The distinction is sometimes made that although the attacks themselves may be classed as epileptic, the patient does not suffer from epilepsy because the convulsions are provoked; but if it is a cerebral tumour that provokes the attacks, the diagnosis of epilepsy is made without question. Experience with electroconvulsive therapy has shown that the ability to suffer attacks of grand mal is a universal attribute and the important problem is not so much why so few people have fits but how the majority manage to avoid them.

The work of Li and of Jasper (Jasper, 1961) has demonstrated clearly that the epileptic process consists fundamentally of hyperactive and hypersynchronous neuronal discharges. The abnormality of the neurone appears to lie in the instability of the cell membrane. An inhibitory feedback mechanism similar to the Renshaw cell system of the spinal cord probably exists in the brain (Eccles, 1965; 1967) and is likely to play an important part in preventing the excessive neuronal discharge that forms the basis of an epileptic attack (Phillips, 1959). The cerebral cortex and perhaps brainstem and cerebellar systems are likely to exert important tonic inhibitory effects upon synapses in the various afferent pathways, particularly those that relay by way of the reticular formation, so that attention can be focused on a small selection of the multitude of afferent stimuli presented at any one moment. Failure of this function might permit an excessive central bombardment by afferent stimuli which in turn could lead to the excessive neuronal discharges associated with epilepsy. Further protection against undue hypersynchronization of neuronal discharges is provided by the presence of γ-aminobutyric acid (GABA) throughout the brain. Primary failure of this mechanism is probably rare but is seen in pyridoxine deficiency, a condition in which convulsions may occur (Symonds, 1959). The effect of inhibition is to increase the degree of cell membrane polarization. Abnormality of the cell membrane may impair its ability to re-establish polarization after cell firing has occurred and the state of persistent depolarization may give rise to continuous excessive firing. Cell membrane stability is influenced by the state of ionic balance across the membrane and appropriate alterations in this due to metabolic disorders may give rise to epileptiform discharges. The epileptic state may then be regarded as one in which hyperdepolarization of certain neurones occurs leading to very rapid neuronal firing which is usually hypersynchronous.

The degree of resistance to the development of attacks varies greatly in different individuals and in regard to the nature of the provocation. Hence the demonstration of a low EEG threshold to leptazol (Metrazol, Cardiazol) or bemegride (Megimide) activation does not necessarily imply that the patient will have spontaneous attacks. There are some individuals whose resistance shows a periodic breakdown for no very obvious reason, although sometimes biochemical changes such as a low blood glucose or hypocapnia, or physiological changes such as drowsiness, menstruation or the effects of fortuitous

71

exposure to flicker and other afferent stimuli, play some part in its failure. These form the group of epileptics sometimes termed 'idiopathic' and the incidence of fits in their relatives demonstrates that a genetic factor plays an important part in their predisposition. Conrad (1937) showed that when one of a pair of dizygotic twins suffered from 'idiopathic' epilepsy, the concordance rate was 4·3 per cent as compared with 86·3 per cent in monozygotic pairs. Lennox (1953) has pointed out the striking similarity in detail of spike and wave discharges in concordant uniovular twins. Considerable support for the suggestion of Lennox, Gibbs and Gibbs (1940) that a single dominant autosomal gene is involved comes from the work of Metrakos and Metrakos (1961) who investigated the EEG findings in the parents and siblings of probands suffering from centrencephalic epilepsy. Their results suggest that the 'EEG trait', that is the presence of bilaterally synchronous spike and wave discharges, is inherited as a dominant but that its penetrance varies with age. Between 5 and 16 years it is almost fully penetrant so that the number of siblings sharing the trait is close to 50 per cent whilst with increasing age the penetrance diminishes, reaching zero at the age of 40 years (*also see* Metrakos *et al.* 1966). Gastaut (1969) reaches very similar conclusions although he believes that the maximum expression rate occurs between the ages of 18 months and 6 years.

It is important to realize that genetic factors also play a part in the 'symptomatic' epilepsies. Patients with brain lesions are more likely to suffer attacks and to experience them at an earlier stage of their illness when there is a family history of epilepsy. This is well shown by the high genetic loading for epilepsy in those patients with cerebral tumours who experience fits, compared with those who have none.

It has been pointed out by Jasper that the EEG abnormalities which may be regarded as characteristic of epilepsy, commonly show certain features. The discharges consist of waves of various forms and frequencies that are of high voltage in relation to the background activity and result from hypersynchrony of individual neuronal discharges. The onset and often the cessation of these discharges tend to be abrupt. Although they may sometimes be provoked in various ways, many of the abnormal discharges arise spontaneously and appear to be self-perpetuating. There is often a tendency for the discharge to spread and this may occur either by conduction along neuronal pathways (trans-synaptic conduction) or by direct spread to contiguous neurones. In the latter case (ephaptic conduction) there appears to be a failure of the inhibitory mechanisms so that neighbouring neurones respond to the electrical field set up by the initial neuronal discharge. Clinically this phenomenon has its counterpart in the jacksonian march. Those neurones giving rise to the epileptiform discharge are no longer able to carry out their normal integrative functions.

The clinical features of an epileptic attack consist therefore of two classes of phenomena: positive effects due to the abnormal neuronal discharge and negative effects due to the abrogation of function of the discharging neurones. In the case of a jacksonian attack, the positive phenomenon is the twitching of the thumb and subsequent march to other segments of the upper limb, while the negative aspect is the patient's inability to use the twitching muscles for any voluntary action. This loss sometimes persists after the attack in the form of a Todd's paralysis.

Epilepsy has been classified in many ways. A classification recommended by the International League against Epilepsy, the World Federation of Neurology, the World Federation of Neurological Societies and the International Federation of Societies for Electroencephalography and Clinical Neurophysiology has been drawn up by a Commission on Terminology (1964; 1969) representative of these bodies. It is essentially an elaborate phenomenological classification alongside which appropriate EEG and aetiological data are listed. The main categories of this classification are:

(1) Partial seizures or seizures beginning locally.
(2) Generalized seizures, bilateral symmetrical seizures or seizures without local onset.
(3) Unilateral or predominantly unilateral seizures.
(4) Unclassified epileptic seizures.

However, it does not appear to the authors that this classification is very helpful from an electro-encephalographic point of view and the older classification of Jasper and Kershman (1949) is preferred. This, too, is based on clinical and EEG observations and in particular on the supposed location of the site of origin of the epileptic discharge.

The principal problem with this classification stems from the uncertainties of anatomical localization particularly in relation to 'epilepsy of cortical origin'; this term makes no allowance for the possibility that focal attacks may originate in areas other than the cerebral cortex (*see* page 91). On the other hand, the term 'partial seizure' which is preferred in the international classification does not seem very appropriate as generalization occurs so frequently; nor is the expression 'seizures beginning locally' sufficiently exclusive if one accepts that attacks of primary subcortical epilepsy may commence locally in the meso-diencephalic region.

The Jasper and Kershman classification has undergone some modification since its introduction (Hill, 1958). There are four groups:

(1) Epilepsy of subcortical origin (primary subcortical epilepsy). Although this group subsumes those cases described as 'idiopathic', other cases are included in which fits occur as the result of generalized cerebral disorders, particularly metabolic disturbances.

(2) Epilepsy of cortical origin (cortical epilepsy). This corresponds closely to the group of focal epilepsies and rather less closely to the group of symptomatic epilepsies.

(3) Secondary subcortical epilepsy.

(4) Epilepsy arising from numerous areas both in the cerebral cortex and subcortical structures.

PRIMARY SUBCORTICAL EPILEPSY

Seizure Patterns in Primary Subcortical Epilepsy

There is considerable evidence that in generalized epilepsy including petit mal and grand mal, the thalamic intralaminar system and the midbrain reticular formation are involved (Gastaut and Fischer-Williams, 1959a). In the view of Penfield and Jasper (1947) the attacks originate in these areas to which they applied the term 'centrencephalic'. Whilst accepting that these areas are involved, Williams (1965) expresses considerable doubt that the attacks originate in them. He points out that tumours involving these structures seldom give rise to epilepsy and indeed that their integrity is necessary for the propagation of generalized epilepsy. He suggests no alternative site of origin. In the 'primary' or 'idiopathic' cases we are considering, the centrencephalic areas are of course intact. While accepting that room for argument remains, the centrencephalic origin of these attacks is the most useful working hypothesis that we have.

Many experimental studies support this view. Jasper and Droogleever-Fortuyn (1947) found that following electrical stimulation of the intralaminar thalamic nuclei of cats, spike and wave activity with a repetition frequency of 3 per second could be recorded from the cerebral cortex. Similar results were obtained by Hunter and Jasper (1949), Hunter (1950), Ingvar (1955) and by Pollen, Perot and Reid (1963). The introduction of alumina cream into the same region (Guerrero-Figueroa *et al.*, 1963; Kopeloff *et al.*, 1950) in kittens and rhesus monkeys, of penicillin (Ralston and Ajmone Marsan, 1956) and of cobalt powder in cats (Mancia and Lucioni, 1966) to establish chronic epileptogenic foci, all gave rise to similar discharges. Pollen (1968) suggests that the surface negative spike results from the generation of EPSP primarily upon apical dendrites of vertically orientated pyramidal type neurones while the slow negative wave is generated by IPSP in the same regions.

Williams (1953), using depth electrodes, has studied spike and wave discharges occuring spontaneously in children. He concluded that the slow waves originated deep in the thalami and could be seen there for nearly a second before appearing in the cortex; they always preceded the initial spike. Localization by a study of phase reversals suggested that the spike had its origin in the deeper layers of the cortex. Following the appearance of the first spike, the site of origin of the slow wave appeared to shift towards the lateral aspect of the thalamus and subsequently spikes and slow waves reciprocated until the slight slowing of the discharge from 3 per second to $2\frac{1}{2}$ per second was associated with decreasing amplitude and disappearance of the spike following which the slow wave activity ceased. This work has not been confirmed. By producing destructive lesions stereotactically in the medial part of the lamina medullaris interna at the level of the commissura media, Spiegel, Wycis and Reyes (1951) obtained marked relief of symptoms in two cases of petit mal.

Although the evidence outlined is very strong and is in accord with clinical observation, some studies, notably those of Bennett (1953) and Gloor (1968), are hard to reconcile with this view. Each was surprised to find that when leptazol was injected into either carotid artery of patients with primary subcortical epilepsy, generalized bilaterally synchronous epileptiform discharges appeared in the

EEG although the territory supplied by the carotid arteries does not include the thalamic intralaminar system. Moreover, in two patients with generalized epileptiform discharges—whether these were examples of primary or of secondary bilateral synchrony is not stated—Gloor found that injection of leptazol into one of the vertebral arteries failed to produce spike and wave activity and indeed was associated with a reduction in the frequency and amplitude of the spontaneous spike and wave discharges even when the dose given was five times that used for the intracarotid injections.

According to the nature of the discharge and the manner of its spread, three types of attack may develop. Two are of minor character—myoclonic epilepsy and petit mal with its variant akinetic epilepsy—and the third is grand mal. Either of the two minor varieties may precede an attack of grand mal. It must be emphasized that as the discharge originates centrally in these attacks, auras never occur.

In both petit mal and grand mal the initial phenomenon, as one would expect from the site of origin of the discharge, is impairment or loss of consciousness. When grand mal follows on a focal attack, as in cortical epilepsy, the same subcortical regions of the brain are activated and from that moment the clinical and EEG phenomena are usually indistinguishable from those of a primary subcortical seizure. The same phenomena occur when fits are induced, whether electrically or by drugs.

Grand Mal

It is seldom that a satisfactory EEG recording is obtained during an attack of grand mal because of the muscle and movement artefacts that occur. Recordings of better quality may be obtained if fits are induced electrically after the administration of thiopentone and a muscle relaxant, but this is a procedure not normally carried out in the EEG laboratory. The best results are obtained by using implanted electrodes which may be extradural, subdural or intracerebral in position. Beautiful tracings free from artefact may be obtained in this way (Chatrian and Petersen, 1960) (*Figure 5.1*).

Preceding a typical attack of grand mal there may be a crescendo of low voltage fast activity which within a few seconds gives way to a generalized rhythmic synchronous discharge of high amplitude

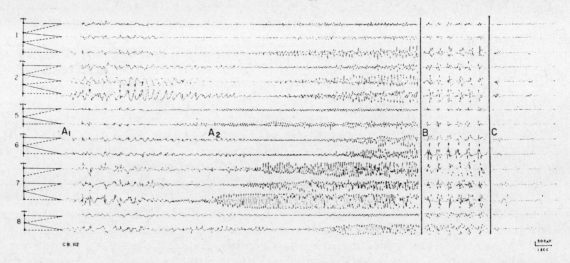

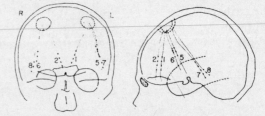

Figure 5.1—Grand mal provoked by intravenous injection of 15 ml leptazol. Depth electrodes. (A_1) *6 s after injection: twitching of mouth and myoclonic jerkings of upper limbs.* (A_2) *Tonic phase.* (B) *Following an interval of 30 s: clonic phase.* (C) *Following an interval of 40 s: beginning of post-ictal coma*

(From Chatrian, G. E. and Petersen, M. C. (1960). 'The convulsive patterns provoked by Indoklon, Metrazol and electroshock: some depth electrographic observations in human patients.' *Electroenceph. clin. Neurophysiol.* **12**, 715, by courtesy of the Editor)

spikes, the frequency lying within the range of 8–12 Hz. This discharge coincides with the tonic phase of the fit during which the amplitude of the spikes tends to increase and their repetition rate progressively to fall. After some 15–30 seconds the spikes become grouped and are sometimes separated by slow waves. This pattern corresponds to the clonic phase of the fit and the groups of spikes coincide with the actual clonic spasms (*Figure 5.2*). The slow activity is at 1·5–3 Hz and becomes more and more prominent; the groups of spikes occur with diminishing frequency and in the later stages of the attack, may be superimposed upon the slow waves. Finally, as the last clonic jerk of the patient gives way to flaccidity, the EEG enters a quiescent phase consisting of very low amplitude *delta* activity often as

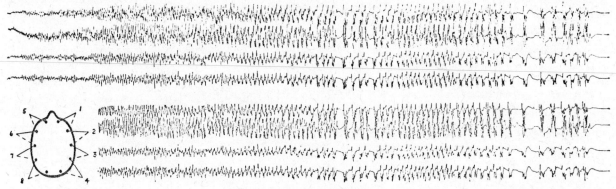

Figure 5.2—Spontaneous grand mal attack. Man aged 28 years. EEG: Initial crescendo of generalized 10 Hz activity obscured by increasing muscle action potentials of tonic phase. Clonic phase associated with slowing of the dominant frequency and synchronized bursts of muscle potentials

slow as 1 Hz. Subsequently, the amplitude increases, faster frequencies appear and gradually the record assumes a normal appearance. Sometimes the slow activity waxes and wanes in such a way as to give a periodic appearance to the record (Cobb and Hill, 1950).

In some cases, slow activity persists for several hours after an attack of grand mal and diagnostic difficulties may be created if it is not known that the patient had a fit prior to the recording.

Petit Mal

Attacks of petit mal are largely confined to children. The term 'minor seizure or attack' should be avoided.

Many akinetic seizures are attacks of petit mal in which generalized muscle relaxation is so profound that the patient falls. On the other hand, Gastaut (1954a) (*see also* Gastaut and Regis (1961)) maintains that the majority of attacks described as 'akinetic' are really violent myoclonic seizures which throw the patient to the ground. In fact, such a distinction may be more apparent than real. Most attacks of petit mal are accompanied by some slight myoclonic twitchings, often restricted to the eyelids, and myoclonic attacks may be accompanied by demonstrable impairment of consciousness.

An attack of petit mal is accompanied by very characteristic EEG findings (*Figure 5.3*). The record is suddenly interrupted by a bilaterally synchronous discharge, often referred to with some accuracy as spike and wave. The discharge is of much higher amplitude than the background EEG and may reach 1,000 μV peak. The paroxysm of abnormal activity is generalized, though usually of higher amplitude in the frontal regions (Chatrian *et al.*, 1968). Recording in a bipolar manner from parasagittal rows of electrodes often shows a phase reversal about the frontal electrodes (F_3 and F_4), indicating a potential maximum in the transverse plane passing through these points. The discharge commonly takes the form of a regular succession of high voltage *delta* waves alternating with spikes of comparable amplitude. Weir (1965) points out that this description is often an evident over-simplification and that frequently the complex can be seen to consist of a small negative spike (c. 10 ms), a positive transient (c. 100–150 ms), a second spike (c. 30–90 ms) which is the one generally observed, and finally the electro-negative wave (c. 150–200 ms). The repetition rate is characteristically 3 per second but at the onset it may be as much as 4 per second, and near its termination a tendency to slow below 3 per second is often apparent. Initially, it may be a little irregular in form. The spike component is commonly electro-negative in the frontal regions. Attacks of petit mal and their EEG concomitants are particularly susceptible to changes in the acid base equilibrium, being provoked by alkalosis caused by overbreathing and inhibited by acidosis, induced for instance by a ketogenic diet or the administration of acetazolamide (Diamox). They are also encouraged by a low blood sugar.

In a few cases, the amplitude of the spike and wave phenomenon is greatest in the occipital regions

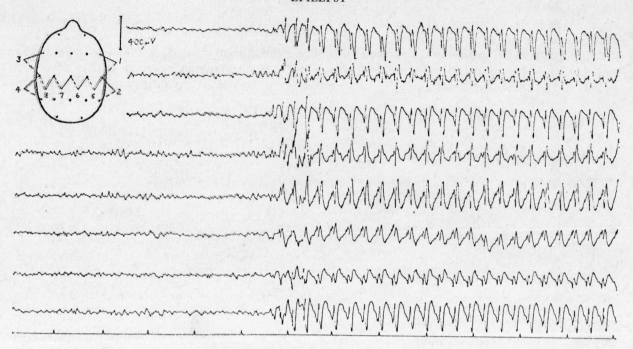

Figure 5.3—Spontaneous petit mal attack. Girl aged 5 years. EEG: Generalized bilaterally synchronous and symmetrical 3 per second spike and wave discharge

and in these the paroxysms often appear when the eyes are closed and disappear on eye opening. Such cases were once referred to as 'pyknolepsy' but there seems little justification for regarding this condition as a distinct entity.

Sleep EEGs are seldom called for in patients with petit mal. Niedermeyer (1965) found that in many patients the typical regular spike and wave episodes seen in the waking state were replaced by polyspike or polyspike and slow wave discharges, their form being distinctly less regular than in the waking state. He also drew attention to the 'spiky' appearance of K-complexes in these patients. Ross *et al.* (1966) confirmed this observation and noted that in most patients the incidence of epileptiform discharges increased progressively with deepening of sleep. At the same time there was a loss of rhythmicity and defective organization of the spike and wave complex. In stage 4 sleep the EEG was irregular with many high voltage spikes, often multiple, interspersed with irregular high amplitude slow waves. With the onset of REM sleep the epileptiform discharges resumed the typical spike and wave appearance but the incidence of the episodes was less than that seen in the waking state.

Myoclonic Attacks

Myoclonic phenomena are a very common experience and epilepsy is only one of their many causes. Many people experience myoclonic jerkings when falling asleep. These are often accompanied by hypnagogic phenomena and a sensation of falling. EEGs taken at these times often show K-complexes, but no epileptiform features are present (Oswald, 1959). Hereditary essential myoclonus is another nonepileptic variety in which the EEG is normal (Daube & Peters, 1966; Mahloudji and Pikielny, 1967).

Myoclonic attacks that are epileptic in nature occur frequently in cases of subcortical epilepsy and have been regarded as fractionated or miniature attacks of grand mal (Gastaut and Fischer-Williams, 1959b). The jerkings are usually bilateral and symmetrical, affecting particularly the face and arms, and are referred to by the patient as 'the jumps'. The EEG accompaniments of such attacks often resemble the spike and wave phenomenon of petit mal, in so far as they consist of an association of high voltage spikes and slow waves which are bilaterally synchronous (*Figure 5.4*), but the episodes seldom have the regularity of true spike and wave: the spikes are frequently multiple, occurring in groups of two to six and are most evident in the central regions. Gastaut (1954b) indeed refers to these complexes as 'polyspikes and waves'. Frequently two or three attacks will be grouped together but even so the whole episode is usually very much briefer than the discharge seen in petit mal. The

76

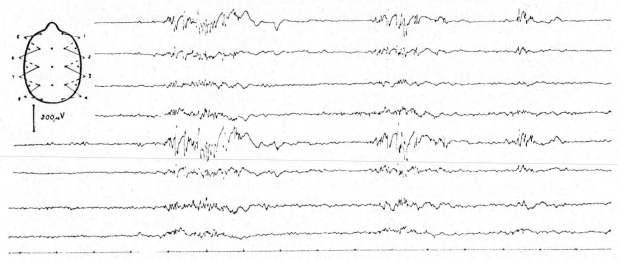

Figure 5.4—*Myoclonic epilepsy. Woman aged 23 years. EEG: Bilaterally synchronous and symmetrical bursts of polyspikes and slow waves. The first was associated with a typical myoclonic attack; the remainder were asymptomatic*

slow waves at 2–3 Hz follow the spikes and are often single, though a brief train of two or three may occur in diminuendo. In epileptic subjects these myoclonic discharges may often be provoked by various stimuli, particularly sudden noises or photic stimulation. Even in normal individuals, similar attacks may be precipitated by photic stimulation (*see* page 64).

Although the origin of the discharge in this type of myoclonic attack is centrencephalic, consciousness in many cases appears to be unaffected. However, this is not always the case and in some attacks a definite amnesia can subsequently be demonstrated. Another factor that may be important is the brevity of most attacks. It is doubtful if very brief interference with the functions of the neurones subserving consciousness would make itself evident to the patient: there is a certain inertia in regard to cerebral mechanisms, as evidenced by flicker fusion, that would tend to mask clinical expression of such brief functional disturbances.

The fact that discharges originating in the centrencephalic areas may produce these dissociated effects suggests that either of two systems may be affected by the abnormal discharge: the centrencephalic system concerned with consciousness and the subcortical motor system projecting to bulbo-spinal motor centres. As myoclonic jerks are sometimes unaccompanied by EEG changes, the latter system may perhaps operate independently of the cerebral cortex. Indeed, the electrical changes recorded from the cerebral cortex, both in myoclonic epilepsy and in petit mal, must be regarded as secondary phenomena that are not essential to the development of the attack.

Unilateral myoclonic attacks may occur with focal cortical lesions (*see* page 85). Myoclonic jerkings are also features of subacute sclerosing panencephalitis (*see* page 144) and the diffuse encephalopathies (*see* page 145). The relationships between various types of myoclonic attacks are reviewed by Halliday (1967a & b).

Interseizure Patterns in Primary Subcortical Epilepsy

It is unusual for a routine EEG recording to coincide with an actual seizure and it is necessary therefore to depend on interseizure patterns for diagnostic assistance in most cases of epilepsy.

Interseizure records may show abnormal discharges which are *formes frustes* or larval forms of seizure discharges and which, in conjunction with an appropriate history, may be accepted as supporting evidence for a diagnosis of subcortical epilepsy. They may show non-specific abnormalities: this is true of 40 per cent of non-activated records taken from epileptics; or they may be within normal limits: this occurs with single routine recordings in 20–30 per cent of cases.

Interseizure epileptiform discharges in subcortical epilepsy are always widespread, bilaterally synchronous and more or less symmetrical. The degree of abnormality of the interseizure record is reflected in the frequency of attacks experienced by the patient. The discharges already described as occurring with petit mal and myoclonic epilepsy are commonly seen as interseizure patterns, the former particularly in children (*Figure 5.5*). The amplitude of these discharges is usually lower than that occurring in actual attacks. The presence of an interseizure spike and wave paroxysm does not necessarily mean that the patient will suffer attacks of petit mal. Such findings have been reported in 50 per cent of cases of subcortical epilepsy having attacks of grand mal only. On the other hand

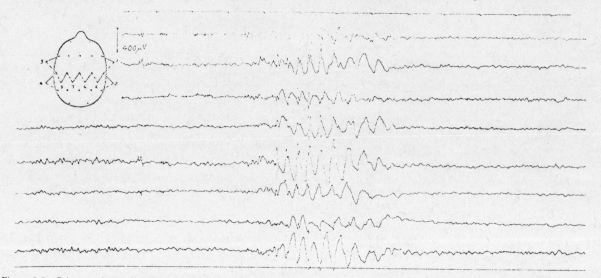

Figure 5.5—Primary subcortical epilepsy—interseizure pattern. Boy aged 14 years. Nine-year history of petit mal attacks; recent occasional grand mal attacks. EEG: Bilaterally synchronous and symmetrical bursts of atypical 3 per second spike and wave activity, unaccompanied by clinical phenomena

in cases known to have petit mal with or without grand mal, the interseizure EEGs show spike and wave episodes in 80 per cent of cases. Faster spike and wave discharges at $3\frac{1}{2}$–$4\frac{1}{2}$ per second (*Figure 5.6*) show an association with attacks of grand mal and in patients having this pattern, petit

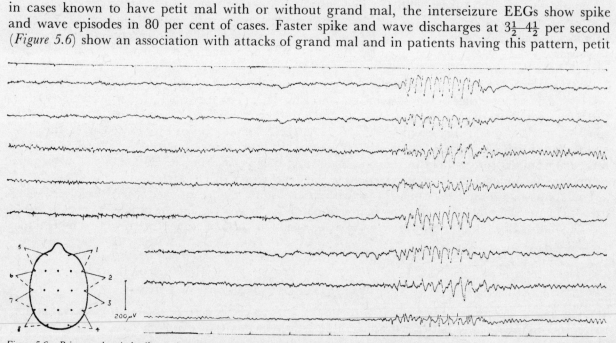

Figure 5.6—Primary subcortical epilepsy—interseizure pattern. Man aged 35 years, had attacks of grand mal only. EEG: Burst of bilateral fast spike and wave activity at 4–5 second unaccompanied by clinical phenomena

mal is relatively uncommon (Kershman, Vásquez and Golstein, 1951). Although these so-called interseizure discharges are unaccompanied by obvious clinical phenomena, more subtle changes may occur. Tizard and Margerison (1963) for instance showed that during spike and wave discharges there was a slowing of response time and an increased numbers of errors when patients were given simple psychological tests.

Sometimes bilateral 3 per second spike and wave discharges occur as the result of cortical lesions: this is secondary subcortical epilepsy (*q.v.*). They have also been recorded from a small number of cases with proven brain tumours arising in predominantly subtentorial or midline structures (Ajmone Marsan and Lewis, 1960). The spike and wave phenomenon therefore is not absolutely diagnostic of primary subcortical epilepsy. Moreover, spike and wave and similar epileptiform discharges are sometimes found in the EEGs of individuals who are not known to have had epileptic attacks of any kind, emphasizing that epilepsy must always be diagnosed on clinical grounds and not solely on EEG evidence. Zivin and Ajmone Marsan (1968) found that of 6,497 non-epileptic patients examined at the National Institutes of Health, Bethesda, 142 (2·2 per cent) had spikes or sharp waves with or without associated slow waves in their EEGs. These were mostly patients with evidence of structural or metabolic disease of the nervous system and on follow-up 20 of the 142 did in fact experience attacks of epilepsy. None of the patients judged clinically to be normal—there were also 142 of these—showed epileptiform discharges in his or her EEG. Metrakos and Metrakos (1961) found that when the siblings of probands with centrencephalic epilepsy were studied, 36·8 per cent showed spike and wave discharges in their EEGs but only 12·7 per cent were known to have suffered from clinical seizures.

An uncommon interseizure discharge takes the form of bursts of spikes similar to those seen in attacks of grand mal (*Figure 5.7*).

Other interseizure abnormalities are frequent in epileptics but also occur commonly in other conditions and on occasion in normal individuals. In the past there has been some danger of electro-encephalography falling into disrepute because of exaggeration of the diagnostic significance of these

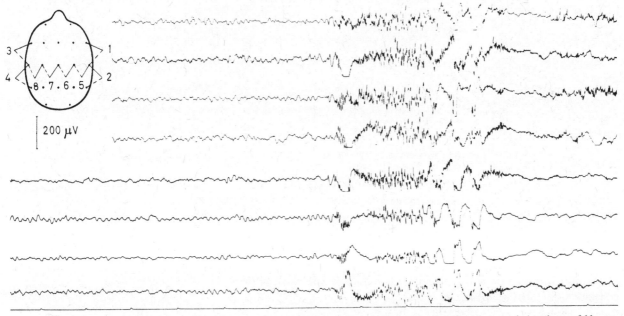

Figure 5.7—Primary subcortical epilepsy—interseizure pattern. Woman aged 18 years. Up to two grand mal attacks per week since the age of 11 years. EEG: Generalized multiple spike discharge terminated by slow waves associated with spikes

abnormalities. Clear-cut paroxysms of symmetrical *delta* activity, particularly at 3 Hz may well be epileptiform discharges in which the spikes are non-existent or masked by the slow activity, but they must not be regarded as having absolute diagnostic significance. Runs of *delta* activity of more gradual onset and cessation and bursts of *theta* activity are also common features in the EEGs of epileptics but carry even less significance. Bursts of 8–12 Hz activity of higher amplitude than the background *alpha* and sometimes of unusual distribution, perhaps limited to the temporal regions, together with runs of faster rhythms, are also seen frequently in these cases, but should not on their own be regarded as diagnostic features. Diffuse abnormalities—an excess of *theta* or *delta* activity—are also more commonly seen in the interseizure records of epileptics than in the normal population but the correlation between these and epilepsy is too low to give them any diagnostic importance.

PROVOCATION TECHNIQUES IN PRIMARY SUBCORTICAL EPILEPSY

In a case of suspected epilepsy provocation techniques may be employed with one of two ends in view: either to precipitate an attack under EEG control, so that both clinical and EEG phenomena can be observed simultaneously, or to produce epileptiform discharges in the EEG unaccompanied by clinical phenomena. The deliberate induction of a major epileptic seizure is very seldom indicated in cases of primary subcortical epilepsy.

Hyperventilation

Reference has already been made to the great variability that is found in the individual responses to hyperventilation; this greatly detracts from its value in the investigation of epilepsy. Nevertheless, there is one clinical group in which it should always be performed: that of children suspected of having petit mal. Occasionally an attack is precipitated before a marked build-up of slow activity occurs, in which

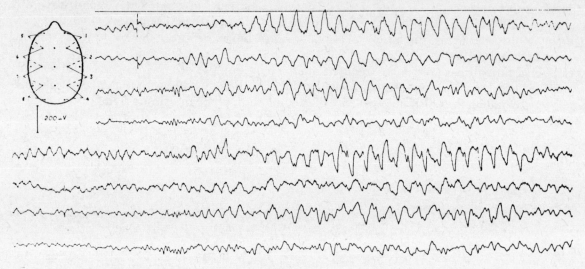

Figure 5.8—Boy aged 9 years with no history of epilepsy. EEG: Frontally predominant 'notched' delta activity at 2·5–3 Hz

case the spike and wave discharge stands out as dramatically as if it were spontaneous. More often there is first a crescendo of bilateral *delta* activity.

In older patients with grand mal or myoclonic epilepsy, relatively brief paroxysms of spikes and slow waves may be evoked, but it is seldom that these are accompanied by clinical manifestations. Occasionally in adults, but much more frequently in children, hyperventilation will evoke bursts or prolonged high voltage runs of notched *delta* rhythm (*Figure 5.8*) sometimes referred to as 'phantom spike and wave'. This is a misnomer: the response is non-specific and must not be taken as conclusive evidence of centrencephalic epilepsy.

Photic Stimulation

The tendency for either major or minor seizures to follow exposure to a rhythmically flashing light is an uncommon but well recognized phenomenon. When photic stimulation is employed as a provocative technique, paroxysmal discharges of two main kinds frequently appear in the EEG (Bickford *et al.*, 1952):

(1) The *photomyoclonic response*, consisting of frontally predominant polyspikes at the flash frequency (*Figure 5.9*) which recruit strongly and which are accompanied by synchronous jerkings, initially of the face and head. The discharge usually ceases when the stimulus is withdrawn and it may be abolished by eye opening. It occurs less often in children than in adults.

(2) The *photoconvulsive response*, consisting of widespread and symmetrical repetitive spike and wave discharges (*Figure 5.10*) which may continue for some seconds after stimulation has ceased and may be accompanied by minor clinical phenomena, including disturbances of consciousness.

Of a group of mixed neurological and psychiatric cases selected because of their known photo-

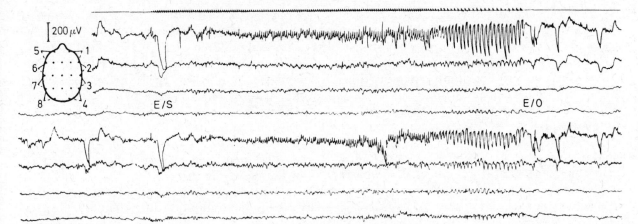

Figure 5.9—Photomyoclonic response. Normal man aged 54 years. EEG: Crescendo of bilateral muscle and eye movement potentials anteriorly synchronized with photic stimuli and terminating with them

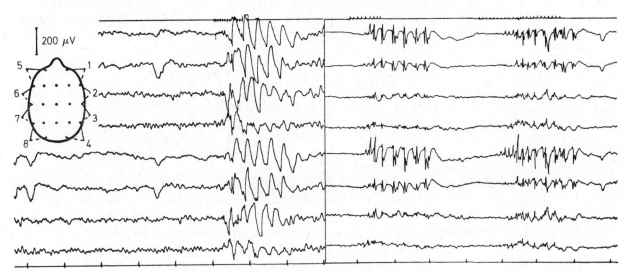

Figure 5.10—Photoconvulsive responses. (a) 'Television' epilepsy. Boy aged 7 years. Occasional 'blackouts' while watching television. EEG: Generalized 3.5 Hz activity associated with spikes evoked by photic stimulation at 16 flashes/second. (b) Man aged 23 years with occasional attacks of grand mal. EEG: Frontally predominant bursts of multiple spike and slow wave activity evoked by photic stimulation at 10 flashes/second

sensitivity, 29 per cent exhibited a purely photomyoclonic response, 57 per cent a purely photo-convulsive response and 14 per cent a mixed response. Half of a normal control group exhibited a photomyoclonic response in some degree, but none a photoconvulsive response. Bickford concluded that the photomyoclonic response is essentially a physiological reaction to high intensity rhythmic photic stimulation and that only when it is pathologically exaggerated, as in certain cases of myoclonic epilepsy, should it be considered significant. Gastaut, Trevisan and Naquet (1958) claimed that the photoconvulsive response is almost confined to patients with primary subcortical epilepsy, and that it occurs in 40 per cent of cases with petit mal and in 20 per cent of cases with grand mal. In view of the form and bilaterally synchronous and symmetrical distribution of this photoconvulsive response, its enhancement by analeptic drugs and its suppression by trimethadione (troxidone: Tridione), Gastaut and Hunter (1950) have suggested that it is subserved by the same mechanisms as those responsible for the irradiation of primary subcortical seizure discharges. Either response may lead to a major convulsion if stimulation is maintained and both are inhibited by intravenous trimethadione.

In childhood and adolescence considerable similarity exists between the EEG responses to inter-mittent photic stimulation in some normals and in epileptics and this has cast considerable doubt as to its validity as a diagnostic test procedure. Brandt, Brandt and Vollmond (1961) found that generalized paroxysmal responses occurred in 16 out of 90 apparently normal children between the ages of 6 and

14 years, although none occurred in 25 children above this age. Jeavons (1969), however, has pointed out that these children were stimulated for periods of up to 6 minutes and that if his own or similar techniques are employed (*see* page 62), 5 per cent of normal children give a paroxysmal response, only about 1 per cent showing true spike and wave (Petersén, Eeg-Olofsson and Sellden, 1968).

A small but interesting group of patients described by Bickford and Klass (1963) showed paroxysmal EEG responses when presented with black and white patterns on a screen. In the majority the discharges comprised diffuse spike and wave activity, but in a few the abnormalities were localized to the occipital areas. A regular pattern of alternating black and white vertical bars appeared to be the most effective stimulus.

Many non-specific patterns of activation occur more frequently in epileptics than in normals, including some rich in harmonics or subharmonics of the flash frequency, or both. Walter (1950) suggested that epileptiform discharges may be contingent on the synchronization of these components in specific phase relationships. The majority of responses to photic stimulation are potentiated by a low blood sugar and they may occur only under particular conditions: by stimulating just as the eyelids are closing, for instance. Carterette and Symmes (1952) have shown that flashes of red light are more effective than those of blue-white in the activation of photosensitive patients. It has also been suggested that the response may vary according to the mental state at the time of examination. In epileptics, it would seem more likely that the variations in mental state and in photic response are both secondary to the spontaneous fluctuations of cerebral excitability to which they are subject.

Sleep

In drowsiness and the early stages of sleep, generalized seizure discharges are sometimes enhanced. Niedermeyer (1965; 1966) claims that patients with primary subcortical epilepsy often show massive irregular bursts of spikes at such times and that these are associated with K-complexes. He feels that these spike discharges can be differentiated from the physiological vertical spikes (*see* page 65).

Leptazol and Bemegride

The analeptic properties of leptazol and bemegride are well known and both drugs have been used to activate the EEGs of suspected epileptics. The value of this procedure in the differential diagnosis of epilepsy is very limited indeed. Since the effect of a given quantity depends upon the rapidity with which it is injected and upon the body weight of the subject, the concentration should be adjusted according to the latter parameter if a standard rate of administration is to be used. Jasper and Courtois

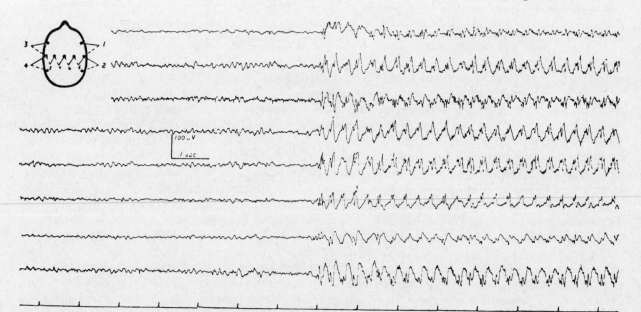

Figure 5.11—Leptazol activation. Man aged 38 years with occasional attacks of grand mal. EEG: Generalized 3 per second multiple spike and slow wave discharge following intravenous injection of a total of 300 mg leptazol

(1953) recommend the dilution of a 10 per cent solution of leptazol with normal saline so that each millilitre of the mixture contains 1 mg/kg of the body weight of the subject. One ml is then given every 30 seconds. With bemegride (standard solution 0·5 per cent) the usual procedure is to give an initial dose of 1 ml (5 mg) per 10 kg of body weight as quickly as possible, followed by further doses of 1 ml every 15 seconds. In different centres, maximum doses varying from 500 to 1,000 mg leptazol or from 100 to 300 mg bemegride are given, but in others injection is continued until a focal or bilateral paroxysmal discharge is elicited in the EEG. The latter may take a variety of forms, of which the principal ones are brief irregular discharges of multiple spikes and slow waves or longer rhythmical discharges of spike and wave activity, usually at about 3 per second (*Figure 5.11*).

Drossopoulo *et al.* (1956) concluded that leptazol and bemegride have similar EEG effects, but that the more gradual action of the latter, at the dosage rate used, is better tolerated and evokes paroxysmal changes in the EEG more readily without causing undesirable sequelae. They regard only the rhythmical spike and wave discharge as indicative of a tendency to have generalized seizures; it never occurred in their normal group. Rodin, Rutledge and Calhoun (1958) confirmed the similar effects of the two drugs, and found that bilateral multiple spike and slow wave discharges sometimes occurred at quite low dosages in chronic epileptics, schizophrenics and in normal controls.

Although this work suggests that the quality of the response, though not the threshold, may carry some significance, it cannot be relied upon clinically as supporting a diagnosis of subcortical epilepsy. Indeed this procedure is seldom indicated in this group of epileptics. Both types of response are facilitated by intermittent photic stimulation. It is recommended that intravenous thiopentone sodium should be given immediately after activation occurs to counteract any further effects of either drug.

Photo-metrazol Activation

The technique of photo-metrazol activation was introduced by Gastaut (1950) who was at pains to stress that its results should be interpreted with caution. It consists of the intravenous injection of 50 mg leptazol every 30 seconds (irrespective of body weight), each dose being followed by exposure of the subject to photic stimulation at about 15 f/s for a period of up to 10 seconds. As the injections proceed, there comes a time when the group of flashes evokes a bilateral myoclonic jerk accompanied by a frontally predominant polyspike discharge in the EEG or by a more prolonged run of irregular spike and wave activity. The quantity of leptazol necessary to produce this result, expressed in mg/kg of body weight, constitutes the photo-metrazol or myoclonic threshold. Subsequent experience of this technique by many workers has confirmed the original finding that low thresholds—of the order of 5 mg/kg or less—are found in centrencephalic epilepsy, but they have also demonstrated similarly low thresholds in a number of other conditions such as schizophrenia and hysteria. Driver's results (1962) suggest that using a refined technique, a clear distinction may be possible between cases of subcortical and cortical epilepsy for when threshold values are obtained from a mixed group of epileptics, they show a bimodal distribution, the lower values corresponding to those with subcortical epilepsy and the higher to those with cortical epilepsy. Any subject in whom paroxysmal discharges occur spontaneously or in whom the photomyoclonic response of Bickford and co-workers is evoked by photic stimulation alone would be classed as having a zero photo-metrazol threshold. Photo-metrazol activation is thus not a satisfactory method of estimating a patient's liability to suffer spontaneous epileptic seizures.

Chlorpromazine

Chlorpromazine (Largactil: Thorazine) has been used extensively for the activation of focal epileptogenic discharges (*see* page 94), but it also has a limited place in the investigation of suspected cases of primary subcortical epilepsy. Occasional seizures have been reported in non-epileptic patients taking the drug therapeutically by mouth, but there do not appear to be any reports of seizures following the intramuscular or intravenous administration of up to 100 mg under EEG control; nor do paroxysmal epileptiform discharges occur in normal controls with the doses so far employed. In this respect it certainly has an advantage over leptazol and possibly over bemegride also. Unfortunately, its comparatively slow action, even when given intravenously, and its hypotensive effect make it unsuitable for the evaluation of an activation threshold.

Stewart (1957), using doses of 50 mg intramuscularly, described the production of bilaterally synchronous spike and wave discharges in 6 out of 8 patients with centrencephalic seizures. He suggested that activation results from hypersynchrony due to the abolition of the desynchronizing effect of the reticular activating system. Further evidence of its value as an activator in this type of epilepsy is advanced by Simons (1958), who gave 100 mg intravenously. Although doses of this order almost invariably induce drowsiness, paroxysmal discharges are usually seen before it is marked and become less apparent as drowsiness deepens and sleep ensues. The optimum safe dose appears to be 50 mg given intravenously over a period of 5 minutes.

CORTICAL EPILEPSY

Seizure Patterns in Cortical Epilepsy

When an area of cerebral cortex is stimulated electrically a spike discharge occurs, which under appropriate conditions is followed by an after-discharge consisting of a succession of spikes. In some circumstances that are far from being fully understood, areas of cerebral cortex affected by a large variety of pathological processes may—seemingly spontaneously—give rise to similar spike discharges. Ward (1961) has put forward evidence suggesting that epileptogenic foci are characterized by a standing (D.C.) negative potential of the order of 7–12 mV which may be attributed to a continuous state of dendritic depolarization. This in turn he relates to the obvious morphological deformities of the dendrites which can be demonstrated in epileptogenic foci. This state of depolarization reduces the threshold to firing of these neurones so that effectively they are hypersensitive and may even respond to normal levels of afferent stimulation with hypersynchronous and sustained discharges.

The transition of sporadic interseizure cortical discharges into the rhythmical sustained discharge that accompanies a clinical seizure may occur in one of two ways. The interseizure spikes may increase progressively in amplitude and frequency until a regular rhythmical discharge develops. Alternatively a single spike discharge may give rise to an after-discharge that continues longer than usual and increases progressively in amplitude until a seizure results. There is evidence that the latter mechanism is the more important (Ralston, 1958). As Ajmone Marsan (1961) has emphasized, the discharge of

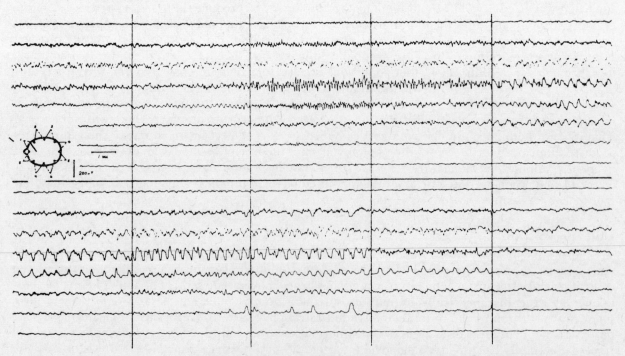

Figure 5.12—Focal seizure pattern. Man aged 30 years, who had a temporal lobe abscess operated upon 16 years previously, followed by occasional attacks in which he experiences blurring of vision on the left accompanied by the sensation of flashing lights. EEG: Consecutive 5-second extracts with intervals of 5 seconds between them. Seizure discharge originates in right occipital lobe, subsequently spreading to left side

the primary epileptic neurones is only the beginning of the process; before a clinical attack develops there must be recruitment of more and more neurones, both locally and at a distance.

Prince and Wilder (1967) have shown in cats that the interictal discharges of an epileptogenic focus with their negative potentials are accompanied by intense inhibitory activity of the neurones in an extensive area of the surrounding cortex. This is likely to be a factor in limiting the spread of the epileptiform discharges. When an attack develops, the inhibitory activity ceases and the same cells are recruited into the epileptiform discharge. It is possible that this mechanism of 'surround inhibition' may operate in clinical attacks of focal epilepsy in man and indeed be the essential mechanism in ensuring that the attacks remain focal.

In a focal seizure the discharge recorded over the scalp may take the form of spikes or sharp waves, spikes and slow waves or, less commonly, rhythmical activity at *alpha*, *theta* or *delta* frequencies. It may be strictly localized, extend widely over one hemisphere or, rarely, be bilaterally synchronous. In focal attacks with a jacksonian march, electrocorticography may show the spread of the discharge; it is less common to be able to demonstrate this at routine electroencephalography. Indeed, in a proportion of jacksonian attacks no abnormality at all may be detected in the EEG. Occasionally, immediately prior to the onset of the seizure, some flattening of the record is evident. This is best seen in temporal lobe attacks but it may also occur with seizures originating elsewhere. Perhaps the most common sequence of events is the appearance of a succession of focal spikes with a repetition rate of about 12 per second; these increase in amplitude and tend to spread. As the attack develops the repetition rate slows progressively, often to as low a frequency as 2 per second (*Figure 5.12*).

It is the bilaterally synchronous discharges, whether ictal or interictal, that give rise to the greatest diagnostic difficulty. Not only is it difficult or impossible to find the site of origin of the discharge in a routine EEG but it may be equally difficult or impossible to decide whether the origin of the discharge is cortical or subcortical. This problem is further considered in the section on secondary subcortical epilepsy (*see* page 96).

Once the seizure discharge has ceased, normal rhythms may return at once. More often there is first a period of low voltage random slow activity. Occasionally, as when a cerebral tumour is present, focal slow activity may be apparent for a period of some hours after a focal attack, although at other times the EEG shows no abnormality.

Psychomotor Epilepsy

The sequence of a focal cortical discharge, its spread to subcortical centres and a subsequent series of generalized spike discharges is a common one and has its clinical counterpart in the form of an aura, followed by loss of consciousness and an attack of grand mal. Another form of spread from a focal cortical discharge is associated with clinical attacks which are now generally called psychomotor epilepsy, although some prefer the term psychoparetic attack or automatism. In 90 per cent of these attacks the origin of the discharge is in one or other of the temporal lobes, particularly when the amygdala, the hippocampus (Ammon's horn), the insula or the temporal pole is involved. In most of the remaining cases the focus is in one of the frontal lobes, most commonly in the orbital gyri. The location of the focus is reflected only in the aura, and the psychomotor attacks which follow cannot be differentiated. Auras are not always described by the patient. Sometimes they are not recalled due to amnesia, but in other cases they fail to occur either because the discharge originates in a 'silent' area or because of the rapidity of its spread. Psychomotor attacks have sometimes been regarded as focal seizures in themselves but this can no longer be accepted and the occurrence of clouding of consciousness in the attack points unmistakably to some centrencephalic involvement. The frequency with which these attacks follow upon temporal lobe discharges implies some particularly close functional relationship of the temporal lobes to the centrencephalic structures. The centres involved in these psychomotor attacks are likely to be the same as those giving rise to attacks of petit mal although there may be quantitative differences. There is a close clinical resemblance between attacks of psychomotor epilepsy and petit mal status (petit mal automatism), and also between very brief psychomotor attacks, when no aura occurs, and ordinary attacks of petit mal. In these brief attacks, the facial expression generally is not as blank as in petit mal and there is frequently some head turning to one or other side. They are usually followed by a spell of confusion, perhaps lasting only a few seconds. It is possible that in some psychomotor attacks the spread of the discharge does not extend beyond the limbic system and the associated clouding of consciousness is more apparent than real. Sudden disturbance of function of the mechanisms subserving memory which lie within the limbic system could well give rise to 'confusion' as occurs in cases of transient global amnesia.

The interictal spike or sharp wave discharges, if present, usually disappear a short time before the onset of a psychomotor attack and there may be a marked diminution in the amplitude of the background activity. In the attack itself the EEG commonly shows bilaterally synchronous discharges at 2–10 Hz, which are best seen in the frontotemporal regions (*Figure 5.13*). Perhaps the most characteristic frequencies fall between 4–6 Hz. In occasional patients this slow activity may be interspersed

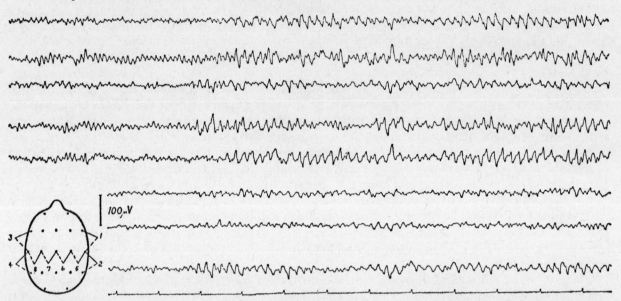

Figure 5.13—Psychomotor epilepsy—commencement of seizure pattern. Man aged 28 years, became vacant and unresponsive during above part of recording: subsequent chewing movements. EEG: Initial 9–10 Hz alpha rhythm replaced by bilateral rhythmical 5–6 Hz theta activity, best seen in the temporal regions and a little more on the right side

with sharp waves or spikes. There is frequently some asymmetry in the record and first one side may be of higher amplitude and then the other. The frequency of the slow activity may vary during the attack and often decreases towards its end, perhaps to 2 Hz.

Changes of this kind have been recorded in 85 per cent of attacks of psychomotor epilepsy. In a few cases the attacks are accompanied by bilateral generalized fast activity at 14–20 Hz. In the remainder a general flattening of the record may be evident (attenuation), while occasionally the record shows no obvious change. After the attack, diffuse random slow activity is seldom seen, but focal slow activity may persist in the affected temporal lobe for hours, days or even longer. This is particularly likely when the lesion responsible is a tumour.

Many patients suffering from psychomotor epilepsy also have attacks of grand mal—70 per cent in Gibbs' series—and sometimes the psychomotor attack itself may give way to a convulsion. Conversely, about 8 per cent of patients with temporal lobe spike foci never experience attacks of psychomotor epilepsy and suffer only attacks of grand mal (Gibbs and Gibbs, 1952b).

The association of personality changes and psychoses with epileptogenic foci in the temporal lobes is of considerable interest. Some authors, notably Bingley (1958), have stressed that personality changes are more likely to occur when bilateral epileptogenic foci are present. In the series of cases of epileptic psychosis studied by Slater, Beard and Glithero (1963) no such trend was apparent; psychiatric abnormalities were seen just as commonly whether one or both temporal lobes were involved or whether the lesion affected the dominant or non-dominant hemisphere. In a proportion of this group of epileptics, progressive dementia occurs and in these patients the dominant posterior rhythm is slowed, sometimes below 8 Hz (Stoller, 1949), and its abundance is diminished. Diffuse *theta* and *delta* activity, usually of low amplitude is present while epileptiform discharges become scanty or disappear. In a more recent study by Flor-Henry (1969) acute organic and schizophrenic-like syndromes were much more commonly associated with dominant hemisphere temporal lobe foci.

INTERSEIZURE PATTERNS IN CORTICAL EPILEPSY

The most characteristic feature of the interseizure EEG in cortical epilepsy is the presence of sporadic spikes which are localized and with a bipolar montage can be shown to have a focal origin. If recorded directly from the cerebral cortex the individual spikes have an amplitude of up to 2,000 μV. On the scalp the amplitude may be 25–500 μV or more and the duration about 20–60 ms. They are usually monophasic and electro-negative at the surface (*Figure 5.14*) but may be diphasic or even triphasic.

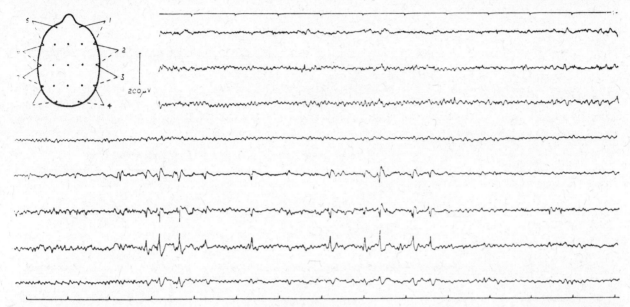

Figure 5.14—Cortical epilepsy—interseizure pattern. Man aged 30 years. Attacks of psychomotor epilepsy. EEG: Left midtemporal focal spikes occurring on an almost normal background

They are sometimes provoked by drowsiness or sleep, occasionally by afferent stimulation and can usually be aggravated by the intravenous injection of analeptic drugs. When these discharges are of adequate amplitude, representing involvement of a large number of neurones, and are repeated rhythmically over a sufficient period, a focal attack of epilepsy may develop. At other times, when only isolated spikes or small groups of spikes appear, there are no obvious clinical concomitants and the EEG provides the only evidence of the epileptic discharge.

Although the site of origin of the discharge and the underlying lesion may be discrete, for a variety of reasons the EEG may show much more widespread abnormalities. In some cases, and this is particularly true of frontal and temporal lobe discharges, owing to the richness of the commissural connections existing between similar areas in the two hemispheres, the discharge, though originating in one hemisphere is reflected as a *mirror focus* in the homologous area of the contralateral cortex (*Figure 5.15*). Oscillographic studies by Ogden, Aird and Garoutte (1956) have shown that such discharges are often so closely synchronized that transcallosal transmission cannot account for them. They postulate that limited activation of a subcortical structure must take place in these cases. However, when such foci are induced experimentally in animals (Morrell, 1960) section of the corpus callosum abolishes the mirror focus. Later the mirror focus achieves autonomy and at this stage commissural section may have little or no effect (Gastaut and Fischer-Williams, 1959a). The amplitude of the mirror discharge is usually smaller but sometimes equal to that of the primary focus. Particularly in cases where the lesion of the affected hemisphere is extensive, the mirror focus may even be the more prominent of the two. In other cases, *independent bilateral foci* are seen (*Figure 5.16*).

When more extensive activation of subcortical structures occurs the discharge is mediated to other cortical areas both of the same and the opposite hemisphere. In such cases the spikes are likely to be associated with slow waves (*see Figure 5.22*). This phenomenon is referred to as secondary bilateral synchrony (*see* page 96). It is particularly likely to occur when the lesion involves the medial aspect of the temporal lobe or the region of the insula.

Another effect of conduction to relatively distant scalp electrodes is a temporal dispersion of the spike

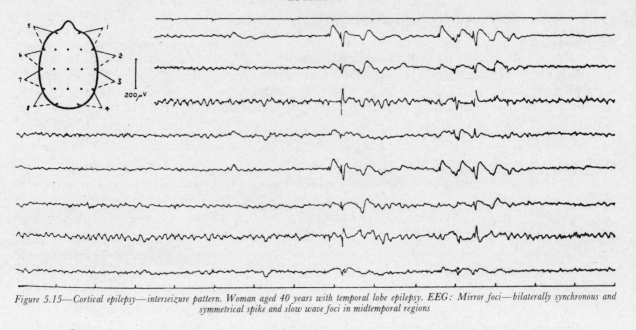

Figure 5.15—Cortical epilepsy—interseizure pattern. Woman aged 40 years with temporal lobe epilepsy. EEG: Mirror foci—bilaterally synchronous and symmetrical spike and slow wave foci in midtemporal regions

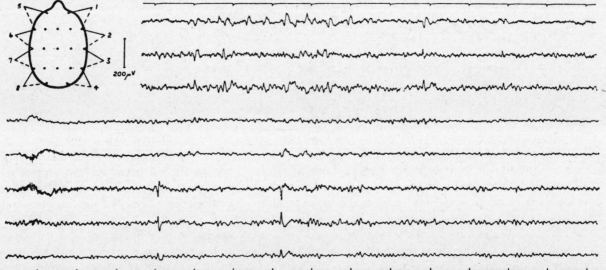

Figure 5.16—Cortical epilepsy—interseizure pattern. Man aged 56 years with temporal lobe epilepsy. EEG: Sharp wave focus in right anterior temporal region with independent spike focus in left midtemporal region

so that its duration is lengthened to between 80 and 200 ms. It is customary for such broadened spikes to be called *sharp waves*.

One characteristic feature of a spike or sharp wave focus is its great inconstancy. An obvious focus may not be evident at a subsequent recording or the amplitude of the sharp waves may be so small in comparison with the background activity that they are overlooked. Provocation techniques not uncommonly fail to evoke a focal discharge which has been seen in a previous recording, or may reveal an apparently unrelated focus, perhaps in the opposite hemisphere.

Not surprisingly, in view of the interposition of soft tissues, cerebrospinal fluid and bone, the spike or sharp wave focus seen in the EEG is seldom as discrete as in an electrocorticogram and even when restricted to one hemisphere, it may be seen, although with varying amplitude and waveform, in all channels recording from that hemisphere. Nevertheless, with care and using closely spaced electrodes, the site of the focus can be identified with some accuracy in many cases by the EEG alone.

Although a spike or sharp wave focus provides the most frequent EEG evidence of a cortical epileptogenic lesion, the discharge may comprise spikes and slow waves or paroxysmal activity in the *alpha*, *theta* or *delta* ranges. There is no relation between the form of the epileptiform disturbances and the structure or functions of the area of cortex involved. There is sometimes a relationship with the type of lesion; spike and slow wave discharges, for instance, appear to be more common with large atrophic lesions.

It is worth remembering that in many cases the area of abnormal cortex may be extensive and the whole of it may be epiloptogenic. At times this may be evident in the EEG when multiple independent foci are seen—the so-called 'shifting foci' (*Figure 5.17*). It may also become apparent after excision of a

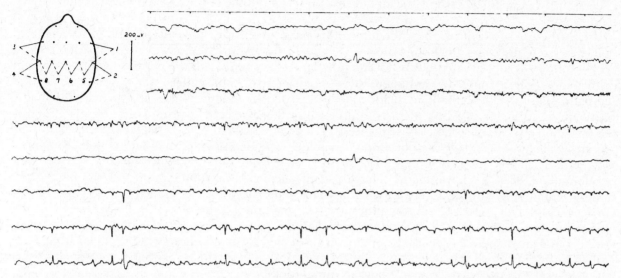

Figure 5.17—Cortical epilepsy—interseizure pattern. Man aged 24 years with temporal lobe epilepsy. EEG: Shifting foci—predominantly left central spike focus, occasionally shifting towards vertex

dominant focus, when it is found that the patient's attacks continue unabated. At subsequent electrocorticography the adjacent cortex may show even more prominent spiking than before. Mirror or secondary conduction foci in normal cortex also appear to obtain a certain autonomy when they have been in existence for some time and may persist following removal of the primary lesion, as Morrell (1960) has demonstrated experimentally in animals.

Migratory foci are found particularly in children when a series of recordings is taken over a number of years. The initial focus may be superseded by another elsewhere in the same hemisphere or occasionally in the opposite hemisphere. The tendency is for the focus to move forwards. An even stronger tendency is for it to disappear (Gibbs and Gibbs, 1953). In a series of children with occipital foci re-examined after the age of 9 years, the focus had disappeared in 40 per cent—all of whom were seizure free—had become occipito-temporal in 18 per cent and midtemporal in 14 per cent. In another series of children with midtemporal foci, subsequent examination after the age of 15 years showed that in 53 per cent the EEGs were normal and in 15 per cent the focus was located in the anterior temporal region; all of those in the first group were seizure free; none of those in the second. In some cases it is likely that migratory foci have the same explanation as shifting foci but in many this is highly improbable and the explanation remains unknown.

The tendency for epileptic attacks to diminish in frequency or disappear with increasing age is paralleled by improvement in the EEG. A corollary of this is that the incidence of epileptiform abnormalities is greater in epileptic children than in epileptic adults. As a rule the clinical improvement whether spontaneous or due to medication occurs first, and for a period, sometimes years, the EEG may continue to show epileptiform features in the absence of clinical attacks.

The interseizure epileptiform discharges described may occur against a background of normal cortical activity (as seen in *Figure 5.14*), but in many cases the lesion responsible for the epileptogenic state of the cortex may give other EEG evidence of its presence. This may take the form of continuous or fluctuating slow wave activity, often focal, or there may be a diminution or loss of normal cortical activity. This latter feature is relatively uncommon in the waking EEG and is likely to be seen only with extensive lesions, whether atrophic, destructive or neoplastic in nature. A comparable phenomenon may occur if oral or intravenous barbiturates are given to the patient to induce widespread fast activity (Pampiglione, 1952). Abolition, or more commonly diminution in amplitude of this fast activity provides very valuable evidence of the location and extent of the lesion. This method is of particular value in the identification of small areas of cortical gliosis which, apart from epileptic attacks, may give no evidence of their presence. It is also useful in identifying which of two mirror foci is the primary and dominant one. A note of caution is suggested by Green and Wilson (1961) who have found that in a small proportion of patients with cortical epilepsy, whether this be determined by an atrophic process or by a tumour, there may be an increase in the amplitude of the *beta* activity over the affected hemisphere.

When the site of origin of the epileptiform discharge is on the convexity of one of the cerebral hemispheres, its discovery and localization are relatively easy. Approximately two-thirds of the cerebral cortex is more deeply situated but is not immune on this account from the multitude of pathological disturbances which trouble its contiguous and superficial neighbour. Indeed, the medial aspect of the temporal lobe is the most common site for epileptogenic foci due to its susceptibility to anoxic damage, particularly at birth (incisural sclerosis) and because the threshold to stimulation of this region is the lowest of any area of cortex. Consequently, if it is affected in a diffuse cortical lesion it is likely that any fits which arise will have their origin in this area. Two interesting cases of temporal lobe epilepsy with well localized anterior temporal spike foci have been described by Falconer, Driver and Serafetinides (1962). Each was found to have a small calcified hamartoma in the posterior part of one middle temporal gyrus but no epileptiform activity could be recorded from its vicinity at electro-corticography. Fits and EEG abnormalities persisted for up to 18 months after local excision of the lesions but finally ceased. The authors suggest that the posterior temporal lesions may have given rise to the distant spike foci, perhaps as the result of subliminal discharges sufficient to trigger off epileptiform discharges. The deep aspect of the temporal lobe might be expected to respond in this way because of its peculiarly low threshold to stimulation.

In 3,271 cases of localized spike foci, Gibbs and Gibbs (1952a) found that in 50 per cent the foci were located in the anterior temporal lobes. In the series of cases reported by Jasper, Pertuisset and Flanigin (1951) the focus was unilateral in 34 per cent, bilaterally synchronous but consistently asymmetrical in 24 per cent, bilaterally synchronous and of equal voltage in 19 per cent, whilst in the remaining 23 per cent bilateral, independent foci were present.

In many patients with foci situated on the inferior or medial aspect of the temporal lobe, localized spikes or sharp waves may be seen at the anterior or midtemporal electrode in a routine recording, particularly if the patient becomes drowsy or if sleep is induced. In other patients, the use of special electrode placements may be required to demonstrate them. Tympanic and nasopharyngeal electrodes are sometimes employed, but more often the sphenoidal (ala magna) electrode (*see* page 218), inserted

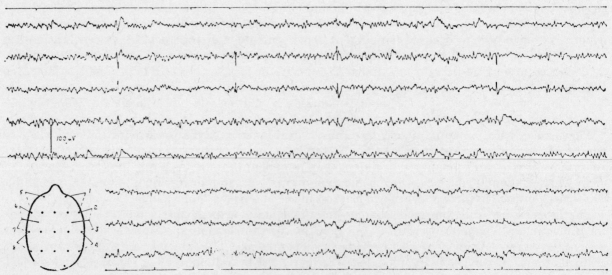

Figure 5.18—Sphenoidal electrodes. Woman aged 31 years with temporal lobe epilepsy. EEG: Focal spikes, right anterior temporal lobe, sometimes seen only in channels recording from sphenoidal electrode

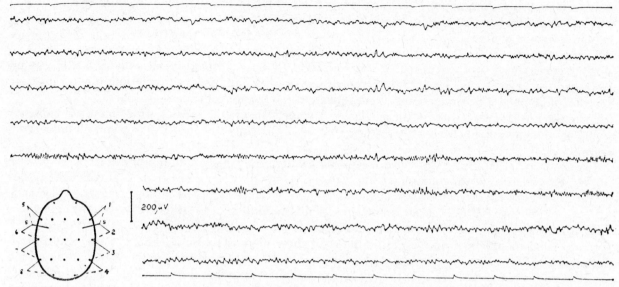

Figure 5.19—Sphenoidal electrodes. Man aged 32 years with temporal lobe epilepsy. EEG: Diminution of beta *activity on right side during pentothal-induced sleep.* Occasional *theta discharges in right anterior temporal region*

to lie under the foramen ovale, is used for this purpose and may prove of great value either in locating a spike focus (*Figure 5.18*) or in detecting asymmetries of barbiturate-induced fast activity (*Figure 5.19*) (Pampiglione and Kerridge, 1956).

More precise localization may sometimes be achieved by using multiple sphenoidal electrodes. Rovit, Gloor and Rasmussen (1961a) have described a technique in which an anterior sphenoidal electrode is placed just anterior and lateral to the pterygopalatine fossa. It is used in conjunction with a sphenoidal needle in the standard placement and a nasopharyngeal electrode. Wire electrodes may be used and if two are twisted together, with their bared tips 1 to 2 cm apart, four electrode placements are achieved under each temporal lobe.

The prognosis following temporal lobectomy is generally better in cases with unilateral or mirror epileptiform foci in the EEG. Some surgeons regard the demonstration of bilateral independent foci as a contra-indication to operation but this is not always the case. Kennedy and Hill (1958) reported that 74 per cent of cases with bilateral foci improved in regard to their epilepsy after operation, compared with 67 per cent of unilateral cases. They point out that the demonstration of bilateral spiking does not preclude a unilateral lesion but it does suggest that if the lesion is unilateral it is likely to affect the medial deep structures of the temporal lobe. Falconer and Kennedy (1961) have again emphasized that bilaterally independent spiking does not always indicate bilateral pathology and they describe 7 such cases all found to have small unilateral tumours of varied pathology and all benefiting from operation. In 4 of these cases the spikes were actually less frequent on the side chosen for operation, the choice being determined by the finding of a diminution of barbiturate-induced fast activity using sphenoidal electrodes.

In the case of mirror foci the choice of the side for operation is greatly aided by studying the effects of the intracarotid injection of sodium amylobarbitone (*see* page 97).

Foci situated on the medial aspect of one hemisphere may produce spike discharges focal at the vertex (Kennedy, 1959), and these must be distinguished from the vertical sharp waves that occur so commonly in sleep and are occasionally seen in the waking records of children (*see Figure 2.4*).

Although it may be accepted that the majority of spike and sharp wave foci are associated with cortical lesions, it is by no means certain that all can be explained in this way. Convincing lesions are sometimes hard to demonstrate in temporal lobe cortex removed at operation in cases of temporal lobe epilepsy. Kaada (1953) suggested that some focal discharges might originate in the subcortical structures projecting to the appropriate area of cortex rather than in the cortex itself. In the case of discharges recorded over the temporal lobe, animal studies indicate that stimulation of subcortical areas may not only cause these but also give rise to physiological responses similar to those that accompany direct cortical stimulation. This work is far from conclusive and no evidence has been advanced that it has any bearing on the problems of human epilepsy. As a hypothesis it has the attraction of explaining some of the failures of surgical treatment of temporal lobe epilepsy.

Gastaut (1954c) has expressed similar views. He believes that it is no longer of value to think of distinct cortical and subcortical regions in relation to epilepsy. Instead he feels that it is more useful to regard the brain as a series of thalamo-cortical systems or sectors, each including the appropriate specific and non-specific projection systems. Focal, or in Gastaut's terminology, partial epilepsy, may be provoked by a lesion either of the cortical or subcortical zone of a sector. In generalized epilepsy, homologous sectors of the two hemispheres become involved simultaneously from a common subcortical centre.

Gastaut *et al.* (1960) have described a syndrome which may develop in infancy in association with an acute febrile illness. The characteristic features comprise the onset of unilateral convulsions and hemiplegia followed several months or years later by attacks of psychomotor epilepsy. They have designated this the *H.H.E. syndrome:* hemiconvulsions, hemiplegia and epilepsy. It is a variant of acute convulsive encephalopathy in the more common form of which the convulsions are generalized. Cortical thrombophlebitis may underlie many of these cases. The initial phase of the syndrome is accompanied by a variety of predominantly unilateral abnormalities in the EEG. Widespread depression of normal activity over the affected hemisphere may precede or follow the occurrence of epileptiform discharges (*Figure 5.20*). Later an ipsilateral spike focus is commonly found in the temporal

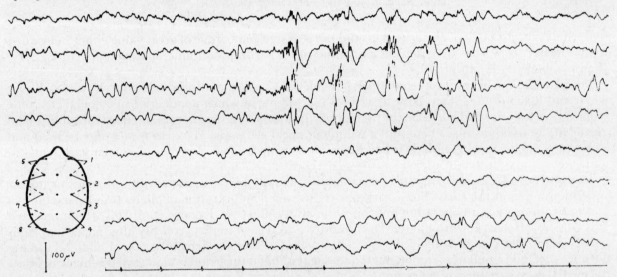

Figure 5.20—H.H.E. syndrome. Boy aged 5 years with left hemiplegia, hemiconvulsions and psychomotor attacks following acute febrile illness at 5 months. EEG : Bursts of polyspikes and associated slow waves originating in the right parietal region. A few independent right central sharp waves. Irregular slow activity and small sharp waves on the left side posteriorly

region, though sometimes generalized epileptiform discharges occur which may be more evident on the contralateral side. Post-mortem examination in the chronic phase of the condition in a few of these cases has revealed the presence of long-standing atrophic lesions in cortical—mainly temporal—and subcortical structures.

PROVOCATION TECHNIQUES IN CORTICAL EPILEPSY

Provocation techniques in patients suspected of suffering from cortical epilepsy may be used with one or more of four aims in view:

(1) To elicit or enhance a focal epileptogenic discharge.
(2) To demonstrate the presence of a focal discharge additional to one already seen in a routine recording.
(3) To demonstrate a localized diminution of a normal component or response of the EEG.
(4) To induce a clinical seizure.

The deliberate induction of a focal seizure is a far more valuable procedure than the provocation of a centrencephalic attack. This is because its clinical pattern, quite apart from the EEG changes, may provide invaluable evidence as to its site of origin. The procedure is justifiable only if there is some possibility of surgical intervention.

Hyperventilation

In general, any pre-existing EEG abnormality is likely to be exaggerated by hyperventilation, though the maximal change may not take place until just after it has stopped. Focal spikes or sharp waves are no exception. Slow wave foci associated with localized lesions may also be aggravated and the response may become rhythmical and more widespread. Abnormalities in the temporal regions are more prone to accentuation than those elsewhere. Occasionally a slow wave focus may be evident only during overbreathing and for a period after its termination. Localized as well as generalized responses are more readily obtained if the blood sugar is low.

Photic Stimulation

Photic stimulation will sometimes activate an epileptogenic lesion in the occipital region, evoking focal sharp waves or slow waves or both, but such lesions are infrequent. Lesions involving one optic radiation or its occipital termination, whether epileptogenic or not, are frequently associated with an ipsilateral diminution or some other anomaly of the photic response: there may be disproportionate harmonics or subharmonics of the flash frequency or a tendency for the discharge to persist on the affected side after the stimulus is withdrawn.

Sleep

The enthusiasm of Gibbs and his co-workers (1958) for sleep as a method of provocation is not shared by all, although there is general agreement that its value is greatest in the investigation of temporal lobe epilepsy. Merlis, Grossman and Henriksen (1951) found that about half their patients with psychomotor epilepsy showed focal epileptiform discharges during sleep, as compared with about one-third in the alert state, but Gloor, Tsai and Haddad (1958) pointed out that in only 7 per cent of their patients was sleep recording necessary to obtain EEG confirmation of the clinical diagnosis of temporal lobe epilepsy. On the other hand, Silverman and Morisaki (1958) found that sleep recording was crucial in confirming the diagnosis in almost 20 per cent of their mixed epileptic group.

As a general rule, any patient suspected of suffering from temporal lobe epilepsy who has a non-specific routine EEG and who does not fall asleep spontaneously, should have a sleep recording carried out before being subjected to the greater ordeals of the insertion of sphenoidal needle electrodes or of activation with bemegride or leptazol. If a barbiturate is used to induce sleep, such as quinalbarbitone sodium (Seconal) by mouth or thiopentone sodium intravenously, the test also provides an opportunity to observe localized diminution of fast activity. Alternatively, sleep recordings can easily be obtained after a period of 24 hours of sleep deprivation (Pratt *et al.* 1968).

Leptazol and Bemegride

The use of leptazol for the activation of epileptogenic lesions was first reported by Kaufman, Marshall and Walker (1947), who found that 44 per cent of a group of post-traumatic epileptics showed evoked or enhanced discharges following a single injection of 200 mg intravenously. Cure, Rasmussen and Jasper (1948) pointed out that slow injection was less likely to precipitate a generalized seizure before local activation took place and suggested a rate of 40 mg/min. They found that 13 out of 14 patients in whom a diagnosis of focal epilepsy had been made on clinical grounds showed selective activation with doses of up to 400 mg. Of these, 10 experienced their habitual auras which gave way in 4 to typical attacks. Bilateral paroxysmal discharges were evoked in 4 out of 27 non-epileptic controls but in none did focal discharges appear.

In contradistinction to centrencephalic epilepsy, Gastaut (1950) found that the photo-metrazol threshold in focal epilepsy was, on average, as high as in normal controls—that is, about 10 mg/kg.

Owing to its milder action there is much to be said for using bemegride in preference to leptazol, although considerable quantities (up to 300 mg=60 ml) may have to be given to achieve a positive result if the procedure recommended on page 83 is adhered to. Drossopoulo *et al.* (1965) claim that when a focal seizure is induced with bemegride it is more likely to develop gradually and to follow the pattern of the habitual attack than when induced with leptazol, which is liable to precipitate a generalized seizure with omission of the introductory phenomena. Danielson and Ellebjerg (1966) felt that bemegride was as good as but no better than leptazol as a provocatant but they confirmed that side-effects were fewer and that generalized seizures were less likely to occur.

Maspes *et al.* (1961) reported that the intravenous administration of mephenesin just prior to activation with leptazol did not increase the amount of leptazol necessary to evoke an epileptiform discharge in the EEG, but did considerably increase the amount needed to precipitate a clinical attack. The period of pre-ictal activation of the EEG was thus prolonged and focal rather than generalized seizures were provoked.

Habitual attacks appear to be more easily initiated when they are prefaced by long auras. It is highly desirable when seizures are provoked that they be recorded cinematographically or on video-tape and that comments are recorded by an observer during the progress of the attack; otherwise many details will be overlooked and errors may arise. Further practical considerations are discussed by Ajmone Marsan and Abraham (1960).

In cases of secondary bilateral synchrony, both drugs are more liable to elicit bilateral than focal discharges.

Chlorpromazine, Imipramine and other drugs

The analeptic properties of chlorpromazine have already been referred to on page 83. Stewart (1957) found that 50 mg, given intramuscularly, activated the EEGs of 17 out of 28 patients with focal epilepsy and Lyberi and Last (1956), using 25 mg intravenously, obtained useful additional information in the same proportion of cases. Chlorpromazine in these doses does not normally induce rhythmical *beta* activity in the EEG, but Lyberi and Last mention its occurrence on the same side as the lesion in a few of their cases. It is possible that drowsiness plays some part in its activating effects.

Imipramine (Tofranil), which is chemically a distant relative of chlorpromazine, was reported by Leyberg and Denmark (1959) to have precipitated seizures in 4 per cent of depressed patients given doses of up to 250 mg per day. There have been no reports of its evoking epileptiform discharges in non-epileptic subjects when given intravenously in doses of up to 100 mg under EEG control.

Imipramine enhances or evokes epileptiform discharges in 60 per cent of patients in whom a diagnosis of temporal lobe epilepsy has been established on clinical or EEG evidence (Kiloh, Davison and Osselton, 1961). A suitable dose is up to 75 mg diluted with saline and injected intravenously over a period of 10 minutes in men and 15 in women. Imipramine appears to be as effective as bemegride in the activation of specific discharges and the effects of the two drugs in the same patient are often very similar. Occasionally imipramine reveals a temporal lobe sharp wave focus when bemegride evokes solely bilateral discharges. It thus seems possible that imipramine may have some advantage as an activating agent in cases of secondary bilateral synchrony. Notwithstanding the slow rate of administration, hypotensive collapse occurred in 4 out of 60 subjects. Cardiovascular disease therefore constitutes a definite contra-indication to imipramine provocation. Mephentermine (Mephine) should always be available to counteract its hypotensive effects.

Davison (1965) found that amitriptyline in doses of 30 mg given over a period of 5 minutes gave similar results to imipramine although Redding (1969) claims that it has no advantage over other drugs that induce drowsiness and sleep. Vas, Exley and Parsonage (1967a; 1967b) have investigated the effects of two other drugs, procyclidine hydrochloride and methixene hydrochloride. The former was given in doses of 10–20 mg and the latter in doses of 10 mg slowly intravenously. Both appeared to be effective activating agents of focal epileptiform activity and were thought to be superior to hyoscine hydrobromide given in doses of 1 mg in 2 ml over 1 minute (Vas, Exley and Parsonage, 1967c) because of the infrequency of side-effects. No epileptiform features were produced in any of the non-epileptic controls.

Pyribenzamine at the rate of 2 mg every 15–20 seconds has been used by King and Weeks (1965) with encouraging results; Verdeaux, Verdeaux and Marty (1954) have described their experiences with alpha-chloralose, while Bercel (1953) has employed mixtures of alpha-chloralose and hyoscine.

Green (1963) and Mosowich (1967) have used hypoglycaemia to provoke epileptiform activity inducing this with tolbutamide in a dosage of 0·5–1·5 g which, it is claimed, has no effect on the EEG of normal individuals.

Hypoxia induced either by breathing mixtures containing 7 per cent oxygen (Meyer and Waltz, 1961) or pure nitrogen (Gastaut *et al*. 1961) has also been used.

Auditory Stimulation

Musicogenic epilepsy is a rare condition and is of exceptional interest because of the specificity of the stimulus by which seizures are precipitated. A patient may be sensitive only to a particular piece of music and, in such a case, it is presumably its associative qualities that provide the crucial stimulus

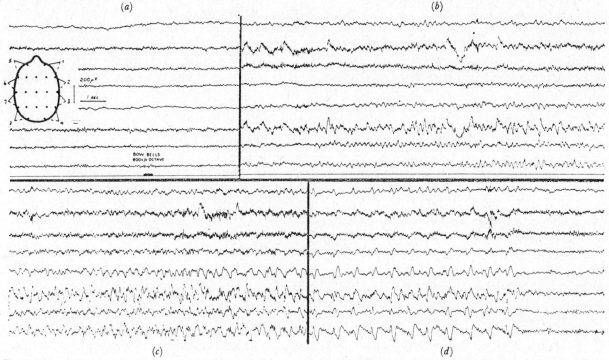

Figure 5.21—Audiogenic epilepsy—seizure pattern. Man aged 62 years with temporal lobe seizures precipitated only by hearing chiming bells. Seizure induced by recorded sound of Bow Bells the frequency spectrum of which had been restricted to a single octave centred about 800 Hz. EEG: (a) Bilateral low voltage fast activity. Onset of auditory stimulation at marker in lowest trace. (b) 25 seconds after onset of stimulation. Emergence of theta rhythm in left temporal region with irregular higher voltage transient discharges more anteriorly. (c) continuous with (b) Crescendo of mixed theta, delta and sharp wave components arising primarily in the left mid- to posterior temporal region. (d) 10 seconds later. Repetitive 1 per second sharp and slow wave complexes of similar distribution terminating abruptly

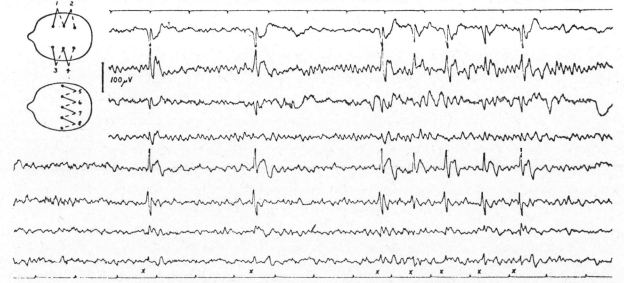

Figure 5.22—Auditory stimulation. Girl aged 5 years with nocturnal attacks of grand mal. EEG: Right parieto-central spike and slow wave complexes in response to tap stimuli (X). The response disappeared following administration of phenobarbitone

95

(Critchley, 1937). In a comprehensive review of 44 previously published cases, Poskanzer, Brown and Miller (1962) noted that of the 22 in which EEG studies had been made, 13 showed abnormalities in one or other temporal lobe. A personal case was sensitive only to a particular recorded chime of bells (*Figure 5.21*).

There are other cases in which attacks follow exposure to non-musical sounds, such as clicks, especially if they be rhythmical. This led Prechtl (1959) to subject a large group of mixed cases to repetitive click stimulation; it was reported to have aggravated pre-existing temporal lobe abnormalities in 37 per cent. The record reproduced in *Figure 5.22* was obtained from a case of nocturnal major epilepsy, not clinically audiogenic, in which random taps evoked individual sharp waves in the right central region. Pure tones have been shown by Arellano, Schwab and Casby (1950) to activate the EEG of a patient with psychomotor epilepsy.

The activation of epileptiform discharges by auditory stimulation is an extremely rare occurrence and it is doubtful whether the testing of a patient is worth while unless there is some clinical indication for this procedure.

SECONDARY SUBCORTICAL EPILEPSY

Secondary subcortical epilepsy is essentially an EEG concept. Examples are not uncommon. They are really varieties of cortical epilepsy showing secondary bilateral synchrony. Foci involving the region of the insula or the medial aspect of either hemisphere are particularly likely to give rise to this phenomenon. The focal epileptiform discharge spreads immediately to subcortical structures and is mediated to all cortical areas, usually in the form of a spike and slow wave discharge. The waveform may be virtually indistinguishable from the spike and wave discharge of petit mal but in most cases the repetition frequency is lower ($2-2\frac{1}{2}$ per second) or greater (4–6 per second) and more variable. In addition it is usually less regular and is frequently asymmetrical, being of higher amplitude over the affected hemisphere although overlying an extensive lesion the discharge may be of lower voltage. Tükel and Jasper (1952) claimed that, when the discharges are symmetrical, they may sometimes be distinguished from those of primary bilateral synchrony by a careful examination of their distribution. Occasional unilateral focal discharges may appear, giving added confirmation of the unilateral origin of the generalized paroxysms (*Figure 5.23*).

Rossi, Walter and Crandall (1968) studied five patients with temporal lobe epilepsy, each of whom at times showed bilaterally synchronous spike and wave complexes of a non-focal type. With depth

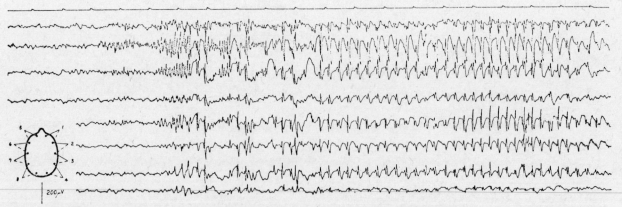

Figure 5.23—Secondary subcortical epilepsy—interseizure pattern. Man aged 20 years with temporal lobe epilepsy. Area of gliosis demonstrated at operation in posterior part of right superior temporal gyrus. EEG: Crescendo of spike discharges in right anterior temporal region followed by generalized spike and slow wave discharges (secondary bilateral synchrony) of higher amplitude on the right side

electrodes the discharge sometimes appeared to originate in the affected temporal lobe subsequently spreading to the thalami and other cortical areas. Sometimes there was no involvement of the thalami at all while on yet other occasions the discharge appeared to originate in the centromedian and anterior thalamic nuclei. On occasion the discharges were limited to the thalami but as the authors point out they were unable to record from every area of the brain and the possibility exists that the discharges may have originated in cortical areas distant from any electrode. When the thalami were involved the discharges tended to be more regular. It is interesting to compare these observations with the experimental findings of Wilder, King and Schmidt (1969). When cortical epileptogenic foci were produced in monkeys, independent secondary foci developed in the contralateral homotopic cortex, the putamen, the subthalamic nucleus, the red nucleus and the nucleus ventralis lateralis of the thalamus.

A review of patients with cerebral tumours showing the phenomenon of secondary subcortical synchrony is presented by Madsen and Bray (1966).

Intracarotid Amylobarbitone

A technique which has proved to be of value in differentiating primary from secondary bilateral synchrony is the intracarotid injection of sodium amylobarbitone during electroencephalography. Wada and Rasmussen (1960) showed this method to be of value in establishing the hemispheric lateralization of speech. Lateralized disturbances of motor and sensory functions occur, while Terzian and Cecotto (1961) have demonstrated the occurrence of such phenomena as astereognosis, anosognosia, asomatognosia, together with tactile, visual and auditory extinction.

The nature of EEG changes varies with the rate of injection. With rates of about 10 mg/second, the first change in the EEG is the appearance of low voltage fast activity on the side of the injection unaccompanied by any change in the clinical state of the patient. This gives way to high amplitude ipsilateral 1·5–3 Hz activity at which stage the appropriate clinical changes occur. This resolves after 1–3 minutes and the fast activity reappears. Slower rates of injection may only give rise to fast activity while if given quickly the slow activity may appear abruptly. In the occasional patient with an unusually large anterior communicating artery or some other vascular anomaly, unilateral injection may give rise to bilateral EEG and clinical changes.

The technical details of the procedure are given by Garretson, Gloor and Rasmussen (1966). Catheters are inserted into each internal carotid artery, care being taken to ensure that they are at the same level. Sodium amylobarbitone, 50 mg in 2 ml normal saline is injected at the rate of 0·3 ml/second on each side with a minimum interval of 30 minutes between the two injections. It is important to give the same quantity of drug at the same rate on both sides. Injection on the side of a unilateral epileptogenic focus produces prompt suppression of epileptiform activity while contralateral injection has no effect. In the case of mirror foci, injection on the side of the primary focus abolishes the activity on both sides, while injection on the side of the secondary focus leads to a cessation of spikes on this side alone (Rovit, Gloor and Rasmussen, 1961b). With bilaterally independent foci, as a rule the ipsilateral focus is suppressed following injection, but Perez-Borja and Rivers (1963) have found that on occasion

In cases of primary subcortical epilepsy, injection on either side has no effect on the frequency of the spike and wave bursts, little or no effect on the slow wave component but may decrease the amplitude of the spike component on the side of the injection. Sometimes epileptiform activity is provoked. In cases with focal lesions showing secondary bilateral synchrony mimicking the EEG picture of primary subcortical epilepsy, very different changes occur. When the injection is made on the side of the focus all the epileptiform activity disappears. When given on the opposite side there is some decrease in the amplitude of the spike component but otherwise there is little effect other than an occasional provocation of bilateral epileptiform discharges. Clearly the method is only worth using when epileptiform discharges are frequent and can be relied on to occur during the procedure. Moderate sedation of the patient is helpful.

Intracarotid Leptazol

The leptazol test is carried out in the same way, generally 30 minutes after the last injection of sodium amylobarbitone (Garretson, Gloor and Rasmussen, 1966). One ml of a solution containing 0·25 mg leptazol is injected every 5 seconds until either activation of the EEG has occurred or a total of 40 ml has been administered. If activation has not occurred a further 40 ml may be given at twice the initial rate and if need be a further 20 ml may be given at a rate of 3 ml every 5 seconds. When an inadequate result is obtained the procedure may be repeated after an interval of 30 minutes using a solution of leptazol containing 1 mg/ml. The purpose of the test is to induce epileptiform discharges for at least 10 seconds with or without clinical epileptic phenomena. Ricci and Silipo (1968) have used bemegride in the same way giving a 0·25 per cent solution at the rate of 1 ml every 2–3 seconds until the seizure commenced. Subsequently 100 mg of amylobarbitone sodium is injected into the carotid artery to prevent spread of the seizure.

EPILEPSY ARISING FROM NUMEROUS AREAS IN THE CEREBRAL CORTEX AND SUBCORTICAL STRUCTURES

Cases falling into this category, suffer from diffuse or scattered brain lesions. Although in many patients birth trauma, infective or toxic processes, cerebral degenerations or widespread vascular disorders can be identified as causal agents, it is important to realize that epileptic attacks themselves, particularly when severe and prolonged as in status epilepticus, can give rise to permanent structural changes both in the cerebral cortex and elsewhere, which in turn may initiate further attacks and give rise to EEG abnormalities.

The interseizure records show widespread bilateral spike and slow wave discharges, often irregular in form and with a frequency varying from 2 to 4 Hz, superimposed upon a background of diffuse slow activity. Spikes are often obvious and may occur in groups but in other cases the slow components are more prominent. Multiple independent foci, either of spikes, sharp waves or spikes and slow waves, are frequent (*Figure 5.24*). Compared with the records of cases of primary or secondary subcortical epilepsy, these records are more continuously abnormal and it is unusual to find even brief

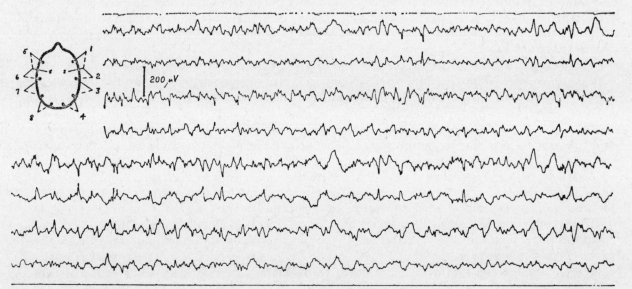

Figure 5.24—Epilepsy arising from numerous areas in the cerebral cortex and subcortical structures—interseizure record. Man aged 18 years. Subnormality, disturbed behaviour and frequent attacks of grand mal. EEG (using sphenoidal electrodes) : Several spike and sharp wave foci on continuously abnormal background of diffuse slow activity

stretches of record that can be accepted as within normal limits. Such cases show a high incidence of abnormal neurological findings and of organic deterioration. Focal seizures, grand mal, psychomotor attacks and myoclonic episodes are accompanied by their usual EEG changes.

A substantial proportion of the cases described by Gibbs and Gibbs (1952c) as showing *petit mal variants* would seem to fall into this group, although others conform more to cortical spike and slow wave foci with or without secondary bilateral synchrony.

HYPSARRHYTHMIA

Cases of hypsarrhythmia (Gibbs and Gibbs, 1952d) would also appear to be best classified in the group of epilepsies arising in the cerebral cortex and subcortical structures. There is nothing specific about hypsarrhythmia, aetiologically, clinically, electroencephalographically or in its response to treatment. The diagnosis is limited to infants and young children and is rarely made after the age of 4 years. These children show the EEG patterns described above although they are, as one would expect, of even higher amplitude with more plentiful slow activity (*Figure 5.25*). They suffer from infantile spasms (salaam attacks; infantile myoclonic spasms) which may be regarded as a variety of tonic attack. Other forms of epileptic attacks may co-exist. Infantile spasms are associated with a

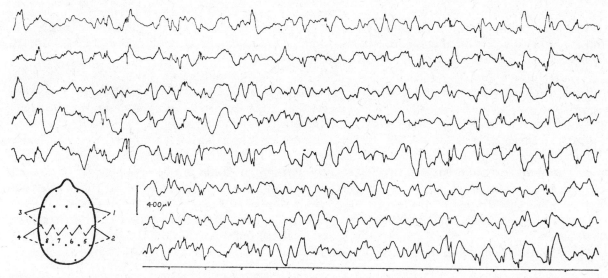

Figure 5.25—'Hypsarrhythmia'—interseizure pattern. Boy aged 14 months with 'jack knife' spasms and subnormality. EEG: Spike and polyspike discharges on continuously abnormal background of diffuse high voltage arrhythmic slow activity

variety of paroxysmal discharges in the EEG or with an overall diminution of electrical activity (Bickford and Klass, 1960). There is a marked tendency for organic deterioration to occur, this feature being reported in up to 95 per cent of cases in various series. A history of brain damage of varied aetiology is frequently obtained and residual neurological signs are commonly present. The attacks show some resistance to the usual anti-epileptic drugs but sometimes respond well to the administration of ACTH.

The so-called hypsarrhythmic EEG is not always accompanied by salaam attacks and about a third of children with salaam attacks do not have this type of EEG abnormality. As the child grows older the pattern changes: the epileptiform discharges tend to diminish and the EEG may even become normal.

A comprehensive review of the aetiology, treatment and prognosis in cases of infantile spasms, with clinical and EEG findings, is given by Jeavons and Bower (1964).

Phenylketonuria

In the first few weeks of life the EEG in phenylketonuria shows only minor abnormalities but by 6 months the EEG generally shows more severe changes. Hypsarrhythmic patterns are not uncommon and occurred in 3 of 19 cases investigated by Fois, Rosenberg and Gibbs (1955) and in 5 of 19 cases described by Low, Bosma and Armstrong (1957). Other cases show high voltage sharp and slow wave discharges, single or multiple sharp wave foci or paroxysmal *delta* discharges. Normal EEGs are infrequent. About half the cases have seizures and even if no fits occur the same EEG abnormalities may be present. Both the fits and the EEG abnormalities show improvement on a phenylalanine-restricted diet; hypsarrhythmic features and multiple spike foci disappear although paroxysms of spikes and waves often persist (Poley and Dumermuth, 1968). In many cases the administration of a loading dose of phenylalanine (0·1 g/kg body weight) leads to a prolonged aggravation of the EEG abnormalities (Clayton *et al.* 1966). Whether treated or untreated there is a tendency for the EEG to improve after the age of 2 years.

MYOCLONUS EPILEPSY

Myoclonus epilepsy (progressive familial myoclonic epilepsy) was first described by Unverricht. The condition is familial and in addition to myoclonic attacks it is characterized by attacks of grand mal, dementia and often by signs of a progressive cerebellar disorder. Examples showing this latter feature were described by Hunt under the title of 'dyssynergia cerebellaris myoclonica'. As a rule the EEG is grossly abnormal, showing background *theta* and *delta* activity which is often ragged in appearance due to the presence of *beta* components. Superimposed upon this are bilaterally synchronous single or multiple spikes, with or without slow waves (Kreindler *et al.* 1959) although between the ages of 4 and 12 years some unstable *alpha* activity is usually evident. In some cases the discharges are periodic and are generally accompanied by myoclonic jerkings, the violence of which may correlate with the number of spikes in the complex (Halliday, 1967b).

Several authors have pointed out that frequently no close relationship exists between the EEG and the clinical phenomena and this fact is claimed by Gastaut and Rémond (1952) to support the view that the myoclonus has its origin in the subcortical structures. It is of interest that in these patients there are widespread degenerative changes involving the reticular formation.

Janeway *et al.* (1967) maintain that progressive myoclonus epilepsy with Lafora inclusion bodies (Lafora's disease) can be distinguished from progressive familial myoclonic epilepsy on histopathological grounds and point out that the EEGs, although similar, differ in that the spike discharges and the myoclonic jerkings are frequently dissociated in Lafora's disease, whereas in the other condition they maintain that the temporal association is close. Kreindler *et al.* stated that in some cases of progressive familial myoclonus epilepsy the spike discharges occurred independently of the myoclonic phenomena but the nosological status of their cases might be questioned. If the claim made by Janeway *et al.* is confirmed, the EEG may be helpful in differentiating these two clinically similar syndromes.

STATUS EPILEPTICUS

CONVULSIVE STATUS

Although the common variety of convulsive status is grand mal, in some patients the repetitive attacks are unilateral, tonic or sometimes myoclonic. Seventeen patients mainly with status grand mal

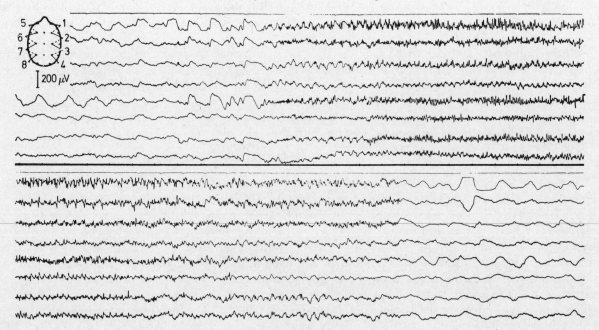

Figure 5.26—Convulsive status epilepticus—subclinical seizure discharge. Man aged 37 years. Repeated major seizures controlled by paraldhyde. EEG: Crescendo of 15 Hz rhythm bilaterally associated with rhythmical theta *and* delta *components and repetitive spikes, emerging from a background of bilateral asynchronous slow activity*

and derived from a mental hospital population have been studied by Bell and Kiloh (1971). During the period of status the background activity in these patients consisted largely of *delta* activity with some fast rhythms probably drug induced. Focal discharges, including spike and wave complexes and slow wave foci, became more prominent than in the pre-status recordings but bilaterally synchronous epileptiform discharges virtually disappeared. Many larval seizure discharges were seen corresponding to the 'after discharges' described in animal studies and during electrocorticography in man, their form varying from patient to patient. The most common variety was a discharge lasting 2–3 seconds commencing with a *delta* wave towards the end of which appeared low voltage rhythmic activity at 14–16 Hz. As the amplitude of this increased, its frequency fell and the bursts terminated with another *delta* wave. These discharges were sometimes focal and sometimes bilaterally synchronous. At times prolonged discharges of the same kind were seen which merged with the convulsive discharge (*Figure 5.26*). In some patients the larval seizure discharge took the form of a series of brief bilaterally synchronous 12–16 Hz bursts resembling low voltage sleep spindles each lasting about 1–2 seconds. Prior to a convulsion each successive burst showed an increase in amplitude and a fall in frequency, the convulsion commencing when the frequency fell within the range 5–10 Hz. The seizure discharges were generally introduced by one of the varieties of 'after discharge', recruitment often continuing during the early part of the convulsion. James and Whitty (1961) have stressed the value of monitoring cases of status grand mal electroencephalographically should the condition require treatment with muscle relaxants and artificial respiration.

PETIT MAL STATUS

Petit mal status was described by Lennox (1945). Each episode may last minutes, hours or even days. The EEG shows continuous 3 per second spike and wave activity which Lennox believed to be as rhythmical as the discharge seen in an 'absence'. The distribution may vary, the complex being predominantly frontal without spread to the occipital areas (*Figure 5.27*). Many papers describe cases of

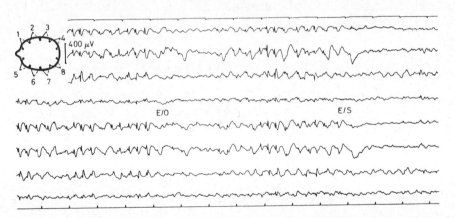

Figure 5.27—Petit mal status. Boy aged 13 years. Repeated petit mal attacks separated by periods of semi-consciousness. EEG: during semi-consciousness: Bilateral 3 per second spike and slow wave activity momentarily interrupted when commanded to open and close eyes

status petit mal in which much more irregular discharges occur. The possible implication of this pattern is discussed below.

PSYCHOMOTOR STATUS

The occurrence of psychomotor status must also be accepted. The possibility was put forward, although without evidence, by Gastaut and Vigouroux (1958) and also forshadowed by Lennox (1960). Bonduelle *et al.* (1964) argued the case strongly in relation to an epileptic aged 55 years who suffered episodes of long-lasting confusion during which his EEG showed generalized irregular polyspikes and sharp waves of variable morphology. Patients with temporal lobe epilepsy have long been known to experience 'fugues', twilight states or epileptic furors and a case can be made that most if not all of these episodes are examples of psychomotor status (Dreyer, 1965). Kroth (1967) described a patient with a right temporal sharp wave focus who suffered a twilight state during which his EEG showed high voltage, continuous, generalized, irregular, convulsive activity. The case described by Rennick and Perez-Borja (1969) had repeated episodes of clouding of consciousness in which his EEG showed 'rhythmic bilateral spikes most evident anteriorly'.

The distinction of such cases from status petit mal on clinical and electroencephalographic grounds during the attacks is not easy, but in view of the relative infrequency of petit mal in adults it seems reasonable to suggest that most cases reported in adults are likely to be examples of psychomotor status. In many of the cases recorded as petit mal status the EEG does not show regular spike and wave activity with a repetition frequency of 3 per second; instead the activity is irregular, often with poly-spikes and slow wave discharges, although generally bilaterally synchronous. On the other hand, one must bear in mind Niedermeyer's (1965) observation of the effect of sleep upon regular spike and wave activity and allow for the fact that persistent clouding of consciousness might sometimes have this kind of effect.

Epilepsia Partialis Continua

There is no reason to regard epilepsia partialis continua as an entity, either clinically or on EEG grounds. The sole feature that characterizes the condition is the almost continuous convulsive activity which occurs of a limb, a segment of a limb or of a group of muscles. This may have a myoclonic quality or be more rhythmical in character. There may or may not be a jacksonian spread. Occasional attacks of grand mal may occur. Similar cases showing continuous or frequently recurring epileptic disturbances of a sensory nature are also well recognized.

In many of these cases the EEG shows continuous focal activity over the appropriate area of cortex, the form of which varies in different patients. Spikes, sharp waves, spikes and slow waves, *theta* or *delta* discharges may all occur (*Figure 5.28*). Juul-Jensen and Denny-Brown (1966) used a

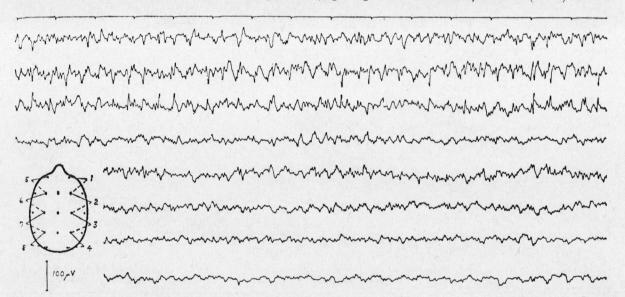

100 μV

Figure 5.28—Epilepsia partialis continua. Man aged 53 years with continuous jerking of left hand. Occasionally, jerking spreads throughout left upper limb and is followed by an attack of grand mal. Condition followed an infected open head injury. EEG: Repetitive focal sharp waves in right central area associated with a preponderance of slow activity in the same area

rather restrictive definition of epilepsia partialis continua and found that in their cases the common EEG accompaniment of the convulsive activity was a 'large blunt wave often polyphasic' of maximal amplitude over the contralateral central area but showing no discrete focus. Sometimes the activity was generalized although never symmetrical. In some cases, and this is particularly true of those showing myoclonic phenomena, the EEG may show no abnormality. It may be that in these cases the discharge originates in the subcortical motor centres without being relayed to the cortex.

102

FEBRILE CONVULSIONS

A febrile convulsion is an attack of epilepsy, generally grand mal. No clear distinction can be drawn between those children whose seizures are associated with high fever and who subsequently remain free of further attacks for the rest of their lives, and those whose attacks are associated with lesser degrees of fever and which recur in later life. If the convulsions have focal or adversive features, recurring attacks—and a diagnosis of epilepsy—are likely to follow. In a follow-up study of a large series of children who suffered febrile convulsions, the incidence of 'true epilepsy' proved to be 5 per cent as compared with 0·5 per cent in the general population; they also showed a high genetic loading for epilepsy. In the majority of cases of febrile convulsions, the interseizure or post-seizure records show no epileptiform discharges, as one would expect in patients who have only one or two attacks and then only as the result of considerable provocation. Even so, in some series of cases, up to 19 per cent of specifically epileptiform records have been reported.

In a series of children with febrile convulsions Millichap (1968) found the EEGs to be normal in 68 per cent, while 12 per cent showed epileptiform discharges. This is similar to Lennox's (1947) findings, 55 per cent of her child patients having normal EEGs and 10 per cent showing epileptiform discharges.

Frantzen *et al.* (1968) found that in children under $2\frac{1}{2}$ years of age the appearance of 1–3 Hz activity mainly in the occipital areas within a few days of the convulsion doubled the chances that the child would subsequently develop a spike focus.

ATTACKS OF EPILEPSY WITH NORMAL ELECTROENCEPHALOGRAMS

It has often been suggested that the EEG is of value in differentiating between epileptic attacks and attacks of other aetiology, particularly those of hysterical origin. Whilst it is true that these other attacks are not accompanied by epileptiform discharges in the EEG, it is unfortunately also true that epileptic attacks may occur without evident changes in the scalp recording. This is quite frequently the case in attacks of jacksonian epilepsy where one presumes that the focus is so discrete and the discharge of such low amplitude that it fails to be conducted to the surface electrodes. With foci less accessible to scalp electrodes this is even more likely to occur. Jasper and Li (1953) have shown, using microelectrodes, that intense epileptiform discharge of cortical units may occur only 1 mm below the surface and yet surface electrocorticography may fail to show any abnormality. In myoclonic epilepsy and epilepsia partialis continua, myoclonic phenomena may occur unaccompanied by EEG changes whilst at other times obvious EEG changes occur without muscle involvement. Occasional attacks of psychomotor epilepsy too may be associated with normal EEGs. The suggestion that some discharges may remain limited to subcortical structures has already been discussed. Another possibility is that in some attacks, although an excessive neuronal discharge occurs, there may be no hypersynchronization, in which case the EEG would tend to be of low voltage.

NARCOLEPSY AND CATAPLEXY

In the past, and notably by Kinnier Wilson, attempts have been made to classify narcolepsy as a variant of epilepsy. The EEG provides no support whatsoever for this view. In a series of 100 cases of narcolepsy (Daly and Yoss, 1957) the waking EEGs were normal. Most of the patients, who were seated during the recordings, became drowsy but the sleep activity showed only momentary responses to the usual alerting measures, such as eye opening, counting and photic stimulation. Nor are epileptiform features found during attacks of cataplexy. Dement, Rechtschaffen and Gulevitch (1966) and subsequently Roth, Brůhová and Lehovský (1969) distinguish sharply between patients with 'independent' narcolepsy and those, who in addition to narcolepsy, suffer attacks of cataplexy, sleep paralysis, hypnagogic hallucinations or nightmares. Both groups believe that in the former condition the attacks are accompanied by synchronous slow wave activity (non-REM sleep) while in the latter a high proportion of patients show REM activity at the onset of the attack. Certainly, as Hishikawa and Kaneko (1965) and Hishikawa *et al.* (1968) have pointed out, the actual attacks of cataplexy and sleep paralysis and the experience of hypnagogic hallucinations occur during REM sleep.

TONIC FITS

Tonic fits, sometimes referred to as midbrain or cerebellar fits, are to be differentiated clearly from epilepsy. They are transient attacks of decerebrate rigidity and the limbs take up the posture characteristic of this condition. Amongst the more common causes are supratentorial tumours with raised intracranial pressure and herniation of one or both temporal lobes; infratentorial tumours, usually with raised intracranial pressure; and head injuries with brainstem damage. The interictal EEGs in these cases will show the changes appropriate to the underlying condition. It is of interest that when Kreindler *et al.* (1958) stimulated the reticular formation in the brainstem of cats and rats the resulting attacks were essentially tonic in nature and were accompanied by a 'desynchronized flat EEG'.

While EEGs have rarely been recorded during the attacks themselves, Strobos and Alexander (1960) have described a boy of 2 years who, following an operation for meningomyelocele, developed raised intracranial pressure with tonic fits. Before an attack the EEG consisted of bilaterally synchronous *delta* activity. During the fit, which was accompanied by loss of consciousness and lasted about one minute, all channels of the EEG showed a remarkably flat trace. After the attack the patient fell into a deep sleep accompanied by generalized slow activity in the EEG.

SYNCOPAL ATTACKS

There have been many suggestions that syncopal attacks bear some relationship to epilepsy. Gowers stated that most people who faint frequently, sooner or later have an attack of grand mal. It is doubtful if this view can any longer be accepted and the work of Gastaut and Fischer-Williams (1957) has done much to disprove it. Syncopal attacks can sometimes be provoked during electroencephalography by eyeball pressure. After some 8–12 seconds of cardiac arrest, rather longer if the patient is recumbent, there is loss of consciousness, pallor and muscle relaxation. Just before the loss of consciousness occurs, runs of bilaterally synchronous slow activity appear and in briefer episodes continue until consciousness is regained. If cardiac arrest is long continued, a period of electrical silence may occur lasting some 6–10 seconds, after which the slow activity reappears, diminishing in amplitude as consciousness returns. Before the period of electrical silence, one or more generalized myoclonic jerks may occur in time with the slow waves, and during the silent period itself there may be a generalized tonic spasm with incontinence. Similar results follow acute cerebral anoxia due to any other cause, including the use of the Valsalva or Weber manoeuvre (Duvoisin, 1962). The picture is clearly similar to that of a tonic fit and the relationship is with transient decerebration rather than with epilepsy. In 100 patients with syncopal attacks investigated by Gastaut and Fischer-Williams, ocular compression caused temporary cardiac arrest in 71 cases. In 20 of these it was of sufficient duration for the clinical and electrical signs of syncope to occur, but epileptiform activity was never seen in the EEG. Tonic seizures due to acute cerebral anoxia can no longer be produced in animals after destruction of the bulbar portion of the reticular formation, and this region appears to mediate this type of attack when deprived of impulses from higher levels of the nervous system.

BREATH-HOLDING SPELLS

As with syncopal attacks, breath-holding attacks in children appear to have no relationship with epilepsy and the great majority of cases (over 90 per cent) have normal EEGs. Very occasionally a convulsion may follow a prolonged attack due to the resulting cerebral anoxia.

REFERENCES

Ajmone Marsan, C. (1961). 'Electrographic Aspects of "Epileptic" Neuronal Aggregates'. *Epilepsia* **2,** 22
— and Lewis, W. R. (1960). 'Pathologic Findings in Patients with "Centrencephalic" Electroencephalographic Patterns'. *Neurology* **10,** 922
— and Abraham, K. (1960). 'A Seizure Atlas'. *Electroenceph. clin. Neurophysiol.* Suppl. 15, 11
Arellano, A. P., Schwab, R. S. and Casby, J. U. (1950). 'Sonic Activation'. *Electroenceph. clin. Neurophysiol.* **2,** 215
Bell, D. S. and Kiloh, L. G. (1971). 'The EEG of Status Epilepticus'. Unpublished observations.
Bennett, F. E. (1953). 'Intracarotid and Intravertebral Metrazol in Petit Mal Epilepsy'. *Neurology* **3,** 668
Bercel, N. A. (1953). 'Experiences with a Combination of Scopolamine and Alpha Chloralose (S.A.C.) in Activating Normal EEG of Epileptics'. *Electroenceph. clin. Neurophysiol.* **5,** 279
Bickford, R. G. and Klass, D. W. (1960). 'Scalp and Depth Electrographic Studies of Electro-decremental Seizures'. *Electroenceph. clin. Neurophysiol.* **12,** 263
— — (1963). 'The EEG in Seizures Induced by Visual Pattern'. *Electroenceph. clin. Neurophysiol.* **15,** 149
— Sem-Jacobsen, C. W., White, P. T. and Daly, D. (1952). 'Some Observations on the Mechanism of Photic and Photo-metrazol Activation'. *Electroenceph. clin. Neurophysiol.* **4,** 275
Bingley, T. (1958). 'Mental Symptoms in Temporal Lobe Epilepsy and Temporal Lobe Gliomas'. *Acta psychiat. neurol. scand.* **33,** Suppl. 120, 1
Bonduelle, M., Sallou, C., Guillard, J. and Gaussel, M. J.-J. (1964). 'L' état de mal psycho-moteur: ses rapports avec les automatismes et les psychoses aigués épileptiques'. *Revue neurol.* **110,** 365
Brandt, H., Brandt, S. and Vollmond, K. (1961). 'EEG Response to Photic Stimulation in 120 Normal Children'. *Epilepsia* **2,** 313
Carterette, E. C. and Symmes, D. (1952). 'Color as an Experimental Variable in Photic Stimulation'. *Electroenceph. clin. Neurophysiol.* **4,** 289
Chatrian, C. A. and Petersen, M. C. (1960). 'The Convulsive Patterns Provoked by Indoklon, Metrazol and Electroshock: Some Depth Electrographic Observations in Human Patients'. *Electroenceph. clin. Neurophysiol,* **12,** 715
Chatrian, G. E., Tassinari, C. A., Somasundaram, M. and Lettich, E. (1968). 'Transcranial Recording of DC Changes during Spike and Wave Discharges in Man. I. Description of a Technique. *Am. J. EEG Technol.* **8,** 101
Clayton, B. E., Moncrieff, A. A., Pampiglione, G. and Shepherd, J. (1966). 'Biochemical and EEG studies in Phenylketonuric Children during Phenylalanine Tolerance Tests'. *Archs Did. Childh.* **51,** 267
Cobb, W. and Hill, D. (1950). 'Electroencephalogram in Subacute Progressive Encephalitis'. *Brain,* **73,** 392
Commission on Terminology (1964). 'A Proposed International Classification of Epileptic Seizures'. *Epilepsia* **5,** 297
— (1969). 'Clinical and Electroencephalographic Classification of Epileptic Seizures'. *Epilepsia* **10,** Suppl. S.2
Conrad, K. (1937). 'Heredity and Epilepsy'. *Z. ges. Neurol. Psychiat.* **159,** 521
Critchley, M. (1937). 'Musicogenic Epilepsy'. *Brain* **60,** 13
Cure, C., Rasmussen, T. and Jasper, H. (1948). 'Activation of Seizures and Electroencephalographic Disturbances in Epileptic and in Control Subjects with "Metrazol" '. *Arch Neurol. Psychiat.* **59,** 691
Daly, D. D. and Yoss, R. E. (1957). 'Electroencephalogram in Narcolepsy'. *Electroenceph. clin. Neurophysiol.* **9,** 109
Danielson, J. and Ellebjerg, J. (1966). 'Comparable EEG Activation by Megimide and Metrazol'. *Epilepsia* **7,** 228
Daube, J. R. and Peters, H. A. (1966). 'Hereditary Essential Myoclonus'. *Archs Neurol.* **15,** 587
Davison, K. (1965). 'EEG Activation after Intravenous Amitriptyline'. *Electroenceph. clin. Neurophysiol.* **19,** 298
Dement, W., Rechtschaffen, A. and Gulevitch, G. (1966). 'The Nature of the Narcoleptic Sleep Attack'. *Neurology* **16,** 18
Dreyer, R. (1965). 'Zur Frage des Status epilepticus mit psychomotorischen Anfällen. Ein Beitrag zum temporalen Status epilepticus und zu atypischen Dämmerzuständen und Verstimmungen'. *Nervenarzt* **36,** 221
Driver, M. V. (1962). 'A study of the Photoconvulsive Threshold'. *Electroenceph. clin. Neurophysiol.* **14,** 359
Drossopoulo, G., Gastaut, H., Verdeaux, G., Verdeaux, J. and Schuller, E. (1956). 'Comparison of EEG "Activation" by Pentamethylenetetrazol (Metrazol) and Bemegride (Megimide)'. *Electroenceph. clin. Neurophysiol.* **8,** 710
Duvoisin, R. C. (1962). 'Convulsive Syncope Induced by the Weber Manœuver'. *Arch Neurol.* **7,** 219
Eccles, J. C. (1965). 'Inhibition in Thalamic and Cortical Neurones and its Role in Phasing Neuronal Discharges'. *Epilepsia* **6,** 89
— (1967). 'Postsynaptic Inhibition in the Central Nervous System'. In *The Neurosciences: A Study Program,* p. 408. Ed. by G. C. Quarton, T. Melnechuk and F. O. Schmitt. New York; Rockefeller University Press
Falconer, M. A., Driver, M. V. and Serafetinides, E. A. (1962). 'Temporal Lobe Epilepsy due to Distant Lesions: Two Cases Relieved by Operation'. *Brain* **85,** 521
— and Kennedy, W. A. (1961). 'Epilepsy due to Small Focal Temporal Lesions with Bilateral Independent Spike-discharging Foci'. *J. Neurol. Neurosurg. Psychiat.* **24,** 205
Flor-Henry, P. (1969). 'Psychosis and Temporal Lobe Epilepsy—A Controlled Investigation'. *Epilepsia* **10,** 363
Fois, A., Rosenberg, C. and Gibbs, F. A. (1955). 'The Electroencephalogram in Phenylpyruvic Oligophrenia.' *Electroenceph. clin. Neurophysiol.* **7,** 596
Frantzen, E., Lennox-Buchtal, M. and Nygaard, A. (1968). 'Longitudinal EEG and Clinical Study of Children with Febrile Convulsions'. *Electroenceph. clin. Neurophysiol.* **24,** 197
Garretson, H., Gloor, P. and Rasmussen, T. (1966). 'Intracarotid Amobarbital and Metrazol Test for the Study of Epileptiform Discharges in Man: A Note on its Technique'. *Electroenceph. clin. Neurophysiol.* **21,** 607
Gastaut, H. (1950). 'Combined Photic and Metrazol Activation of the Brain'. *Electroenceph. clin. Neurophysiol.* **2,** 249
— (1954). *The Epilepsies: Electro-clinical Correlations.* (a) p. 12, (b) p. 32, (c) p. 59. Springfield, Illinois; Thomas
— (1969). 'On Genetic Transmission of Epilepsies'. *Epilepsia* **10,** 3
— and Hunter, J. (1950). 'An Experimental Study of the Mechanism of Photic Activation in Idiopathic Epilepsy'. *Electroenceph. clin. Neurophysiol.* **2,** 263
— and Rémond, A. (1952). 'Etude électroencéphalographique des myoclonies'. *Revue neurol.* **86,** 596
— and Fischer-Williams, M. (1957). 'Electroencephalographic Study of Syncope, its Differentiation from Epilepsy'.

Lancet **2,** 1018

— — (1959). 'The Physiopathology of Epileptic Seizures'. In *Handbook of Physiology*. Ed. by J. Field, H. W. Magoun and V. E. Hall. (a) p. 329, (b) p. 346. Washington; Am. Physiol. Soc.

Gastaut and Vigouroux, M. (1958). 'Electro-clinical Correlations in 500 Cases of Psychomotor Seizures'. In *Temporal Lobe Epilepsy*, p. 118. Ed. by M. Baldwin and P. Bailey. Springfield; Thomas

— and Regis, H. (1961). 'On the Subject of Lennox's "Akinetic" Petit Mal. In Memory of W. G. Lennox'. *Epilepsia* **2,** 298

— Trevisan, C. and Naquet, R. (1958). 'Diagnostic Value of Electroencephalographic Abnormalities Provoked by Intermittent Photic Stimulation'. *Electroenceph. clin. Neurophysiol.* **10,** 194

— Bostem, F., Fernandez-Guardiola, A., Naquet, R. and Gibson, W. (1961). 'Hypoxic Activation of the EEG by Nitrogen Inhalation'. In *Cerebral Anoxia and the Electroencephalogram*. pp. 343, 355. Ed. by H. Gastaut and J. S. Meyer. Springfield; Thomas

— Poirier, F., Payan, H., Salamon, G., Toga, M. and Vigouroux, M. (1960). 'H.H.E. Syndrome. Hemiconvulsions, Hemiplegia, Epilepsy'. *Epilepsia* **1,** 418

Gibbs, F. A. (1958). 'Abnormal Electrical Activity in the Temporal Regions and its Relationship to Abnormalities of Behaviour'. *Res. Publ. Ass. nerv. ment. Dis.* **36,** 278

— and Gibbs, E. L. (1952). *Atlas of Electroencephalography*. Vol. 2 *Epilepsy*. Cambridge, Mass.; Addison-Wesley Press. (a) p. 163, (b) p. 168, (c) p. 31, (d) p. 24

— — (1953). 'Changes in Epileptic Foci with Age'. *Electroenceph. clin. Neurophysiol.* Suppl. 4, 233

— — and Lennox, W. G. (1937). 'Epilepsy: A Paroxysmal Cerebral Dysrhythmia'. *Brain* **60,** 377

Gloor, P. (1968). 'Generalized Cortico-Reticular Epilepsies. Some Considerations on the Pathophysiology of Generalized Bilaterally Synchronous Spike and Wave Discharge'. *Epilepsia* **9,** 249

— Tsai, C. and Haddad, F. (1958). 'An Assessment of the Value of Sleep-electroencephalography for the Diagnosis of Temporal Lobe Epilepsy'. *Electroenceph. clin. Neurophysiol.* **10,** 633

Green, J. B. (1963). 'The Activation of Electroencephalographic Abnormalities by Tolbutamide-induced Hypoglycemia'. *Neurology* **13,** 192

Green, R. L. and Wilson, W. P. (1961). 'Asymmetries of Beta Activity in Epilepsy, Brain Tumour and Cerebrovascular Disease'. *Electroenceph. clin. Neurophysiol.* **13,** 75

Guerrero-Figueroa, R., Barros, A., de Balbian Verster, F. and Heath, R. G. (1963). 'Experimental "Petit Mal" in Kittens'. *Archs Neurol.* **9,** 297

Halliday, A. M. (1967a). 'The Clinical Incidence of Myoclonus'. In *Modern Trends in Neurology*—4, p. 69. Ed. by D. Williams. London; Butterworths

— (1967b). 'The Electrophysiological Study of Myoclonus in Man'. *Brain* **90,** 241

Hill, D. (1958). 'Value of the EEG in Diagnosis of Epilepsy'. *Br. med. J.* **1,** 663

Hishikawa, Y. and Kaneko, Z. (1965). 'Electroencephalographic Study on Narcolepsy'. *Electroenceph. clin. Neurophysiol.* **18,** 249

— and Nan'No, H., Tachibana, M., Foruya, E., Koida, H. and Kaneko, Z. (1968). 'The Nature of Sleep Attack and Other Symptoms of Narcolepsy'. *Electroenceph. clin. Neurophysiol.* **24,** 1

Hunter, J. (1950). 'Further Observations on Subcortically Induced Epileptic Attacks in Unanesthetized Aminals'. *Electroenceph. clin. Neurophysiol.* **2,** 193

— and Jasper, H. H. (1949). 'Effects of Thalamic Stimulation in Unanesthetized Animals'. *Electroenceph. clin. Neurophysiol.* **1,** 305

Ingvar, D. H. (1955). 'Reproduction of the 3 per Second Spike and Wave EEG Pattern by Subcortical Electrical Stimulation in Cats'. *Acta physiol. scand.* **33,** 135

James, J. L. and Whitty, C. W. M. (1961). 'The Electroencephalogram as a Monitor of Status Epilepticus Suppressed Peripherally by Curarization'. *Lancet* **2,** 239

Janeway, R., Ravens, R. J., Pearce, L. A., Odor, D. L. and Suzuki, K. (1967). 'Progressive Myoclonus Epilepsy with Lafora Inclusion Bodies'. *Archs Neurol.* **16,** 565

Jasper, H. (1961). 'General Summary of "Basic Mechanisms of the Epileptic Discharge" '. *Epilepsia* **2,** 91

— and Courtois, G. (1953). 'A Practical Method for Uniform Activation with Intravenous Metrazol'. *Electroenceph. clin. Neurophysiol.* **5,** 443

— and Droogleever-Fortuyn, J. (1947). 'Experimental Studies on the Functional Anatomy of Petit Mal Epilepsy'. *Res. Publ. Ass. nerv. ment. Dis.* **26,** 272

— and Kershman, J. (1949). 'Classification of the EEG in Epilepsy'. *Electroenceph. clin. Neurophysiol.* Suppl. 2, 123

— and Li, C. L. (1953). 'Microelectrode Studies of "Spontaneous" and Evoked Potentials of Cerebral Cortex'. *Fed. Proc.* **12,** 73

— Pertuisset, B. and Flanigin, H. (1951). 'The EEG and Cortical Electrograms in Patients with Temporal Lobe Seizures'. *Archs Neurol. Psychiat.* **65,** 272

Jeavons, P. M. (1969) 'The Use of Photic Stimulation in Clinical Electroencephalography'. *Proc. electrophysiol. Technol. Ass.* **16,** 225

— and Bower, B. D. (1964). *Infantile Spasms*. Clinics in Developmental Medicine No. 15. London; Heinemann

Juul-Jensen, P. and Denny-Brown, D. (1966). 'Epilepsia Partialis Continua'. *Archs Neurol.* **15,** 563

Kaada, B. R. (1953). 'Temporal Lobe Seizures'. *Electroenceph. clin. Neurophysiol.* Suppl. 4, 235

Kaufman, I. C., Marshall, C. and Walker, A. E. (1947). 'Activated Electroencephalography'. *Archs Neurol. Psychiat.* **58,** 533

Kennedy, W. A. (1959). 'Clinical and Electroencephalographic Aspects of Epileptogenic Lesions of the Medial Surface and Superior Border of the Cerebral Hemisphere'. *Brain* **82,** 147

— and Hill, D. (1958). 'The Surgical Prognostic Significance of the Electroencephalographic Prediction of Ammon's Horn Sclerosis in Epileptics'. *J. Neurol. Neurosurg. Psychiat.* **21,** 24

Kershman, J., Vásquez, J. and Golstein, S. (1951). 'The Incidence of Focal and Non-focal EEG Abnormalities in Clinical Epilepsy'. *Electroenceph. clin. Neurophysiol.* **3,** 15

Kiloh, L. G., Davison, K. and Osselton, J. W. (1961). 'An Electroencephalographic Study of the Analeptic Effects of Imipramine'. *Electroenceph. clin. Neurophysiol.* **13,** 216

REFERENCES

King, G. and Weeks, S. D. (1965). 'Pyribenzamine Activation of the Electroencephalogram'. *Electroenceph. clin. Neurophysiol.* **18,** 503

Kopeloff, N., Whittier, J. R., Pacella, B. L. and Kopeloff, L. M. (1950). 'The Epileptogenic Effect of Subcortical Alumina Cream in the Rhesus Monkey'. *Electroenceph. clin. Neurophysiol.* **2,** 163

Kreindler, A., Crighel, E. and Poilici, I. (1959). 'Clinical and Electroencephalographic Investigations in Myoclonic Cerebellar Dyssynergia'. *J. Neurol. Neurosurg. Psychiat.* **22,** 232

— Zuckermann, E., Steriade, M. and Chimion, D. (1958). 'Electroclinical Features of Convulsions Induced by Stimulation of the Brain Stem'. *J. Neurophysiol.* **21,** 430

Kroth, N. (1967). 'Status with Psychomotor Attacks'. *Electroenceph. clin. Neurophysiol.* **23,** 183

Lennox, M. A. (1947). 'Febrile Convulsions in Childhood'. *Proc. Ass. Res. nerv. ment. Dis.* **26,** 342

Lennox, W. G. (1945). 'The Treatment of Epilepsy'. *Med. Clins. N. Am.* **28,** 1114

— (1960). *Epilepsy and Related Disorders*, Vol. 1, p. 372. London; Churchill

— (1953). 'Characteristics and Significance of Seizure Discharges: Introductory Remarks'. *Electroenceph. clin. Neurophysiol.* Suppl. 4, 215

— Gibbs, E. L. and Gibbs, F. A. (1940). 'Inheritance of Cerebral Dysrhythmia and Epilepsy'. *Archs Neurol. Psychiat* **44,** 1155

Leyberg, J. T. and Denmark, J. C. (1959). 'The Treatment of Depressive States with Imipramine Hydrochloride (Tofranil)'. *J. ment. Sci.* **105,** 1123

Low, N. L., Bosma, J. F. and Armstrong, M. D. (1957). 'EEG Findings in Phenylketonuria'. *Electroenceph. clin. Neurophysiol.* **9,** 159

Lyberi, G. and Last, S. L. (1956). 'The Use of Chlorpromazine as an Activating Agent'. *Electroenceph. clin. Neurophysiol.* **8,** 711

Madsen, J. A. and Bray, P. F. (1966). 'The Coincidence of Diffuse Electroencephalographic Spike-wave Paroxysms and Brain Tumors'. *Neurology* **16,** 546

Mahloudji, M. and Pikielny, R. T. (1967). 'Hereditary Essential Myoclonus'. *Brain* **90,** 669

Mancia, M. and Lucioni, R. (1966). 'EEG and Behavioural Changes Induced by Subcortical Introduction of Cobalt Powder in Chronic Cats'. *Epilepsia* **7,** 308

Maspes, P. E., Infuso, L., Migliore, A., Marossero, F. and Pagni, C. A. (1961). 'Emploi de la Myanésine associée au Métrazol comme méthode d'activation en électroencéphalographie'. *Epilepsia* **2,** 318

Merlis, J. K., Grossman, C. and Henriksen, G. F. (1951). 'Comparative Effectiveness of Sleep and Metrazol-activated Electroencephalography'. *Electroenceph. clin. Neurophysiol.* **3,** 71

Metrakos, K. and Metrakos, J. D. (1961). 'Is the Centrencephalic EEG Inherited as a Dominant?' *Electroenceph. clin. Neurophysiol.* **13,** 289

Metrakos, J. D., Metrakos, K., Polizos, P. and Valle, F. (1966). 'Genetics and Ontogenesis of the Centrencephalic EEG'. *Electroenceph. clin. Neurophysiol.* **21,** 404

Meyer, J. S. and Waltz, A. G. (1961). 'Relationship of Cerebral Anoxia to Functional and Electroencephalographic Abnormality'. In *Cerebral Anoxia and the Electroencephalogram*, p. 307. Ed. by H. Gastaut and J. S. Meyer. Springfield; Thomas

Millichap, J. G. (1968). *Febrile Convulsions*, p. 37. New York; Macmillan

Morrell, F. (1960). 'Secondary Epileptogenic Lesions'. *Epilepsia*, **1,** 538

Mosowich, A. (1967). 'The Role of Oral Hypoglycaemiants as Activators in Epilepsy'. In *Neurological Problems*. Ed. by J. Choróbski. Oxford; Pergamon

Niedermeyer, E., (1965). 'Sleep Electroencephalograms in Petit Mal'. *Archs Neurol.* **12,** 625

— (1966). 'Generalized Seizure Discharges and Possible Precipitating Mechanisms'. *Epilepsia* **7,** 23

Ogden, T. E., Aird, R. B. and Garoutte, B. C. (1956). 'The Nature of Bilateral and Synchronous Cerebral Spiking'. *Acta psychiat. neurol. scand.* **31,** 273

Oswald, I. (1959). 'Sudden Bodily Jerks on Falling Asleep'. *Brain* **82,** 92

Pampiglione, G. (1952). 'Induced Fast Activity in the EEG as an Aid in the Location of Cerebral Lesions'. *Electroenceph. clin. Neurophysiol.* **4,** 79

— and Kerridge, J. (1956). 'EEG Abnormalities from the Temporal Lobe Studied with Sphenoidal Electrodes'. *J. Neurol. Neurosurg. Psychiat.* **19,** 117

Penfield, W. and Erickson, T. C. (1941). *Epilepsy and Cerebral Localization.* p. 12. London; Baillière, Tindall & Cox

— and Jasper, H. (1947). 'Highest Level Seizures'. *Res. Pubs Ass. nerv. ment. Dis.* **26,** 252

Perez-Borja, C. and Rivers, M. H. (1963). 'Some Scalp and Depth Electrographic Observations on the Action of Intracarotid Sodium Amytal Injections on Epileptic Discharges in Man'. *Electroenceph. clin. Neurophysiol.* **15,** 488

Petersen, I., Eeg-Olofssen, O. and Sellden, U. (1968). 'Paroxysmal Activity in the EEG of Normal Children'. In *Clinical Electroencephalography of Children*, p. 167. Ed. by P. Kellaway and I. Petersen. Stockholm; Almqvist and Wiksell

Phillips, C. G. (1959). 'Actions of Antidromic Pyramidal Volleys on Single Betz Cells in the Cat'. *Q. Jl. exp. Physiol.* **44,** 1

Poley, J. R. and Dumermuth, G. (1968). 'EEG Findings in Phenylketonuria before and during Treatment with a Low Phenylalanine Diet'. In *Some Recent Advances in Inborn Errors of Metabolism*, p. 61. Ed. by K. S. Holt and V. P. Coffey. Edinburgh; Livingstone

Pollen, D. A. (1968). 'Experimental Spike and Wave Responses and Petit Mal Epilepsy'. *Epilepsia* **9,** 221

— Perot, P. and Reid, K. H. (1963). 'Experimental Bilateral Wave and Spike from Thalamic Stimulation in Relation to Level of Arousal'. *Electroenceph. clin. Neurophysiol.* **15,** 1016

Poskanzer, D. C., Brown, A. E. and Miller, H. (1962). 'Musicogenic Epilepsy Caused only by a Discrete Frequency Band of Church Bells'. *Brain* **85,** 77

Pratt, K. L., Mattson, R. H., Weikers, N. J. and Williams, R. (1968). 'EEG Activation of Epileptics Following Sleep Deprivation: a Prospective Study of 114 Cases'. *Electroenceph. clin. Neurophysiol.* **24,** 11

Prechtl, H. F. R. (1959). 'Provocation of Electroencephalographic Changes in the Temporal Region by Intermittent Acoustic Stimuli'. *Electroenceph. clin. Neurophysiol.* **11,** 511

Prince, D. A. and Wilder, B. J. (1967). 'Control Mechanisms in Cortical Epileptogenic Foci: "Surround Inhibition"'. *Archs Neurol.* **16,** 194

Ralston, B. L. (1958). 'Mechanisms of Transition of Interictal Spiking Foci into Ictal Seizure Discharges'. *Electroenceph. clin. Neurophysiol.* **10,** 217

— and Ajmone Marsan, C. (1956). 'Thalamic Control of Certain Normal and Abnormal Cortical Rhythms'. *Electroenceph. clin. Neurophysiol.* **8,** 559

Redding, F. K. (1969). 'EEG Activation with Amitriptyline'. *Electroenceph. clin. Neurophysiol.* **26,** 634

Rennick, P. M. and Perez-Borja, C. (1969). 'Recurrent Epileptic-Clouded State: A Case Study'. *Electroenceph. clin. Neurophysiol.* **26,** 110

Ricci, G. B. and Silipo, P. (1968). 'Megimide and Intracarotid Amytal in Epileptic Subjects and the Comparison of the Convulsive Threshold of the Two Cerebral Hemispheres'. *Electroenceph. clin. Neurophysiol.* **25,** 83

Rodin, E. A., Rutledge, L. T. and Calhoun, H. D. (1958). 'Megimide and Metrazol'. *Electroenceph. clin. Neurophysiol.* **10,** 719

Ross, J. J., Johnson, L. C. and Walter, R. D. (1966). 'Spike and Wave Discharges during Stages of Sleep'. *Archs Neurol.* **14,** 399

Rossi, G. F., Walter, R. D. and Crandall, P. H. (1968). 'Generalized Spike and Wave Discharges and Nonspecific Thalamic Nuclei'. *Archs Neurol.* **19,** 174

Roth, B., Brůhová, S. and Lehovský, M. (1969). 'R.E.M. Sleep and N.R.E.M. Sleep in Narcolepsy and Hypersomnia'. *Electroenceph. clin. Neurophysiol.* **26,** 176

Rovit, R. L., Gloor, P. and Rasmussen, T. (1961a). 'Sphenoidal Electrodes in the Electrographic Study of Patients with Temporal Lobe Epilepsy'. *J. Neurosurg.* **18,** 151

— — — T. (1961b). 'Intracarotid Amobarbital in Epileptic Patients'. *Archs Neurol.* **5,** 606

Silverman, D. and Morisaki, A. (1958). 'Re-evaluation of Sleep Electroencephalography'. *Electroenceph. clin. Neurophysiol.* **10,** 425

Simons, A. J. R. (1958). 'EEG-activation by Means of Chlorpromazine'. *Electroenceph. clin. Neurophysiol.* **10,** 356

Slater, E., Beard, A. W. and Glithero, E. (1963). 'The Schizophrenia-like Psychoses of Epilepsy'. *Br. J. Psychiat.* **109,** 95

Spiegel, E. A., Wycis, H. T. and Reyes, V. (1951). 'Diencephalic Mechanisms in Petit Mal Epilepsy'. *Electroenceph. clin. Neurophysiol.* **3,** 473

Stewart, L. F. (1957). 'Chlorpromazine: Use to Activate Electroencephalographic Seizure Patterns'. *Electroenceph. clin. Neurophysiol.* **9,** 427

Stoller, A. (1949). 'Slowing of the Alpha Rhythm of the Electroencephalogram and its Association with Mental Deterioration and Epilepsy'. *J. ment. Sci.* **95,** 972

Strobos, R. R. J. and Alexander, E. (1960). 'The Electroencephalogram in Cerebellar or Tonic Fits'. *Electroenceph. clin. Neurophysiol.* **12,** 491

Symonds, C. (1959). 'Excitation and Inhibition in Epilepsy'. *Brain* **82,** 133

Terzian, H. and Cecotto, C. (1961). 'Intracarotid Sodium Amytal in Man for the Study of Cerebral Dominance'. *Electroenceph. clin. Neurophysiol.* **13,** 130

Tizard, B. and Margerison, J. H. (1963). 'The Relationship between Generalised Paroxysmal EEG Discharges and Various Test Situations in Two Epileptic Patients'. *J. Neurol. Neurosurg. Psychiat.* **26,** 308

Tükel, K. and Jasper, H. (1952). 'The Electroencephalogram in Parasagittal Lesions'. *Electroenceph. clin. Neurophysiol.* **4,** 481

Vas, C. J., Exley, K. A. and Parsonage, M. J. (1967a). 'Activation of the EEG by Procyclidine Hydrochloride in Temporal Lobe Epilepsy'. *Epilepsia* **8,** 241

— — — (1967b). 'Methixene Hydrochloride as an EEG Activating Agent.. *Epilepsia* **8,** 252

— — — (1967c). 'An Appraisal of Hyoscine as an EEG Activating Agent'. *Electroenceph. clin. Neurophysiol.* **22,** 373

Verdeaux, G., Verdeaux, J. and Marty, R. (1954). 'L'activation des électroencéphalogrammes par le chloralose'. *Electroenceph. clin. Neurophysiol.* **6,** 19

Wada, J. and Rasmussen, T. (1960). 'Intracarotid Injection of Sodium Amytal for the Lateralization of Cerebral Speech Dominance: Experimental and Clinical Observations'. *J. Neurosurg.* **17,** 266

Walter, W. G. (1950). 'Epilepsy'. In *Electroencephalography.* 1st Edn. p. 228. Ed. by D. Hill and G. Parr. London; Macdonald

Ward, A. A. (1961). 'The Epileptic Neurone'. *Epilepsia* **2,** 70

Weir, B. (1965). 'The Morphology of the Spike-Wave Complex'. *Electroenceph. clin. Neurophysiol.* **19,** 284

Wilder, B. J., King, R. L. and Schmidt, R. P. (1969). 'Cortical and Subcortical Secondary Epileptogenesis'. *Neurology* **19,** 643

Williams, D. (1953). 'A Study of Thalamic and Cortical Rhythms in Petit Mal'. *Brain* **76,** 50

— (1965). 'The Thalamus and Epilepsy'. *Brain* **88,** 539

Zivin, L. and Ajmone Marsan, C. (1968). 'Incidence and Prognostic Significance of "Epileptiform" Activity in the EEG of Non-epileptic Subjects'. *Brain* **91,** 751

CHAPTER 6

SPACE-OCCUPYING LESIONS

CEREBRAL TUMOURS

As long ago as 1931 Berger described the occurrence of slow activity in the EEGs of patients suffering from cerebral tumours (Gloor, 1969). His findings were confirmed and elaborated by Walter (1936) who established the concept of a slow wave focus and formulated a technique for its localization.

The point must be made that cerebral tumours do not give rise to specific EEG abnormalities. It is always necessary to read the record in conjunction with the clinical details of the case and to base any interpretation on a full knowledge of the patient. Serial recordings are frequently more valuable than single examinations. Provocative techniques seldom provide any additional information of significance.

A cerebral tumour itself produces no electrical activity. The only abnormal EEG feature attributable directly to it is a suppression of normal rhythms. All other abnormalities are produced by neurones in the vicinity of the lesion or at a distance, whose functions are disturbed either directly or indirectly by the tumour.

INFRATENTORIAL TUMOURS: RAISED INTRACRANIAL PRESSURE

Routine electroencephalography of patients with infratentorial tumours will reveal only those changes in electrical activity that occur in the cerebral cortex. In most published series, between 75 per cent and 85 per cent of cases show such abnormalities at the time the diagnosis is made. Although the changes produced by posterior fossa tumours are similar whatever their precise location, the incidence of these abnormalities varies considerably according to the site and nature of the neoplasm. With tumors of the cerebellopontine angle, at least 50 per cent of records are normal when the patients are seen for the first time.

The most characteristic abnormality associated with posterior fossa tumours is the appearance of rhythmic, almost sinusoidal slow activity commonly at 2–3 Hz (*Figure 6.1*) or 4–7 Hz (*Figure 6.2*). It may be continuous, or occur in runs: sometimes, particularly when at 4–7 Hz, it may have a paroxysmal appearance. Less frequently—in perhaps 15 per cent of cases—arrhythmic slow activity, irregular in form and of variable amplitude may occur. Associated with either of these abnormalities there may be changes in the background activity, particularly a reduction in the amplitude or slowing of the frequency of the *alpha* rhythm. Bagchi *et al.* (1961) emphasize that *alpha* activity may occur in bursts, both anteriorly and posteriorly, which may shift from side to side. Some general increase in the amount of fast activity may also occur.

The distribution of the rhythmic slow activity varies considerably in different cases. In the series described by Daly *et al.* (1953), 4–7 Hz activity was diffuse in 20 per cent, situated posteriorly in 40 per cent, anteriorly in 30 per cent and was restricted to the temporal areas in 10 per cent. In records showing 2–3 Hz activity this was diffuse in 60 per cent, distributed posteriorly in 20 per cent, anteriorly in 10 per cent and limited to the temporal regions in 5 per cent. Some reduction of the slow activity on eye opening is frequently seen and it may be augmented by hyperventilation.

The arrythmic slow activity shows similar variations in its distribution. It was diffuse in 25 per cent of Daly's cases, confined to the temporal areas in 20 per cent and to the posterior regions of the hemispheres in 50 per cent. It is little affected by eye opening or hyperventilation.

In the majority of cases the slow activity is symmetrical and synchronous but in an appreciable number (17 per cent in Daly's series) it is of greater amplitude on one or other side. It has been suggested (Bagchi *et al.*, 1952; 1961) that the incidence, amplitude and duration of the runs of slow

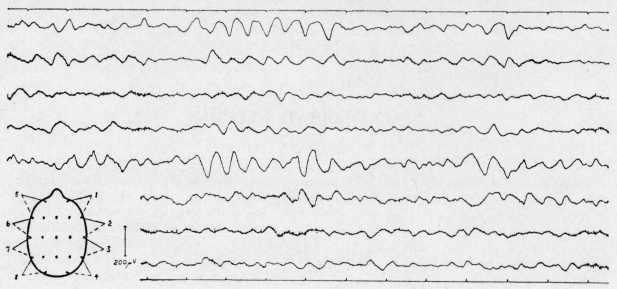

Figure 6.1—Medulloblastoma. Boy aged 9 years. Raised intracranial pressure and ataxia for 2 months. EEG: Generalized rhythmical delta *activity at 2 Hz with marked frontal predominance. Complete absence of normal rhythms*

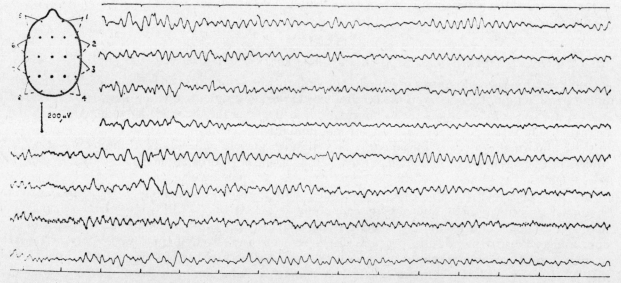

Figure 6.2—Astrocytoma, left cerebellar hemisphere. Woman aged 18 years. Vomiting and double vision for 4 months; ataxia for 1 month. EEG: Rhythmical frontally predominant 5–6 Hz theta *activity and less persistent irregular* delta *activity, the latter a little more marked on the left side*

activity are greater over the contralateral cerebral hemisphere and that this observation has localizing value. Other observers claim that the slow activity is more evident over the ipsilateral hemisphere. Neither of these views can be maintained, even in the case of cerebellopontine angle tumours. Homolateral and contralateral slow activity occur with much the same incidence and in many cases the site of maximal amplitude shifts from side to side in the same or in subsequent recordings. Nor does lateralization of the slow activity rule out the presence of a midline tumour.

When the slow activity is not only predominantly unilateral but is also largely confined to one area of the hemisphere, there is clearly room for a mistaken diagnosis of a supratentorial tumour. In the series of patients described by Bagchi *et al.* (1961) such an incorrect localization was made in 10 per cent.

Although the majority of patients with posterior fossa tumours show some of these various abnormalities, the converse is not necessarily true. Immature EEGs in particular may show bilaterally distributed slow activity of a similar kind, and in normal children occipital slow activity is a not infrequent finding.

The problem is why these changes should occur. Raised intracranial pressure, often with some clouding of consciousness, is an early feature of cerebellar and midbrain tumours, but is a relatively late occurrence with cerebellopontine angle tumours and with tumours of the pons. The incidence of EEG abnormalities in these latter groups is relatively low. Moreover, the EEG abnormalities so often associated with posterior fossa tumours frequently occur with third ventricle tumours and these, too, show an early onset of raised intracranial pressure. More significantly, the same changes may occur in cases of obstructive hydrocephalus due to arachnoiditis in which there is no destruction or infiltration of cerebral tissues.

Of Daly's cases with raised intracranial pressure, 82 per cent had abnormal EEGs, whereas those cases in which there was no papilloedema—though some may still have had raised intracranial pressure—the EEG was abnormal in only 38 per cent. Procedures such as Torkildsen's operation, which relieve raised intracranial pressure without affecting the underlying lesion, frequently lead to a dramatic improvement both of clouding of consciousness and of the EEG abnormalities. When raised intracranial pressure is present there is no precise relationship between the pressure measured during lumbar puncture and the degree of EEG abnormality, but there is a rough relationship between the latter and the level of consciousness.

Raised intracranial pressure is therefore highly correlated with these EEG abnormalities but as it happens the relationship is not a direct one. The presence of any space-occupying lesion within the confines of a virtually closed space such as the cranium inevitably results in displacement and distortion of intracranial structures. This in turn causes obstruction to the flow of cerebrospinal fluid and consequent raised intracranial pressure. At the same time it commonly leads to stretching and spasm of the perforating arteries supplying the brainstem and diencephalon so that ischaemia of these structures occurs. Of the constituents of the 'diencephalic ischaemic syndrome' so well described by Dott (1960) it is impairment of function of the reticular formation and the resulting disturbances of function of the diffuse projection systems that gives rise to the EEG abnormalities. In some cases similar abnormalities may result from direct invasion of these structures. It is possible too that distant tumours may sometimes distort this region of the brain by such mechanical effects as upward herniation of the brainstem. It is highly improbable, as has been suggested, that pressure on one or both occipital lobes due to upward bulging of the tentorium cerebelli can be responsible for the slow activity occurring in these areas.

Although the value of the EEG in the investigation of posterior fossa tumours is limited, certain points emerge. Arrhythmic slow activity, particularly if asymmetrical or confined to the frontal areas, is unlikely to be associated with an infratentorial lesion and is more suggestive of a supratentorial tumour. Symmetrical bilaterally synchronous rhythmical slow activity, whether generalized or not, is more likely to result from an infratentorial than a supratentorial neoplasm. This is particularly true when the slow activity is localized to the occipital areas but a temporal localization has little significance. In the presence of a posterior fossa tumour a normal EEG is likely to be associated with a tumour of the cerebellopontine angle or of the pons.

It will be clear that the EEG changes associated with posterior fossa tumours are indirect effects due to involvement of the upper brain stem and diencephalon and that any lesion of these structures whatever its nature will give rise to similar abnormalities. Conversely, until the function of these structures is disturbed directly or indirectly the EEG is likely to remain normal.

SUPRATENTORIAL TUMOURS

Tumours Involving the Third or Lateral Ventricles

Tumours involving the third ventricle, including those extending upwards from the suprasellar region, produce EEG changes similar to those associated with tumours in the posterior fossa. Raised intracranial pressure is an early feature but even when absent, similar EEG changes may occur due to invasion, ischaemia or distortion of basal structures. In spite of their central position, it is not uncommon to find that the slow activity to which they give rise is asymmetrical; the laterality of the asymmetry may vary in successive recordings. The slow activity is commonly at 4–7 Hz and Arfel and Fischgold (1961) have noted that in some cases this *theta* activity can be recorded only from a midline row of electrodes or is markedly predominant in this plane. Disorganization or disappearance of the *alpha* rhythm is common, particularly when tumours involve the floor of the third ventricle.

Cobb and Gassel (1961) described ten patients with meningiomas in either of the lateral ventricles, the majority arising from the region of the trigone. Great variety and inconstancy were noted in the clinical symptoms, but the EEG abnormalities were largely confined to the appropriate temporal area; in some cases these provided the first clue that the lesion was supratentorial.

Pituitary tumours do not give rise to EEG abnormalities unless they extend beyond the pituitary fossa or give rise to hypopituitarism (*see* page 161).

Tumours Involving the Thalamus

Tumours involving the thalamus, particularly the anterior mesial portion, are often associated with slowing, disorganization, diminution in amplitude or absence of the *alpha* rhythm on the same side. The response of any remaining *alpha* activity and of the contralateral *alpha* rhythm to eye opening, is not affected (Jasper and Van Buren, 1953).

The other changes depend very much on the manner in which the tumour extends. Involvement of the third ventricle, which is frequent, will lead to the changes described in the preceding section. Extension of the tumour laterally to involve the white matter of the hemisphere is likely to be associated with prominent, irregular *delta* activity which may be present over the entire ipsilateral hemisphere.

Tumours of the Cerebral Hemispheres

It is pertinent to consider the way in which a space-occupying lesion comes to be associated with electrical activity that takes the form of slow waves, sharp wave discharges or both together. As was demonstrated by Walter (1936), the tumour itself does not give rise to the abnormal electrical activity. Only neurones can do this and those in the neighbourhood of a tumour become abnormal in such a way that hypersynchronization of the electrical discharges of thousands or millions of nerve cells produces the form of a slow wave or a spike in the EEG. It is likely that the tumour gives rise to metabolic abnormalities of adjacent neurones, perhaps by direct pressure, by oedema or by interference with their blood supply. Oedema is probably the most important mechanism and this would explain why rapidly growing tumours are more likely to produce EEG abnormalities than those of slower growth. This view is strengthened by the observation of Silverman *et al.* (1961) that a focus of slow activity may become less obvious and even disappear after an intravenous infusion of urea.

Tumours that are producing clinical evidence of their presence are accompanied by abnormal EEGs in 75–85 per cent of cases. The fact that 15–25 per cent of patients with cerebral tumours have normal EEGs emphasizes the important point that a normal record does not exclude the presence of such a lesion. In some of these cases the character of the EEG is probably in the process of change without having reached the point at which it is regarded as abnormal. In various series of cases that have been published, correct localization has been achieved by means of electroencephalography in 50–90 per cent of cases. Detailed figures of successful localization of tumours in various regions of the cerebral hemispheres, together with comparative figures for correct clinical and arteriographic localization, are given from Van der Drift's (1957) series in Table 6.1.

TABLE 6.1
COMPARATIVE FIGURES FOR CORRECT LOCALIZATION OF SUPRATENTORIAL TUMOURS
(after Van der Drift, 1957)

Site of tumour	Total No. of cases	Correctly localized clinically (per cent)	Correctly localized by EEG (per cent)	Correctly localized by arteriography (per cent)
Frontal	79	63	89	83
Temporal	103	78	91	90
Rolando-parietal	40	87	65	78
Occipital	7	86	71	—

Note: percentages are quoted because, although cases assessed clinically all had EEG studies, only 196 out of the total of 229 cases had arteriograms

Focal delta activity—The classical EEG abnormality associated with a cerebral tumour is a focus of *delta* activity. The discharge may vary in frequency between 0·5 and 4 Hz and is commonly at 2–3 Hz. It is usually irregular in form and amplitude (*Figure 6.3*), often being intermixed with *theta* activity and

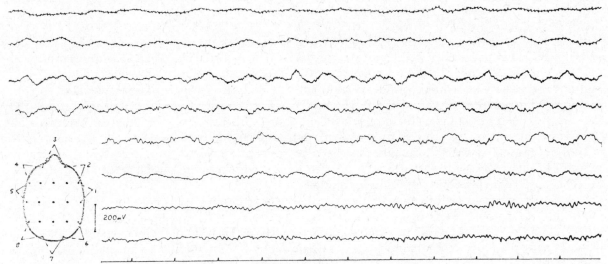

Figure 6.3—Glioblastoma, left frontal region. Man aged 56 years. Three-month history of headache; recent expressive dysphasia and papilloedema. EEG: Focal low frequency delta *activity in left fronto-temporal region. Preservation of* alpha *rhythm posteriorly*

residual background rhythms. Less often it may be more sinusoidal in form, particularly in the frontal regions, where it may be bilateral. In such cases differentiation from a tumour in the posterior fossa may be impossible.

The focal slow activity may be continuous, fluctuant or episodic. Sometimes it may occupy only brief stretches of the record and its amplitude may be so low that it can easily be overlooked or dismissed as artefact. Its voltage in adults is usually less than 150 μV but in some cases, particularly in children, it may reach 500 μV. The voltage is usually greatest in the immediate vicinity of the lesion, but this does not necessarily mean, when using a bipolar montage, that the greatest amplitude of deflection will occur in that channel recording from the pair of electrodes nearest to it (*see* page 42). The slow activity may occasionally be accentuated on eye closure and rather more often by hyperventilation.

Silverman and Groff (1957) claimed that during sleep the focal slow activity may undergo various alterations depending on the distance of the tumour from the surface of the brain. With superficial

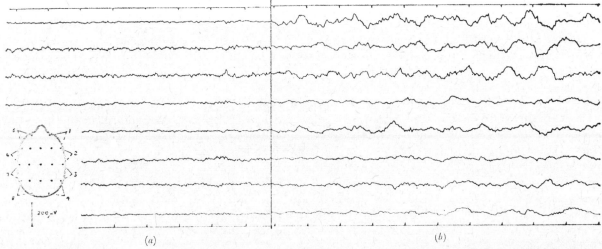

(*a*)   (*b*)

Figure 6.4—Astrocytoma, right frontal region. Man aged 18 years. No neurological signs; occasional attacks of grand mal. (a) Awake. EEG: Low voltage theta *activity in right midtemporal region. (b) Asleep. EEG: Focal arrhythmic* delta *activity in right midtemporal region extending anteriorly*

tumours the slow wave focus persists during sleep and occasionally may be accentuated (*Figure 6.4*); somewhat less superficial tumours show a persistent slow wave focus without suppression of sleep potentials, while with tumours at depths greater than 3 cm from the surface the focus may disappear so that the sleep EEG may show no obvious abnormality.

Gibbs and Gibbs (1964), however, were unable to establish any constant relationship between the depth of the tumour and persistence or disappearance of the *delta* activity during sleep. The whole question has been reviewed by Daly (1968). When a discharge takes the form of polymorphic *delta* activity this may disappear in sleep but is just as likely to do so with superficial as with deep tumours. On the other hand when the abnormality consists of unilateral or bilateral rhythmic slow activity— and this was usually associated with deeper tumours, many in the posterior fossa— the abnormalities disappeared in nearly every case. Daly also found that 13 of 24 patients with polymorphic *delta* activity showed asymmetry of spindle discharges in sleep; those with tumours involving the thalamus also showed spindle asymmetry. In general those with rhythmic slow activity showed normal sleep spindles.

In some cases the focal abnormality may become apparent or be accentuated after air encephalo-graphy (Riehl and Ansel, 1969) although this procedure is not generally to be recommended in such cases because of the possibility of brain herniation and death.

If a definite phase-reversal cannot be established with a bipolar technique, the area of maximal amplitude of the slow activity may be taken as an indication of the location of the tumour, but this is not as reliable a guide as phase-reversals established in two orthogonal planes. When using a unipolar technique the point of maximal amplitude of the slow activity may usually be taken as indicating the site of the lesion.

Nevertheless, a focus, even when accurately established, may prove misleading as an indication of the tumour site. Rarely, indeed, the focus may be found over the opposite hemisphere. When there is raised intracranial pressure this may be due to contralateral uncal herniation but when the pressure is normal such a finding may be difficult to explain. One possibility is that the cerebral haemodynamics are disturbed so that a relative circulatory insufficiency arises in the opposite hemisphere. This appears to have been the explanation in four patients with intracranial arteriovenous aneurysms described by Loeb and Favale (1962). Each showed contralateral EEG abnormalities and there was also clinical evidence of involvement of the contralateral hemisphere. Against such cases one must offset those with false localizing signs that are correctly localized or at least lateralized by the EEG. Of 26 cases of meningiomas with false localizing signs, Gassel and Diamontopoulos (1961) were able to localize or lateralize 23 correctly.

It appears to be a general rule that if there is displacement of the *delta* focus away from the region of the tumour, it is found in front of and perhaps lateral to the actual tumour site. This is particularly the case with tumours in the parietal and temporal regions. Posterior temporal tumours are frequently associated with anterior temporal foci, while anterior temporal tumours may be accompanied by foci in the lateral frontal region. In some medial frontal tumours the foci are evident in the prefrontal areas. In such cases a study of those areas in which there is suppression of *alpha* or fast activity may suggest the correct localization of the lesion.

Other EEG abnormalities—Even when the tumour produces a discrete *delta* focus, other EEG abnormalities are present as a rule. Some random *theta* activity may be evident over the affected hemisphere and sometimes over the opposite hemisphere as well. Occasionally the slow wave focus itself may consist of activity in the *theta* range (*Figure 6.5*). Loss of normal rhythms is frequent in the vicinity of the slow wave focus. Reduction or loss of the *alpha* rhythm due to thalamic tumours has been referred to already and may occur with tumours elsewhere in the hemisphere, particularly in the posterior parietal, posterior temporal and occipital regions. Sometimes the *alpha* frequency may be lower over the ipsilateral hemisphere and occasionally there may be a loss or diminution of the response at *alpha* frequencies on photic stimulation. A rare abnormality is a failure of the *alpha* rhythm to block over the affected hemisphere; the asymmetry is apparent only when the eyes are open, the higher amplitude being on the same side as the tumour. In such cases Bancaud (1959; 1961) has noted that there is always present some disturbance of symbolic functions—a degree of dysphasia, dyspraxia or agnosia. Conversely when such functional disturbances were present, unilateral failure of the *alpha* rhythm to block was evident in 78 per cent of his cases.

Bagchi (1955) has pointed out that overlying some tumours the amplitude of the *alpha* activity may

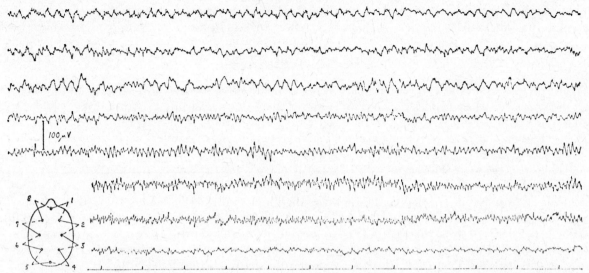

Figure 6.5—Meningioma, right parietal region. Man aged 42 years. Left-sided jacksonian epilepsy—interseizure pattern. EEG: Well-developed 10–11 Hz alpha rhythm more evident on left side. Widespread 4–5 Hz theta activity with occasional delta waves in right fronto-parietal region

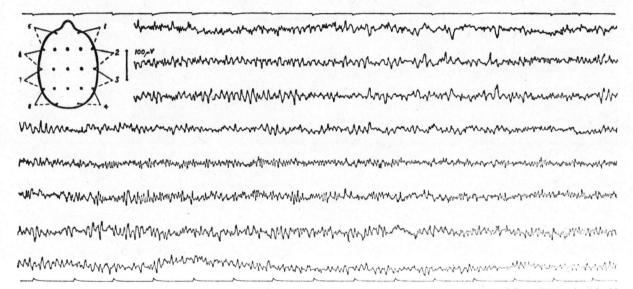

Figure 6.6—Cystic astrocytoma, right fronto-temporal region. Man aged 32 years. EEG: Diminution of thiopentone-induced fast activity on the right side anteriorly. Well-marked 7–8 Hz rhythm in right midtemporal region and occasional possible sharp waves in right anterior temporal region

be persistently increased; he regards a localized increase of 40 per cent or more in comparison with the contralateral homologous area as suggestive of a focal lesion. This may prove to be the first sign of a cerebral tumour. If *delta* activity is present locally or nearby, the greater the significance of the increased *alpha* activity.

A localized slowing, diminution or absence of fast activity, either spontaneous or pentothal induced, is a further valuable indication of an underlying disturbance of cerebral function (*Figure 6.6*). However, in many cases this feature cannot be demonstrated. Occasionally the fast activity in the vicinity of a tumour or over the ipsilateral hemisphere is found to be of greater amplitude than elsewhere (Green and Wilson, 1961). The use of barbiturates may be of value for these drugs usually have little effect on abnormal fast activity whereas normal fast rhythms are considerably augmented.

Attenuation—In a few cases, all frequencies are diminished or absent over the tumour and a channel recording from a pair of electrodes in its vicinity may show relative electrical silence. This is quite different from the situation (*see Figure 3.5*) in which a channel records from a pair of electrodes symmetrically placed on either side of a focus—and therefore equally affected by it—so that the

115

potential difference between them approaches zero. The resolution of this ambiguity is discussed on page 43. In both these cases slow activity is usually present in adjacent channels. The finding of diminished activity in a single channel of the EEG is most often due to recorder or electrode artefacts, and these possibilities must be excluded before the observation is regarded as having clinical significance.

Arfel and Fischgold (1961) have emphasized the fact that in many cases with superficial tumours an area showing 'flat polymorphic *delta* activity' without any faster background rhythms may be identified which appears to be an early stage in the development of an area of 'electrical silence'. From neighbouring regions the usual higher amplitude polymorphic slow activity with intermixed faster frequencies is found.

Spike or sharp wave foci—The occurrence of spike or sharp wave foci has been discussed in the chapter on epilepsy. Amongst the many pathological states associated with such foci, tumours are frequently represented. Astrocytomas, oligodendrogliomas, angiomas and meningiomas are particularly likely to give rise to such abnormalities. In 100 patients with cerebral tumours reported by Kirstein (1953), localized sharp waves were present in 23. Of cases subsequently shown to have astrocytomas, sharp waves were present in 40 per cent, in patients with meningiomas they were present in 22 per cent and with glioblastomas in 17 per cent. Sharp wave discharges are particularly likely to occur with tumours of the temporal lobe (40 per cent), are less frequent with tumours of the frontal lobe (12·5 per cent) and appear rarely with tumours of the parietal lobe. Figures giving the incidence of epileptiform discharges in Van der Drift's series according to the pathological nature of the tumour are given in Table 6.2. When the sharp wave focus is accompanied by focal *theta* or *delta* activity, the possibility of the underlying lesion being a tumour is strengthened. Not all cases showing sharp waves in the EEG experience attacks of epilepsy. Of the 23 patients with sharp waves referred to by Kirstein, only 13 suffered such attacks.

TABLE 6.2

INCIDENCE OF EPILEPTIFORM DISCHARGES IN THE EEG AND OF ATTACKS OF EPILEPSY
IN CASES OF CEREBRAL TUMOUR ACCORDING TO THE PATHOLOGICAL FINDINGS
(after Van der Drift, 1957)

Tumour	No. of cases	No. with epileptiform discharges in EEG		No. with epilepsy	
			Per cent		Per cent
Meningiomas	33	15	45	17	52
Astrocytomas	57	36	63	21	37
Oligodendrogliomas	12	12	100	8	67
Glioblastomas	90	27	30	24	27
Metastases	27	4	15	14	52
Angiomas	10	10	100	6	60
Total	229	104	45	90	39

K-complexes—An occasional finding in patients with cerebral tumours is an asymmetry of K-complexes or of sleep spindles. Rarely, this may be the only indication of the presence of the lesion.

Relation to intracranial pressure—Sooner or later many tumours of the cerebral hemispheres give rise to the features of the diencephalic ischaemic syndrome (Dott, 1960) and to raised intracranial pressure and these in turn will be associated with the diffuse abnormalities already described as associated with posterior fossa tumours. In addition to the slow activity that occurs, there may be some general slowing of the frequency of the *alpha* rhythm which may fall below 8 Hz. For a time the *delta* focus may remain discrete and obvious against a background of generalized abnormality but sooner or later it becomes obscured. In such cases an intravenous injection of 50 ml or more of 50 per cent sucrose or of 1 g of urea per kg body weight made up as a 30 per cent solution with 5 per cent dextrose, may disclose the focal abnormality.

Flodmark (1965) has described an interesting technique that may prove to have some value in differentiating between tumours and atrophic lesions. The test depends on the fact that progressive lesions such as cerebral tumours are associated with an alteration in the blood-brain barrier, whereas atrophic lesions are not. Normally the passage of lipid-insoluble drugs such as neostigmine is prevented by lipid structures in the blood-brain barrier, whereas lipid-soluble drugs such as physostigmine can pass readily. Apart from the differences in their lipid solubility the two drugs have similar neuropharmacological effects. Physostigmine tends to aggravate focal abnormalities whether associated with tumours or atrophic lesions whilst neostigmine aggravates only those associated with tumours. Both drugs are given in doses of 0·75 to 1 mg I.V. over a period of 5–8 minutes.

Sequential studies of the EEGs of cases of cerebral tumour do not invariably show the steady and relentless progress that might be expected. Sometimes the abnormal activity may disappear—temporarily at any rate. Such improvements may be related to changes in cerebral circulation, to the resolution of areas of infarction within or adjacent to the tumour, or to a reduction of the surrounding oedema (Daly and Thomas, 1958).

Van der Drift and Magnus (1962) have pointed out that in elderly patients the EEG abnormalities accompanying cerebral tumours tend to differ in certain respects from those seen in younger age groups. Variations in the *alpha* amplitude are more common; *mu* rhythm contralateral to the tumour is seen more frequently; paroxysmal sharp and slow wave activity is relatively more common; bilateral frontal rhythmic *delta* activity is more frequent but arrhythmic *delta* is seen less often. These differences may be attributable to the greater incidence of ischaemic changes in elderly patients both locally and at a distance from the cerebral tumour.

After successful operations in which total removal of the tumour has been achieved it is usual to find that the EEG is of higher amplitude on the side of the skull defect. The increase may be of the order of 50 to 150 per cent. Prior (1968) has shown that when meningiomas have been removed, although there is usually an improvement in the localized slow wave activity this often fails to disappear. Stability is reached in 3–6 months and if subsequently the slow activity becomes more prominent a recurrence of the tumour or a new lesion should be suspected.

RELATION OF EEG FINDINGS TO LOCALIZATION OF THE TUMOUR

Frontal lobe tumours—A focus of arrhythmic *delta* activity is the most common indication of a frontal lobe tumour (*Figure 6.3*). There is a tendency, even though the tumour is strictly confined to one side, for the slow activity to appear bilaterally and it is sometimes difficult to decide the laterality of the tumour from the EEG alone.

Rhythmic or sinusoidal slow activity similar to that seen with some posterior fossa tumours may also occur (*Figure 6.7*). It may be ipsilateral, bilateral or even contralateral in distribution. It is particularly

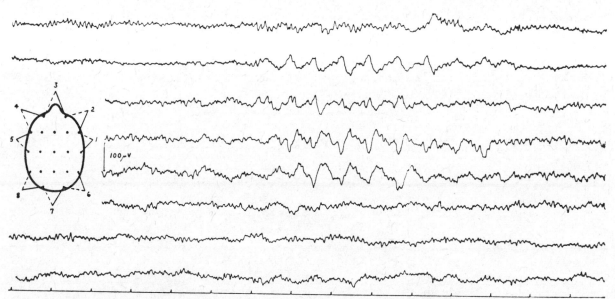

Figure 6.7—Glioblastoma, left frontal region. Man aged 24 years with headaches for 3 months. EEG: Bilateral rhythmical delta discharge in frontal regions, more evident on left side. More 10 Hz rhythm in right temporal region than in left

frequent with tumours in the medial and inferior regions of the frontal lobe. The interpretation of such rhythmic slow activity calls for considerable caution.

Frontal lobe tumours with normal intracranial pressure are not usually associated with changes in the *alpha* rhythm but local suppression of faster rhythms may occur.

Temporal lobe tumours—In view of the displacement of the *delta* focus that occurs with so many temporal lobe tumours, it is often worth paying attention to abnormalities of the *alpha* rhythm. With tumours of the anterior temporal lobe, the *alpha* is seldom affected but tumours of the posterior part of the lobe cause depression, disorganization or loss of the *alpha* rhythm in many cases. In Van der Drift's material such diminution was present in 35 out of 56 cases. In 42 cases in which a homonymous hemianopia was present, the *alpha* rhythm was absent on the side of the tumour in 37 cases and its amplitude diminished in the other 5.

Asymmetry of fast activity demonstrable sometimes only in a sphenoidal recording may be a valuable indication of a temporal lobe tumour.

Rolando-parietal tumours—Foci of *delta* activity occur less frequently with rolando-parietal tumours than with tumours elsewhere in the cerebral hemispheres. Although they sometimes appear with tumours in other areas, foci of activity at 5–9 Hz are particularly likely to occur, especially with tumours near the midline (*Figure 6.5*) (Cobb and Muller, 1954). The most common frequency is 7 Hz and the discharge may be either episodic or continuous. It is unaffected by eye opening and when its frequency extends into the *alpha* range, this failure to block provides a useful distinction from the normal *alpha* rhythm. Cobb and Muller described 37 patients with parietal lobe lesions presenting with this type of EEG abnormality. Of these, 26 had tumours of varied pathology and in all cases the lesion involved the roof and body of the lateral ventricle. Local *delta* activity was also present in some cases and when this was prominent the *theta* activity tended to be obscured. An occasional finding is an increase in the amplitude of the ipsilateral *mu* rhythm.

Occipital lobe tumours—Tumours of the occipital lobe are uncommon. They are usually accompanied by *delta* foci and a total ipsilateral absence of *alpha* rhythm occurs sooner or later in most, if not all, cases. Significant asymmetries of fast activity are seldom found in this area.

Relation of EEG Findings to Pathological Nature of the Tumour

It is seldom wise or justifiable to make any dogmatic deduction from the EEG in an individual case as to the pathological nature of the tumour, though Van der Drift and Magnus (1961) view the situation more optimistically. Certain trends are apparent with different types of tumour and in occasional cases a shrewd guess may be possible.

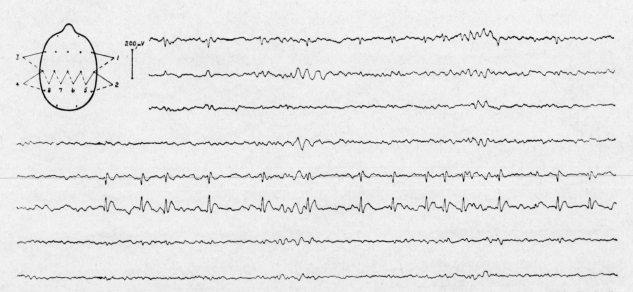

Figure 6.8—Meningioma, right parieto-temporal region. Woman aged 27 years with nocturnal attacks of grand mal—interseizure pattern. EEG: Focal spike and slow wave complexes in right central region

118

Meningiomas

Meningiomas often fail to give rise to EEG abnormalities even though clinical signs are well developed. When *delta* foci do occur—they are most likely to be seen with meningiomas involving the frontal lobes—they are relatively discrete and well localized, and the electrical activity recorded over the opposite hemisphere is usually within normal limits. The more vascular the meningioma the more prominent the *delta* activity (Millar, 1955). Epileptiform discharges are frequent (*see* Table 6.2) (*Figure 6.8*).

Astrocytomas

As with meningiomas, the abnormal slow activity is usually restricted to the ipsilateral hemisphere. The degree of abnormality is greater in the more rapidly growing varieties of astrocytomas including those cases in which cysts develop, containing fluid under pressure. Epileptiform discharges are very frequent (*see* Table 6.2).

Oligodendrogliomas

Epileptiform discharges are particularly common in oligodendrogliomas and localized *theta* activity may also be very prominent.

Glioblastomas

Probably because of their rapid rate of growth, the destruction of brain tissue and the presence of oedema, glioblastomas show EEG abnormalities of a degree more marked than other types of tumour, except for some cases with metastases. The abnormalities may approach in severity those associated with cerebral abscesses. The *delta* activity tends to be lower in frequency, higher in amplitude and more widespread than with other tumours but epileptiform discharges are less common. Abnormal activity in the *theta* or *delta* range, random in its distribution, is often present over the contralateral hemisphere. A normal EEG in the presence of localizing clinical signs makes a glioblastoma unlikely.

Metastases

If a single cerebral metastasis occurs it generally produces effects comparable to those of an astrocytoma, although they may be severe enough to suggest a glioblastoma. Although foci of arrhythmic *delta* activity may be seen, rhythmic *delta* and *theta* activity are frequent. Epileptiform discharges are uncommon in spite of the fact that fits often occur. In most cases the metastases are multiple and the abnormalities widespread.

Angiomas

Epileptiform discharges are particularly common in the case of angiomas (*see* Table 6.2) and may be associated with *delta* foci, particularly if there has been a recent haemorrhage from the tumour. Persistent pulse artefact that cannot be eradicated by moving the electrodes has been described (Chavany, David and Lérique, 1949), but such a finding clearly demands cautious interpretation.

TUBEROUS SCLEROSIS

In tuberous sclerosis with cerebral involvement, numerous glial nodules may be found, mainly in the cerebral cortex and adjacent to the ventricles. Argument continues as to the neoplastic or teratomatous nature of these nodules and of the other varieties of tumour that are found in many organs, but there is no difficulty in accepting them as examples of space-occupying lesions. Mental subnormality is very frequent though not invariable and fits—of every variety—occur almost without exception.

In cases of tuberous sclerosis without evidence of cerebral involvement showing perhaps nothing more than adenoma sebaceum, the EEG is likely to be normal.

Very occasionally, as with cerebral metastases, one cerebral nodule may prove dominant, and clinically and electroencephalographically the case presents as a typical cerebral tumour, perhaps with raised intracranial pressure.

Of the other more usual cases, the majority show abnormal EEGs. No specific abnormality occurs

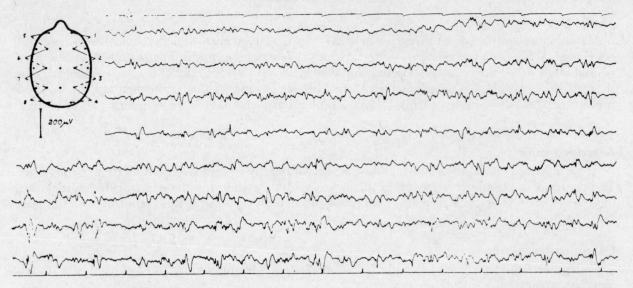

Figure 6.9—Tuberous sclerosis. Woman aged 18 years. Adenoma sebaceum; severely retarded; occasional major seizures. EEG: Scattered sharp waves and small spikes superimposed upon a background of widespread irregular slow activity more marked on the left side

and different patients may show single or multiple spikes, spikes and slow waves or slow wave foci (Dickerson and Hellman, 1952; Harvald and Hauge, 1955) (*Figure 6.9*).

Infantile spasms with hypsarrhythmic EEG patterns are frequent in the first year or so of life (Krauthammer, 1966; Pampiglione, 1968).

CEREBRAL ABSCESS

Electroencephalographically, cerebral abscesses behave in a similar fashion to cerebral tumours. Acute abscesses produce abnormalities that one would expect only with the most rapidly growing glioblastomas. Chronic abscesses mimic the effects of slower growing tumours such as astrocytomas. Abnormalities, often of gross degree, are present in 90–95 per cent of cases, but they are not always easy to localize accurately. This is because focal activity may be obscured by diffuse abnormalities, because

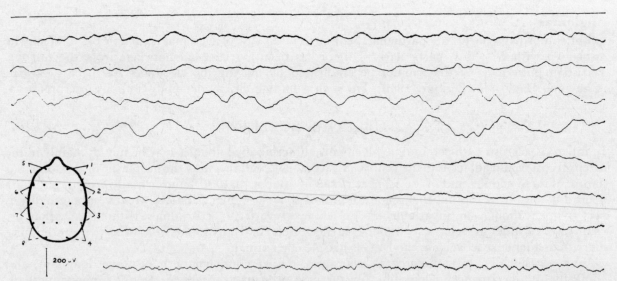

Figure 6.10—Cerebral abscess, right posterior temporal region. Boy aged 5 years. Increasing headache, drowsiness and delirium following penetrating brain injury 10 days previously. EEG: Arrhythmic very low frequency delta activity focal in right posterior temporal region. Generalized absence of normal rhythms. Recording made with a time constant of 1 second in all channels

cerebellar abscesses are not infrequent and because temporal lobe abscesses often show an anterior displacement of the accompanying slow wave focus.

Infratentorial abscesses usually involve one or other of the cerebellar lobes and the changes they produce are identical with those already described as resulting from the presence of a rapidly expanding infratentorial tumour.

A typical EEG record of a supratentorial cerebral abscess shows generalized random *theta* and *delta* activity with a focus of the lowest frequency components overlying the abscess (*Figure 6.10*). This focal *delta* activity is often of very low frequency, sometimes as low as 0·3 Hz, and may be of high voltage, perhaps reaching 500 μV. Ipsilateral slowing or loss of *alpha* rhythm is frequent when the abscess involves the posterior half of the hemisphere. The generalized slow activity is often associated with clouding of consciousness and may be due to widespread oedema, to meningitis or to an ischaemic-diencephalic syndrome. Reasonable localization of supratentorial abscesses can be achieved by means of the EEG in about 70 per cent of cases. Multiple abscesses may show multiple foci.

Spike or sharp wave discharges are rarely seen in pre-operative records although a third of the cases give a history of fits. Post-operatively, fits occur in rather more than half the survivors. These cases frequently show spike or sharp wave discharges with or without slow waves. There is little relation between pre-operative and post-operative epilepsy.

In a number of cases abnormalities of the same quality but of lesser severity are seen: this is particularly likely with the more chronic forms of abscess. An occasional case may be encountered in which the EEG is within normal limits.

CHRONIC SUBDURAL HAEMATOMA

In about 90 per cent of cases of chronic subdural haematoma, the EEG is abnormal. Thus the finding of a normal EEG in a suspected case makes the presence of a haematoma unlikely, but does not exclude it.

As with glioblastomas and abscesses, subdural haematomas tend to give rise to bilateral abnormalities but the slow activity is generally of much lower amplitude than that produced by these lesions (*Figure 6.11*). In some cases this widespread abnormality is a correct indication of a bilateral haematoma,

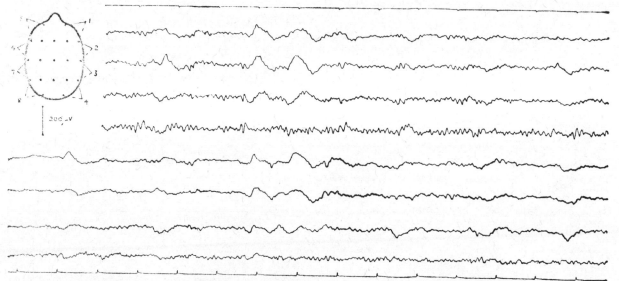

Figure 6.11—Subdural haematoma—left. Man aged 20 years. Increasing drowsiness and right hemiparesis for 2 days following a head injury of only moderate severity. EEG: Bilateral frontally predominant delta *activity with attenuation of* alpha *rhythm on the left side*

but in the majority it is associated with raised intracranial pressure and clouding of consciousness. Just as the level of consciousness fluctuates from day to day, so also may the degree of EEG abnormality.

In various published series, correct lateralization of the haematoma is claimed in about 75 per cent of the cases and accurate localization in about 50 per cent. In up to 20 per cent of cases, incorrect lateralization is reported, and it is of interest to consider the reasons for this. Of all space-occupying lesions, subdural haematomas are most frequently associated with diminution in amplitude or suppression of normal cerebral rhythms. The cerebral cortex is distorted and compressed and at the same time is separated from the scalp electrodes by an increasing thickness of membrane and blood-stained fluid. Whether attenuation secondary to the compression, or diminished conduction due to the presence of the haematoma, is the more important factor, remains debatable. In some of these cases, particularly when generalized slow activity is present, attenuation of all rhythms over the haematoma and sometimes over the entire ipsilateral hemisphere leads to the paradoxical situation that the EEG appears more abnormal over the contralateral hemisphere (*Figure 6.12*). In other patients the reverse is the case—over the affected hemisphere the amplitude of the slow activity is greater, and in many cases a focus can be established (*Figure 6.13*). Close examination of the relative frequency and amplitude of the *alpha* and other background rhythms on the two sides, both of which may be diminished over the affected hemisphere, may provide a highly significant clue to the correct location of the lesion. A

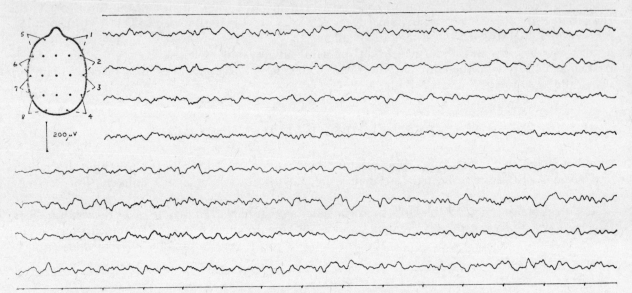

Figure 6.12—Subdural haematoma—right. Woman aged 45 years. Minor head injury 3 weeks previously, followed by headaches and drowsiness. EEG: Generalized irregular delta *activity of higher voltage on the left side with diminution of faster frequencies on the right side*

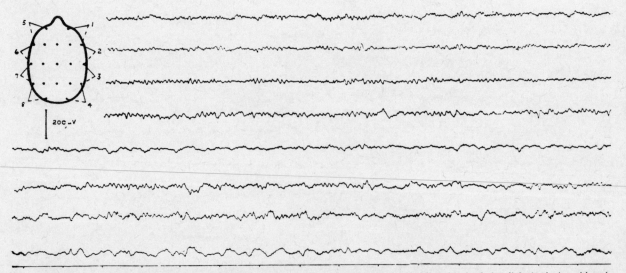

Figure 6.13—Subdural haematoma—left. Woman aged 66 years. Minor head injury 2 weeks previously, followed by headache, slight dysphasia and latterly drowsiness and vomiting. EEG: Widespread arrhythmic delta *activity over left hemisphere with suggestion of a focus in the posterior temporal region. Suppression of* alpha *rhythm in left occipital region*

122

diminished response to photic stimulation may also be found on the ipsilateral side. Mistakes are still likely in cases where the *alpha* rhythm remains symmetrical and are inevitable in the occasional case where the *alpha* rhythm is of lower amplitude over the normal hemisphere, perhaps due to pre-existing *alpha* asymmetry. Spike or sharp wave discharges are rarely seen with subdural haematomas.

Some of the these difficulties are illustrated by the EEG findings in 23 cases of chronic subdural haematoma reported by Millar (1959). In 10 cases there was unilateral slow activity; in 8, the haematoma was on the same side as the slow activity and in 2 it was on the opposite side. In 8 cases the *alpha* rhythm was asymmetrical; in 7 of these it was diminished in amplitude on the same side as the haematoma and in 1 on the opposite side. Bilateral slow activity was present in 10 cases; in 3 the amplitude was equal on the two sides, in 5 the haematoma was on the side of the lower amplitude, while in 2 it was on the side of the higher amplitude slow activity.

Watson, Flynn and Sullivan (1958) have reported two cases of chronic subdural haematoma each showing bursts of slow waves which recurred periodically. They comment on the resemblance of the pattern to the periodic EEG sometimes found in hepatic coma.

From the EEG alone it is not possible to distinguish with confidence between chronic subdural haematomas and cerebral tumours. Strictly localized foci of *delta* activity are more suggestive of tumours. In some cases of chronic subdural haematoma the EEG changes are indistinguishable from those found with posterior fossa tumours.

EXTRADURAL HAEMATOMA

Although nearly always the result of a severe head injury, it is convenient to discuss the EEG changes due to extradural haematomas at this point as these constitute another variety of space-occupying lesion. In a typical case, perhaps stuporose with a large fixed pupil on the side of the lesion, the EEG shows widespread high amplitude slow activity at 1–3 Hz or less which is commonly sinusoidal in form. In those cases running a subacute course in which as long as a week may have elapsed between the injury and the onset of coma, a *delta* focus overlying the lesion may be evident, with loss of the normal rhythms in its vicinity. Occasionally there may be an area of attenuation over the haematoma. Some generalized slow activity is likely to be present and this increases in amount and submerges the focal abnormalities as the clinical state of the patient deteriorates.

BENIGN INTRACRANIAL HYPERTENSION (PSEUDO TUMOR CEREBRI)

Most authors (Foley, 1955; Davidoff, 1956) have commented that in contradistinction to cases with obstructive hydrocephalus those with benign intracranial hypertension frequently have normal EEGs. In the 16 cases described by Sidell and Daly (1961) the EEGs were normal in 11 and unquestionably abnormal in only two, both showing bilateral bursts of *theta* activity. In this condition there is free ventricular communication, air studies show no distortion or dilatation of the ventricular system and presumably there is no distortion or displacement of the brainstem. Mani and Townsend's (1964) findings seem contradictory but as their 14 cases were carefully selected they cannot be ignored. They found abnormalities to be common, several patients showing slowing of the background rhythms while 12 showed bursts of activity often of *alpha* frequency but sometimes of *theta* or even *delta* frequency. Mani and Townsend felt that it was hard to distinguish between the EEGs of patients with obstructive hydrocephalus and those with benign intracranial hypertension. They believed that the burst activity might be directly related to the raised intracranial pressure.

REFERENCES

Arfel, G. and Fischgold, F. (1961). 'EEG Signs in Tumours of the Brain'. In *Electroencephalography and Cerebral Tumours. Electroenceph. clin. Neurophysiol.* Suppl. 19, 36

Bagchi, B. K. (1955). 'Preoperative Electroencephalographic Localization of Brain Tumours'. In *Electrochemistry in Biology and Medicine.* p. 335. London; Chapman and Hall

Bagchi, B. K., and Kooi, K. A., Selving, B. T. and Calhoun, H. D. (1961). 'Subtentorial Tumours and Other Lesions: An Electroencephalographic Study of 121 Cases'. *Electroenceph. clin. Neurophysiol.* **13**, 180

— Lam, R. L., Kooi, K. A. and Bassett, R. C. (1952). 'EEG Findings in Posterior Fossa Tumours'. *Electroenceph. clin. Neurophysiol.* **4**, 23

Bancaud, J. (1959). *Utilisation de l'Examen Neuro-psycho-pathologique dans l'Interprétation de l'EEG des Tumeurs Intracraniennes.* Paris; R. Foulon

— (1961). 'Correlations of Neuro-psycho-pathological and EEG Findings in Cases with Cerebral Tumours'. In *Electroencephalography and Cerebral Tumours. Electroenceph. clin. Neurophysiol.* Suppl. 19, 204

Berger, H. (1931). 'Über das Elektrenkephalogramm des Menschen III'. *Arch. Psychiat. NervKrankh.* **94**, 16 Translated by P. Gloor (1969). In 'Hans Berger on the Electroencephalogram of Man'. *Electroenceph. clin. Neurophysiol.* Suppl. 28, 95

Chavany, J. A., David, M. and Lérique, Mme. (1949). 'Pouls cérébral, manifestation électroencéphalographique focale d'un angiome hémisphérique avec épilepsie, gaucherie et écriture en miroir'. *Revue neurol.* **81**, 63

Cobb, W. A. and Gassel, M. M. (1961). 'The EEG with Lateral Ventricle Meningiomas'. In *Electroencephalography and Cerebral Tumours. Electroenceph. clin. Neurophysiol.* Suppl. 19, 111

— and Muller, G. (1954). 'Parietal Focal Theta Rhythm'. *Electroenceph. clin. Neurophysiol.* **6**, 455

Daly D. D. (1968). 'The Effect of Sleep upon the Electroencephalogram in Patients with Brain Tumours'. *Electroenceph. clin. Neurophysiol.* **25**, 521

— and Thomas, J. E. (1958). 'Sequential Alterations in the Electroencephalogram of Patients with Brain Tumours'. *Electroenceph. clin. Neurophysiol.* **10**, 182

— Whelan, J. L., Bickford, R. G. and MacCarty, C. S. (1953). 'The Electroencephalogram in Cases of Tumours of the Posterior Fossa and Third Ventricle'. *Electroenceph. clin. Neurophysiol.* **5**, 203

Davidoff, L. M. (1956). 'Pseudotumor Cerebri (Benign Intracranial Hypertension)'. *Neurology* **6**, 605

Dickerson, W. W. and Hellman, C. D. (1952). 'Electroencephalographic Study of Patients with Tuberous Sclerosis'. *Neurology* **2**, 248

Dott, N. M. (1960). 'Brain, Movement and Time'. *Br. med. J.* **2**, 12

Drift, J. H. A. Van der (1957). *The Significance of Electroencephalography for the Diagnosis and Localization of Cerebral Tumours.* Leiden; Stenfert Kroese

— and Magnus, O. (1961). 'The Value of the EEG in the Differential Diagnosis of Cases with Cerebral Lesions'. In *Electroencephalography and Cerebral Tumours. Electroenceph. clin. Neurophysiol.* Suppl. 19, 183

— — (1962). 'The EEG with Space Occupying Intracranial Lesions in Old Patients'. *Electroenceph. clin. Neurophysiol.* **14**, 664

Flodmark, S. (1965). 'Clinical Detection of Blood-Brain Barrier Alteration by Means of EEG'. In *Technical Progress in Neurological Diagnostics*, p. 163. Ed. by O. Gilland. Amsterdam; Elsevier

Foley, J. (1955). 'Benign Forms of Intracranial Hypertension—"Toxic and Otitic" Hydrocephalus'. *Brain* **78**, 1

Gassel, M. M. and Diamontopoulos, E. (1961). 'EEG in Supratentorial Meningiomas Falsely Localized on Clinical Grounds'. *Acta neurol. scand.* **37**, 41

Gibbs, F. A. and Gibbs, E. L. (1964). *Atlas of Electroencephalography. Vol. 3, Neurological and Psychiatric Disorders*, p. 339. Reading, Mass.; Addison-Wesley

Gloor, P. (1969). 'Hans Berger on the Electroencephalogram of Man.' *Electroenceph. clin. Neurophysiol.* Suppl. 28, 95

Green, R. L. and Wilson, W. P. (1961). 'Asymmetries of Beta Activity in Epilepsy, Brain Tumour and Cerebrovascular Disease'. *Electroenceph. clin. Neurophysiol.* **13**, 75

Harvald, B. and Hauge, M. (1955). 'The Electroencephalogram in Patients with Tuberous Sclerosis'. *Electroenceph. clin. Neurophysiol.* **7**, 573

Jasper, H. and Buren, J. Van (1953). 'Interrelationship between Cortex and Subcortical Structures: Clinical Electroencephalographic Studies'. *Electroenceph. clin. Neurophysiol.* Suppl. **4**, 168

Kirstein, L. (1953). 'The Occurrence of Sharp Waves, Spikes and Fast Activity in Supratentorial Tumours'. *Electroenceph. clin. Neurophysiol.* **5**, 33

Krauthammer, W. (1966). 'EEG Observations in Children with Tuberose Sclerosis'. *Electroenceph. clin. Neurophysiol.* **21**, 201

Loeb, C. and Favale, E. (1962). 'Contralateral EEG Abnormalities in Intracranial Arteriovenous Aneurysms'. *Archs Neurol.* **7**, 121

Mani, K. S. and Townsend, H. R. A. (1964). 'The EEG in Benign Intracranial Hypertension'. *Electroenceph. clin. Neurophysiol.* **16**, 604

Millar, J. H. D. (1955). 'Some Observations on the Electroencephalogram in Cerebral Tumour'. *J. Neurol. Neurosurg. Psychiat.* **18**, 68

— (1959). 'The EEG in Chronic Subdural Haematomata'. *Electroenceph. clin. Neurophysiol.* **11**, 603

Pampiglione, G. (1968). 'Some Inborn Metabolic Disorders Affecting Cerebral Electrogenesis'. In *Some Recent Advances in Inborn Errors of Metabolism*, p. 80. Ed. by K. S. Holt and V. P. Coffey. Edinburgh; Livingstone

Prior, P. F. (1968). 'Electroencephalographic Studies in Patients after Removal of Intracranial Meningiomas'. *Acta neurol. scand.* **44**, 107

Riehl, J.-L. and Ansel, R. (1969). 'EEG Changes Following Air Encephalography'. *Acta neurol. scand.* **45**, 270

Sidell, A. D. and Daly, D. D. (1961). 'The Electroencephalogram in Cases of Benign Intracranial Hypertension'. *Neurology* **11**, 413

Silverman, D. and Groff, R. A. (1957). 'Brain Tumour Depth Determination by Electrographic Recordings During Sleep'. *Archs Neurol. Psychiat.* **78**, 15

— Parandian, S., Shenkin, H. and Mellies, M. (1961). 'Effect of Intravenous Urea on the EEG of Brain Tumour Patients'. *Electroenceph. clin. Neurophysiol.* **13**, 587

Walter, W. G. (1936). 'The Location of Cerebral Tumours by Electroencephalography'. *Lancet* **2**, 305

Watson, C. W., Flynn, R. E. and Sullivan, J. F. (1958). 'A Distinctive Electroencephalographic Change Associated with Subdural Haematoma Resembling Changes which Occur with Hepatic Encephalopathy'. *Electroenceph. clin. Neurophysiol.* **10**, 780

CHAPTER 7

HEAD INJURIES AND VASCULAR LESIONS

HEAD INJURY

The term head injury is now employed so universally that it would be unduly pedantic to substitute the more accurate term 'brain injury'. The EEG changes seen after head injuries are extremely varied and this is due in the main to three facts. First, the general diagnostic label of head injury encompasses a number of different types of lesion, the character, extent and distribution of which vary widely from patient to patient. Secondly, a head injury gives rise to an illness which is a dynamic process with an evolution and devolution which vary greatly in form and timing in different patients. Thirdly, certain features of the illness, notably alterations of consciousness, may in their own right produce EEG abnormalities. Other factors such as age influence the degree of abnormality, and it seems that there is also an individual variation in the response to brain trauma.

It is customary to follow Williams' (1941) method of assessing the severity of a head injury from the duration of the post-traumatic amnesia. There are some exceptions, notably those cases of injury due to high velocity projectiles in which consciousness may be retained, but nevertheless it is a good working rule and is largely followed in this text when referring to mild and severe head injuries.

In closed head injuries rapid linear or rotational acceleration or deceleration of the head due to impact gives rise to violent movement of the brain relative to the skull. The mesencephalon and adjacent diencephalon are particularly vulnerable because of the peculiarity of their vascular supply. These regions are supplied by perforating arteries that arise from the basilar artery and its major branches which enter the brain stem perpendicularly. As the basilar artery is tethered firmly to the base of the skull by the meninges, any movement of the brainstem will lead to stretching and spasm of these vessels or even to rupture should the movement be sufficiently severe and sudden (Dott, 1960). Ischaemia of these areas occurs (diencephalic ischaemic syndrome) the most obvious effect being loss of consciousness. In milder cases it is unlikely that shearing strains or a sudden rise in intracranial pressure (Gurdjian, Webster and Lissner, 1955) exert any significant effect although these may play a part in more severe cases. Williams and Denny-Brown (1941) found that in cats subjected to experimental head injuries there was an almost immediate reduction in amplitude of the EEG, sometimes amounting to complete attenuation. After some 10–80 seconds *delta* activity appeared and remained evident for 10–160 seconds following which the record returned to its premorbid state. Walker, Kollros and Case (1944) confirmed these findings and noted additionally that the period of suppression was preceded by a generalized high voltage discharge. Denny-Brown believes that this is a cortical injury potential but it seems more likely that it is an artefact.

Mild Head Injuries

In mild injuries, the duration of the post-traumatic amnesia amounts to seconds or at most to a few minutes. Patients with such injuries are commonly described as suffering from 'concussion' though this is a term to which exception may be taken on a number of grounds. There is no clinical evidence of focal brain damage and recovery is uncomplicated, speedy and complete.

In man it is impossible to obtain records at such an early stage as in animals, but remarkably Dow, Ulett and Raaf (1944) (*also see* Ulett, 1955), by setting up an EEG laboratory in a shipyard, obtained a number of records from men with mild head injuries within 10 minutes of their accidents and in all, they examined 213 such cases within 24 hours of injury. Many of these cases were not even concussed and in a large proportion the EEGs were within normal limits. The EEG changes when present

125

consisted of diffuse *theta* or *delta* activity. Some cases were seen in which the injury was sufficient to give rise to retrograde amnesia, yet the EEGs obtained 15 minutes after injury were within normal limits. In other cases the EEG abnormalities disappeared within a few minutes. If impairment of consciousness was still evident at the time of the recording, the EEG was usually abnormal.

Boxers form another group in which it is relatively easy to obtain early recordings following head injury and in these a general diminution or attenuation of cortical electrical activity similar to that seen in animals has been noted. Pampus and Grote (1956) for instance, examined several boxers shortly after being knocked out and found relatively low voltage, slow records with a marked diminution or complete absence of *alpha* rhythm. Further recordings after 3 days showed that although the *alpha* rhythm had returned, the amplitude of the slow activity had increased.

SEVERE HEAD INJURIES

A head injury may be regarded as severe when the period of impaired consciousness and that of the post-traumatic amnesia are prolonged. The same acceleration and deceleration mechanisms are involved as in concussion but they are of greater magnitude. In addition to mass movements of the brain there may be distortion of the skull and dural septa. Violent fluctuations of intracranial pressure may occur; a sudden increase may cause shearing stresses, while a sudden reduction can produce cavitation effects. These various mechanisms may give rise to cerebral contusions or areas of maceration, cerebral lacerations, intracerebral haematomas and to extradural or acute subdural collections of blood. Such clinical indices of the severity of the injury as the presence of a skull fracture, of blood in the cerebrospinal fluid, of open injury, particularly with penetration of the dura, show a rough correlation with the degree of EEG abnormality.

The literature concerning the EEG effects of head injury abounds with large series of cases in which single recordings have been made at varying intervals, often months or years after the accident. It is not unfair to say that the value of such studies is limited and it must be emphasized that they are little more than studies of scarred brains. Several workers have made successful attempts to obtain recordings soon after the injury and to trace the development of the changes in relation to the clinical progress of the patient (Dawson, Webster and Gurdjian, 1951; Whelan, Webster and Gurdjian, 1955). Although there is generally a fairly close correlation between the degree of EEG abnormality and the level of consciousness, in a few cases, even though the patient is comatose, the EEG taken shortly after the injury may show normal basic rhythms. Such records are reminiscent of those described as resulting from vascular lesions of the pons and lower midbrain by Lundervold, Hauge

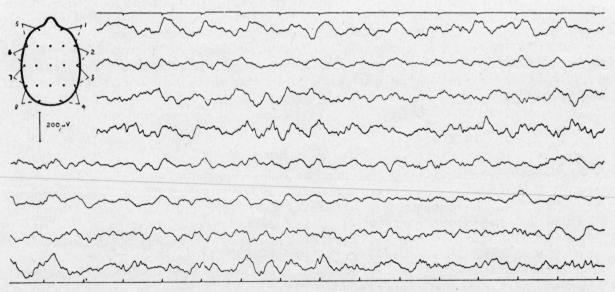

Figure 7.1—Severe head injury suffered 2 days previously. Man aged 18 years. Stuporose, responding only to painful stimuli. Left plantar extensor response. EEG: Dominated by diffuse random delta activity mainly at 1–2 Hz

126

and Löken (1956) (*see* page 130). Although the basic rhythms in these cases are normal, focal abnormalities are commonly present and the distribution of the *alpha* frequencies may be unusual, perhaps being maximal in the frontal regions. As a rule, subsequent deterioration of the EEG occurs with the appearance of generalized slow activity (*Figure 7.1*).

Generalized Abnormalities

Immediately after any head injury sufficiently severe to cause loss of consciousness some degree of generalized attenuation of cortical electrical activity of the kind reported in animals is probable, but in the majority of cases this phase is over by the time EEG recordings are carried out. Complete and persistent attenuation carries a bad prognosis and is usually accompanied by deep coma giving way to death. Attenuation appearing after an interval of several days or after surgical intervention is not uncommon and coincides with returning consciousness and a period of restless and confused behaviour; this variety has a good prognosis. Such attenuation may be related to the spreading depression of Leão that may follow electrical, mechanical or pharmacological stimulation of the cortex in animals (Marshall, 1959).

Infrequently, records obtained soon after injury may show continuous activity at 12–15 Hz. In the series reported by Dawson, Webster and Gurdjian (1951) this finding proved to carry a poor prognosis and of 4 patients with this abnormality, 3 died.

The initial attenuation gives way to a higher amplitude EEG in which disorganized slow activity is dominant—frequently no *alpha* rhythm is detectable. In the less severe injuries the basic frequency may be at 7–8 Hz returning to normal over a period of hours or days. In the more severe injuries the basic frequency slows to 4–6 Hz (*Figure 7.2*). The rate at which this occurs is of prognostic significance.

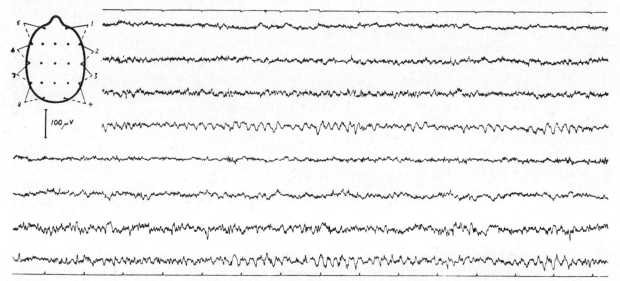

Figure 7.2—Moderately severe head injury suffered 7 days previously. Woman aged 25 years. Unconscious for 4 hours. Clouding of consciousness evident at time of recording. EEG: Dominant posterior rhythm at 5 Hz

The outlook is poor when it occurs within 48 hours and better if it takes place more slowly. Dawson *et al.*, found that cases were rarely seen with a basic frequency below 4 Hz as at this level practically all activity ceased. However, there is no doubt that many cases do occur in which the basic rhythm may be as slow as 1 Hz and though the amplitude may be low, this is by no means always the case (*Figure 7.1*).

The progressive slowing of the EEG rhythms is presumably related to secondary effects of the injury and may continue for as long as 20 days. Having reached its minimum frequency, the usual course is for the slow activity progressively to increase in frequency and amplitude, sometimes acquiring a paroxysmal quality, and finally to become more regular. The *alpha* activity which first appears is slower than the premorbid rhythm but gradually regains its former frequency. Stability of the EEG pattern may not be achieved for weeks or many months and in some patients remains abnormal. There is a reasonably good correlation between the EEG and clinical improvement but occasionally the paradoxical situation occurs in which the EEG abnormalities increase although the clinical state is improving.

Although they remain stuporose and unrousable, in some patients there may be a period in which the EEG shows a fairly typical sleep pattern with spindles, vertical sharp waves and K-complexes (Chatrian, White and Daly, 1963). Bergamasco *et al.* (1968) have shown that such patterns with a circadian distribution indicate a favourable prognosis.

Localized Abnormalities

Although patients with closed head injuries frequently show only generalized EEG abnormalities, in a substantial proportion localized changes are also present. These sometimes indicate local lesions—contusions, macerations or haematomas—but are sometimes transient and variable and are then likely to result from vascular changes or oedema. Sometimes a localized abnormality may be disclosed as the general abnormality diminishes. Penetrating injuries may give rise to severe localized changes alone.

If an area of cortex has been damaged a corresponding area of attenuation of electrical activity may be seen. This may be absolute but more often its degree falls in the range of 50–80 per cent of the overall amplitude of the record. The area may be small or extend over an entire hemisphere and it may vary as regards its location and extent in successive recordings. If an *alpha* rhythm is detectable its frequency is usually slowed. Although contusions, areas of cortical maceration or intracerebral haematomas are frequently related to these areas of attenuation, in 40 per cent of such cases described by Dawson *et al.* no macroscopic lesions could be demonstrated. Similar areas of localized attenuation are common with acute subdural or epidural collections of blood providing these have been present for 2–3 days. In the first 24 hours, even though a large amount of blood is present, attenuation is rarely seen; it may be unilateral even though the haematoma is bilateral.

Foci of irregular slow activity at frequencies of 0·5–7 Hz are commonly seen. The slow activity may be continuous, random or intermittent and often shifts from place to place in successive recordings. In 45 per cent of Dawson's series of slow wave foci, there was no other evidence of a localized lesion but in the others, subdural haematomas, intracerebral haematomas or areas of contusion or maceration were present. In all but two subdural haematomas there was a reasonable correlation between the EEG localization and the actual site of the lesion; in each of the two exceptions the *delta* focus was contralateral.

Epileptiform Activity after Recent Head Injury

In patients suffering from early post-traumatic epilepsy, the development of attacks is prefaced by groups of high amplitude spikes in the EEG (Jasper, Kershman and Elvidge, 1945). Isolated or continuous spike or sharp wave discharges are occasionally seen in addition to the other abnormalities already described, even though no fits are experienced. Such discharges have been noted within an hour of the injury, but more commonly they appear after an interval of days or weeks. They occur more commonly in children. It is difficult to be sure in some of these cases that similar discharges did not antedate the injury.

Late or post-traumatic epilepsy, the effects of birth injury and incisural sclerosis are considered in Chapter 5.

Late Changes after Head Injuries

Although in the mildest of injuries the evolution of the whole process is completed within a few minutes, in the more severe injuries, as judged by continuing improvement in the EEG, it may take from a few months to as long as two years.

In many cases—even of severe head injury—the EEG may return to normal. As a rule this is associated with clinical recovery but it may occur when neurological or psychiatric abnormalities persist. In these cases the existence of a normal EEG indicates that the disabilities have a poor prognosis, for it implies the presence of areas of irreversible destruction of brain tissue that are incapable of giving rise to electrical activity and therefore of modifying the normal EEG produced by the intact regions of the brain. Such a situation in which a normal EEG indicates a poor prognosis, is sometimes referred to as 'Williams' paradox'.

As with the early EEG changes due to head injury, residual EEG abnormalities may be generalized, localized or a combination of the two. As might be expected the incidence of abnormalities is greater the more severe the initial injury, rising as one goes from closed to open non-penetrating and to open penetrating injuries. The incidence is also greater when permanent neurological signs persist or if post-traumatic epilepsy develops. In a series of 324 cases with a history of severe penetrating head injuries described by Kaufman and Walker (1949), of which 241 suffered from epilepsy, 91·3 per cent of those with epilepsy and 77·1 per cent of those without epilepsy had abnormal EEGs. In the majority the abnormality consisted of a slow wave focus.

From a medico-legal point of view it is important to realize that slow activity noted after a head injury may have been present before the accident. This is particularly true in certain categories of head injury and reference to Table 9.1 will indicate some of the groups of individuals in whom this is especially likely.

HEAD INJURIES IN CHILDREN

The EEGs of children are notoriously labile and the effects of head injuries are often more dramatic than the clinical state would seem to warrant (*Figure 7.3*). The changes are similar in character to those

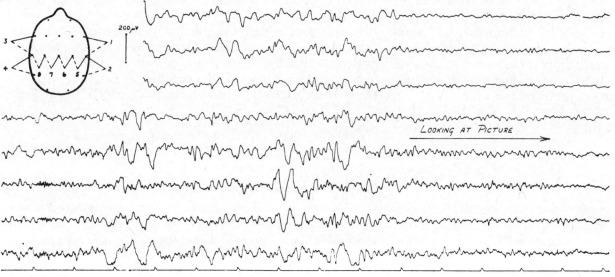

Figure 7.3— Moderate head injury. Boy aged 2 years. Unconscious for about 2 minutes 36 hours previously; two major fits in following hour. EEG: Widespread irregular theta *and* delta *activity greatly reduced by visual attention. Eyes open throughout*

described above but tend to be more severe being more widespread and of higher amplitude than in adults. Although occasionally very marked foci may disappear with remarkable speed, resolution of the abnormalities after severe injury usually takes considerably longer than in adults and, as has been mentioned, in infants hypsarrhythmic patterns may occur. Epileptiform discharges are more common.

WHIPLASH INJURIES

Following accidents which result in sudden and excessive hyperextension-flexion movements of the neck, many patients are found to show clinical evidence of brain damage even though consciousness may not have been lost. Generalized and even focal EEG abnormalities of the kind described above are frequent and in a group of such cases compared with a series of patients with closed head injuries the incidence and nature of the abnormalities proved to be similar (Torres and Shapiro, 1961).

Progressive Traumatic Encephalopathy

Some residual intellectual deficit after a severe head injury is not uncommon but a progressive dementia is a rare sequel to a single injury. It occurs more frequently after repeated episodes of concussion, notably in boxers. The incidence of abnormal EEGs in boxers is high. Larsson *et al.* (1954) found that 52 per cent of EEGs recorded after fights were abnormal while Nesarajah *et al.* (1961) reported that in 60 per cent of cases they found bursts of high amplitude slow activity sometimes with sharp waves, compared with 8 per cent of a control group. Blonstein (1961) found that of 100 boxers, 48 showed posteriorly distributed slow activity when examined before fights and stressed that this might be related to the personality traits likely to occur in this group, namely immaturity and aggressiveness.

In cases with progressive traumatic encephalopathy, the EEGs commonly show generalized 4–6 Hz activity sometimes with focal or bilaterally synchronous sharp waves. Occasionally the EEG may be within normal limits. The brains of such patients show degenerative changes similar to those of Alzheimer's disease (Corsellis and Brierley, 1959) or Pick's disease (Neubuerger, Sinton and Denst, 1959). Pampus and Grote (1956) have pointed out that the demonstration of a normal EEG after a series of fights is no guarantee against the later development of a progressive encephalopathy.

Conclusions

In general, the EEG abnormalities found in cases of head injury correspond both in severity and localization with those of the brain damage. Sometimes the EEG proves to be a more sensitive index of the degree of brain damage than the clinical state. The EEG is helpful in assessing prognosis but it is essential to beware of records taken too soon after the injury: EEGs obtained after several days are a much more reliable guide than those obtained within a few hours. When the record is normal or shows slight abnormalities only it suggests a good prognosis. Obvious abnormalities at this time suggest a more protracted recovery. A persistent EEG abnormality does not preclude a return to full activity.

VASCULAR LESIONS

Cerebrovascular Disease

As in the case of traumatic brain damage, a cerebrovascular catastrophe is a dynamic process. Electroencephalographically, the region of the brain affected and the extent of its involvement are more important than the precise nature of the causal lesion. Cerebral haemorrhage, it is true, can produce more severe and widespread abnormalities than a cerebral embolus or thrombosis, but this is an expression of the fact that the former usually gives rise to a much more extensive lesion. Secondary effects of infarction, particularly local oedema and vascular spasm, may exert a considerable influence upon the EEG. Complications such as shock, cardiac failure or renal failure, may also be reflected in the EEG picture.

Extensions of the lesion due to spreading vascular insufficiency or to the occurrence of further areas of infarction may also contribute to the variety and extent of the EEG abnormalities.

Vascular Lesions of the Brainstem

Infarction confined to the medulla, pons, the lower midbrain and the lateral portions of the upper midbrain produces little or no effect upon the EEG (Titeca, 1956). An example is the case described by Lundervold, Hauge and Löken (1956). Following vertebral angiography, a male patient of 63 years became unconscious and remained so until his death from coronary thrombosis 18 months later. Necropsy showed an obliterated aneurysm at the top of the basilar artery but communication between the posterior cerebral arteries and the internal carotid artery system was unaffected. There was severe damage to the pontine region and the sixth, seventh and eighth cranial nerve nuclei could not be identified. The pyramidal tracts, cerebellar cortex, dentate nuclei and roof nuclei were destroyed. The midbrain with the third and fourth nerve nuclei and the cerebral cortex remained intact. A total of 17 EEGs was obtained, two before angiography. The only change after the catastrophe was that no response could be obtained to painful stimuli. The frequency and amplitude of the *alpha* rhythm were unaffected and sleep produced the usual changes.

Many similar cases have since been described. In those recorded by Loeb, Rosadini and Poggio (1959) reactivity of the EEG to sensory stimulation was retained but in Radermecker's (1967) case the EEG although normal, failed to react to afferent stimulation. Such lack of reaction was also noted by Chase, Moretti and Prensky (1968) and these authors believe that the failure of the *alpha* activity to react to afferent stimuli is a pathognomonic feature of pontine involvement. In the 3 similar cases described by Otomo (1966) fast activity became prominent after the onset of coma. Boonstra and Notermans (1967) have shown that the rostral limit of a brainstem lesion can be determined by the abnormality or apparent normality of the EEG.

These observations may be viewed in the light of the work of Lindsley, Bowden and Magoun (1949). Elimination of the bulbar segment of the brainstem of cats had little effect upon the EEG. Some changes occurred when the pons was sectioned but to produce profound effects it was necessary to transect the midbrain or to produce a discrete injury to the mesencephalic tegmentum or to the basal diencephalon. When such injuries were inflicted the EEG activation pattern of low voltage fast activity was reduced or abolished and the record became dominated by bursts of high amplitude *delta* activity.

Infarction of the upper midbrain and adjacent diencephalon with involvement of the reticular activating system in man has similar effects upon the EEG. The normal basic rhythm is replaced by bilaterally synchronous and symmetrical slow activity, sometimes of maximal amplitude in the frontal regions (*Figure 7.4*). These findings are associated clinically with vascular lesions affecting the territory

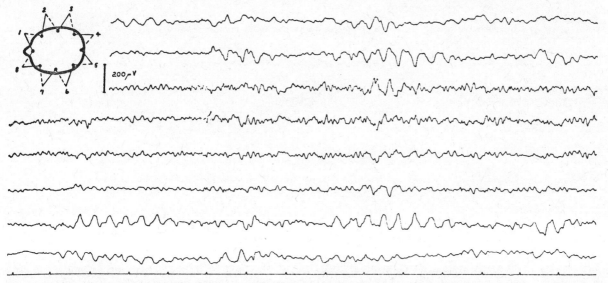

Figure 7.4—Basilar artery thrombosis 7 days previously. Woman aged 68 years with episodes of vertigo for 2 years. Thrombosis left posterior inferior cerebellar artery 3 months previously. EEG: Bilaterally synchronous, frontally predominant runs of 2–5 Hz delta activity

supplied by the rostral portion of the basilar artery and its branches. In cases of basilar artery disease, EEG may be helpful in determining the longitudinal extent of the vascular disorder and may indicate the involvement of the upper midbrain and diencephalon before any clinical evidence of this is present.

In patients with vertebrobasilar insufficiency low voltage records are frequent. Many of these fall within the accepted limits of normality but their incidence—80 per cent in the series described by Niedermeyer (1963)—is very much greater than that found in an age-specific sample of the general population. Van der Drift (1961) has drawn attention to the occurrence of temporo-occipital slow activity on one or both sides which he attributes to an insufficient blood supply from the posterior cerebral arteries. Phillips (1964) found such slow activity at frequencies varying from 2–7 Hz in different patients in 13 of 40 cases; it was frequently asymmetrical and was strictly unilateral in 4 and focal in 1 of these. The slow activity may sometimes be provoked or aggravated by table tilting (Meyer, Leiderman and Denny-Brown, 1956), by rotation or hyperextension of the neck or by overbreathing which accentuates the relative hypoxia in these areas; it may disappear on breathing a mixture of 93 per cent oxygen and 7 per cent carbon dioxide.

Thrombosis of the Internal Carotid Artery

In recent years a great deal of interest has been shown in the syndromes associated with thrombosis of one or both internal carotid arteries, particularly as there is evidence that ingravescent obstruction of these vessels may be associated with progressive dementia. The clinical diagnosis of internal carotid artery obstruction—particularly from cerebral tumour—is seldom easy and as a rule it is necessary to resort to arteriography, a procedure not without danger in these patients. Any contribution made by electroencephalography to the diagnosis is therefore likely to be valuable.

In patients with carotid artery occlusion but no symptoms or signs the EEG is unaffected or virtually so. When intermittent symptoms and signs occur in the distribution of the affected vessel, the amplitude of the basic rhythms over the whole of the ipsilateral hemisphere is diminished and low amplitude polyrhythmic *delta* activity may become evident in the temporal and parieto-temporal areas (*Figure 7.5*). Runs of rhythmic *delta* activity may appear over one or both frontal regions. The slow activity

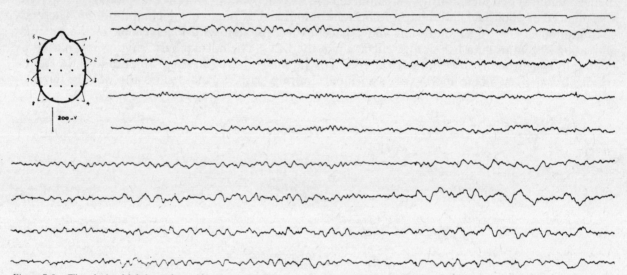

Figure 7.5— Thrombosis of left internal carotid artery two weeks previously. Man aged 67 years. Followed by progressive aphasia and hemiplegia. One previous thrombotic episode. EEG: Widespread theta and delta activity over the left hemisphere with loss of normal components

may sometimes be exaggerated by table tilting, the inhalation of nitrogen, hypocapnia or compression of the opposite carotid artery. These abnormalities may fluctuate in accord with the episodic clinical picture.

In florid cases with a dramatic onset of focal signs, slow wave foci are obvious. Focal *theta* and *delta* activity, usually frontotemporal or temporal in distribution, is superimposed upon a background of widespread lower amplitude irregular slow activity which may extend to the opposite hemisphere. The EEG changes tend therefore to be more widespread as well as more persistent than those due to obstructive lesions of smaller vessels, though in individual cases it is seldom possible to be dogmatic about the diagnosis from the EEG alone (Hass and Goldensohn, 1959).

The effects of carotid compression on the EEG in patients with cerebrovascular abnormalities have been studied extensively by Gastaut's group (Paillas *et al.* 1961; Roger *et al.* 1961) and by Solomon (1966). In normal individuals this rarely produces any EEG effects. Solomon used the test in 200 individuals with suspected cerebrovascular disease, 71 of whom ultimately were considered to have carotid or vertebrobasilar occlusive disease. In many, the resting EEG showed appropriate abnormalities. During carotid compression many of the patients developed focal or diffuse abnormalities or both together. Focal abnormalities were more likely to occur if the ipsilateral artery were compressed and diffuse abnormalities when pressure was applied to the contralateral artery. When focal abnormalities occurred they were usually followed after a few seconds by diffuse slow activity. Such abnormalities occurred in over half of the patients with major artery disease but in less than a quarter of those with disease of the more peripheral vessels. No difference was noted in the EEG effects whether the patients had vertebrobasilar or carotid artery disease.

Minor transient neurological phenomena including focal or generalized attacks of epilepsy occurred in one-third of the patients. Permanent neurological sequelae and even death have occurred as the result of carotid compression and although carrying out the procedure under EEG control probably makes it safer in that compression can be discontinued as soon as EEG abnormalities appear, the dangers should be borne in mind.

Vascular Lesions of the Cerebral Hemispheres

Any acute vascular lesion of a cerebral hemisphere of sufficient magnitude to give rise to apoplexy has clearly caused displacement of the upper brainstem with impairment of function of the reticular activating system. In such cases there is usually a loss of the normal background rhythms, which are replaced by widespread bilaterally synchronous slow activity. Focal abnormalities may be apparent in such cases but are often obscured by the generalized slow activity.

When the onset is less dramatic and the abrogation of consciousness is less complete the most striking EEG abnormality is a focus of slow activity. This is usually polyrhythmic *delta* activity but the frequency may fall within the *theta* range and in a proportion of cases—rather higher than in the case of space-occupying lesions—the *delta* activity may be sinusoidal in form. The focus appears as a rule within a few hours of the ictus. With ingravescent infarcts the EEG changes may herald the clinical signs. The site of the focus is often more anteriorly placed in early recordings than would be expected from the clinical picture, but subsequently there is a more precise coincidence. The amplitude of the focal discharge may increase during the first few days, probably due to perifocal oedema, and may resolve at a similar rate. Speedy resolution may also occur in those cases in which vasospasm is an important

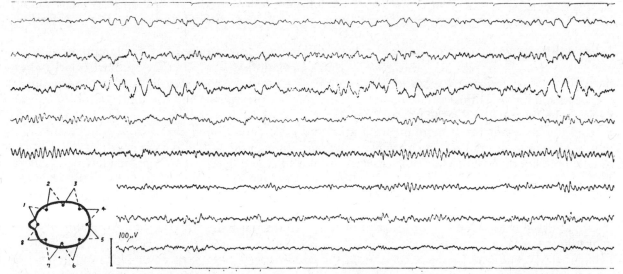

Figure 7.6—Thrombosis of the right middle cerebral artery 18 months previously. Man aged 65 years with residual severe left hemiplegia. EEG: Prominent delta *activity on right side, focal in the anterior temporal region. Amplitude of the* alpha *rhythm diminished on the right side*

feature. When tissue necrosis is prominent, the focus resolves slowly. Such foci may often disappear in a few weeks or months, but some persist for years (*Figure 7.6*).

There is some evidence that cortical, as compared with subcortical, infarcts give rise to foci of slow activity which are more prominent and much more persistent. The position is complicated by the fact that an infarct confined to the white matter may still be accompanied by oedema or vasomotor disturbances involving the overlying cortex. Nevertheless, it can be argued that in the presence of focal neurological signs due to a cerebral infarct, the absence of a corresponding slow wave focus suggests that the lesion lies deeply in the hemisphere.

Occasionally slow activity is diffusely distributed over the entire ipsilateral hemisphere without any clear focus being apparent (*Figure 7.7*). In at least some of these cases deep lesions involving the

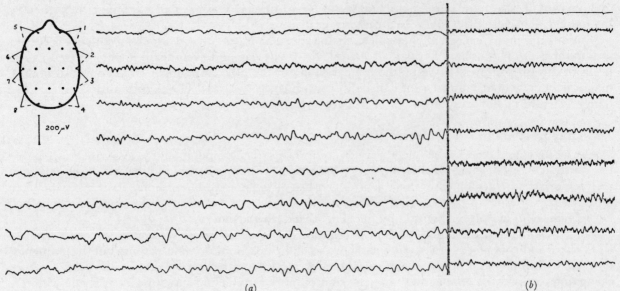

(a)   (b)

Figure 7.7—Thrombosis of the left middle cerebral artery. Woman aged 67 years. Right hemiplegia with dysphasia. (a) 3 days after infarction—EEG: Widespread random delta *activity over left cerebral hemisphere more evident posteriorly. Slowing of the basic rhythms with some random* theta *activity on the right side. (b) 6 months after infarction—EEG:* Theta *activity persists in the left temporal region and the* alpha *rhythm is of reduced amplitude on the left side*

thalamus are present (Grünthal and Remy, 1952). In other cases attenuation of electrical activity over the region of the infarct may be seen. With massive infarcts attenuation may extend over the entire hemisphere with or without low amplitude *delta* activity (Birchfield, Wilson and Heyman, 1959). In these cases there may be medium or high amplitude slow activity over the opposite hemisphere. Lavy, Carmon and Schwartz (1964) have emphasized the poor prognosis indicated by this form of abnormality.

In addition to slow wave foci, other less dramatic changes occur in the EEG. Ipsilateral diminution of the frequency or amplitude of the *alpha* rhythm—or both together—is common, particularly when the infarct is sited posteriorly. Occasional exceptions occur in which the *alpha* rhythm is more prominent on the affected side. Diffuse random *theta* activity may be present beyond the limits of the *delta* focus and is often most evident in the frontotemporal areas.

Amplitude asymmetry of spontaneous and induced fast activity may occur though less commonly than with cerebral tumours. When affected, the amplitude of the fast activity is nearly always diminished on the side of the lesion and only rarely—in contradistinction to space-occupying lesions—is there an ipsilateral increase (Green and Wilson, 1961). Such changes are more likely to be present when the infarct involves the cortex. The asymmetry of fast activity may not become evident until several weeks after the ictus.

Providing consciousness is not disturbed or has been regained, the EEG pattern over the opposite hemisphere is relatively unaffected.

Particularly with small areas of infarction, the EEG may show little or no change, and in a series of acute cerebrovascular lesions in which EEGs were obtained within two weeks of the onset by Cohn (1949), 25 per cent were normal or showed only minimal abnormalities.

Bruens, Gastaut and Giove (1960) found that in many elderly patients with chronic vascular insufficiency of the Sylvian region, rhythmical paroxysmal *delta* activity was present in one or both temporal regions. The slow activity was aggravated by ipsilateral carotid compression or by inhaling nitrogen and diminished following the inhalation of oxygen and carbon dioxide. The risk of cerebral infarction is high in these patients and the recognition of these EEG abnormalities has prognostic value. Van der Drift (1961) comments that the association of marked focal EEG signs with minimal clinical signs often heralds a stroke.

Late Changes after Cerebral Infarction

In a large number of cases—around 50 per cent in most series—the EEG becomes normal even though neurological deficits persist.

Even though the EEG does not return to normal, considerable or complete resolution of the *delta* focus is common. Random *theta* activity in the vicinity of the infarct and asymmetries of the *alpha* and of fast activity are more persistent. In an otherwise normal EEG pentothal-induced sleep may activate a focal abnormality or disclose asymmetry of the fast activity. Improvement in the EEG may be complete in a few days or weeks and rarely continues beyond 3–6 months.

Epileptiform discharges are very unusual in the acute phase of a vascular lesion but become more and more common with the passage of time; sharp wave or spike foci are well-recognized sequelae of cerebral infarction. Chatrian, Shaw and Leffman (1964) described a number of patients in whom repetitive unilateral epileptiform discharges appeared within hours or days of the infarct. Several showed epilepsia partialis continua.

In the subacute and chronic stages of a superficial cerebral infarct, in contradistinction to the acute phase of such a condition, a close correlation exists between the slow activity in the EEG and the regional cerebral blood flow (Ingvar, 1967).

With single recordings it is not possible with any confidence to differentiate between a vascular lesion and a cerebral tumour. Vascular lesions tend to produce more discrete changes and when a focus is present the *delta* activity tends to be more sinusoidal in form. Asymmetry of fast activity is less frequent than in the case of tumours and ipsilateral fast activity, when present, tends to be of greater frequency (20–30 Hz), perhaps due to the absence of raised intracranial pressure. On the other hand, depression of ipsilateral *alpha* activity is rather more prominent (Van der Drift, 1957). Serial EEGs provide a more sure foundation for making the differentiation, though as a rule little more information is provided than can be obtained from the clinical progress of the patient. Rapid improvement in the EEG with resolution of an obvious *delta* focus is very unusual in cases of tumour and is always suggestive of a vascular lesion. Occasional exceptions to this rule have been referred to on page 117.

Serial records also have more prognostic value than single EEGs. Absent or minimal changes early in the course of the ictus suggest a good prognosis, as does rapid resolution of such EEG changes as may have appeared. Only a rough correlation exists between the intensity of the clinical signs and the degree of EEG abnormality even in the acute phase of the disorder. In the later stages some cases occur in which the EEG abnormalities disappear but the severe neurological deficits persist, whilst in others the EEG may remain quite abnormal even though clinical signs ameliorate or vanish. To some extent this latter phenomenon may be explained in terms of the functional importance of the particular areas of the brain destroyed by the infarct. As with head injuries, whilst slow activity persists, the possibility of clinical improvement remains. In the presence of continuing neurological signs, a normal EEG indicates that these are likely to persist. Residual cortical atrophy may be indicated by a persistent decrease in the amplitude of the normal spontaneous activity.

Diffuse cerebral arteriosclerosis is considered on page 186.

Transient Global Amnesia

Transient global amnesia described by Fisher and Adams (1964) is an episodic condition occurring in elderly individuals in whom for a few hours the ability to form long-term memory traces is lost. Previously learned activities are performed normally.

Few EEGs have been recorded during the actual attacks, although these were obtained in 5 of Jaffe and Bender's (1966) 51 cases. Four of these were normal and 1 showed bursts of 3–5 Hz activity in both temporal areas which were more obvious on the left side; the abnormality persisted after the attack subsided. In Tharp's (1969) case bursts of sharp waves occurring independently in either temporal lobe were intermixed with runs of *theta* activity; after recovery the EEG became normal. In a case described by Lou (1968) focal slow activity was evident in the left temporal region with sharp waves during the attacks which persisted after clinical recovery. One of the 3 cases described by Evans (1966) showed slowing of the dominant rhythm to below 8 Hz and a sedation record showed a few small sharp waves in both temporal areas, more obviously on the left side. In this second case the symmetrical *alpha* rhythm was associated with brief runs of 7–8 Hz activity.

Recovery is generally complete although amnesia for the period of the illness persists. The clinical and EEG features are compatible with transient ischaemia of the hippocampal areas due to spasm of the basilar artery.

135

Subarachnoid Haemorrhage

Before a subarachnoid haemorrhage occurs it is very unusual to find EEG abnormalities attributable to an intracranial aneurysm unless it is causing interference to the cerebral circulation. The same is true of cerebral angiomas unless they are epileptogenic.

In the acute phase of the illness the EEG changes are very similar to those seen with closed head injuries. The record is diffusely abnormal, containing generalized slow activity which increases in frequency and diminishes in amplitude as the clinical state and particularly the level of consciousness improve.

After the first day or two of the illness the EEG may provide an indication of the laterality of the ruptured vessel (*Figure 7.8*). Roseman, Bloor and Schmidt (1951) noted that in a proportion of cases

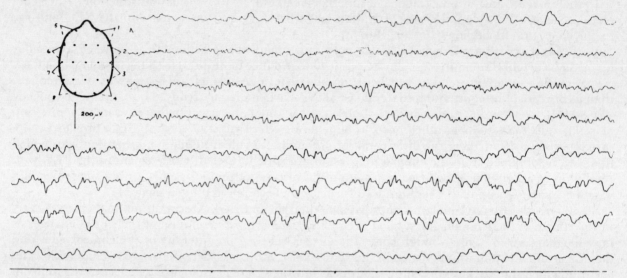

Figure 7.8—Subarachnoid haemorrhage. Woman aged 31 years. Rupture of aneurysm of the left anterior cerebral artery 10 days previously. Headache, dsyphasia and clouding of consciousness. EEG: Irregular delta and theta activity over the left anterior quadrant of the head. Absence of alpha rhythm on the same side

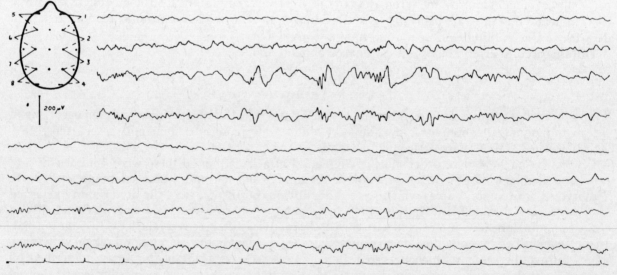

Figure 7.9—Subarachnoid haemorrhage 3 years previously. Man aged 45 years. Occasional focal sensory seizures by day; less frequent major seizures at night. EEG: Irregular focal slow activity and groups of sharpish waves in the right parietal region

there is an ipsilateral decrease in overall amplitude of the record and sometimes slowing of the *alpha* rhythm. A few cases show a well-marked *delta* focus due to vascular spasm, with or without frank infarction, or to an intracerebral or, less commonly, a subdural haematoma. In such cases the abnormalities are likely to indicate the laterality of the aneurysm or at any rate to suggest on which side carotid arteriography may be most profitably carried out.

In a series of 70 patients in whom subarachnoid haemorrhage was due to rupture of an intracranial aneurysm, Margerison *et al.* (1970) claimed that EEG investigations commenced within a few days of bleeding, enabled location of the aneurysm to be made with some confidence. They examined serial EEG tracings in respect of 180 possible features and selected 35 as being of most value in localization. They point out that no one feature is characteristic of bleeding from a particular site, but that certain clusters of features provide reliable evidence of location in the great majority of cases. For instance, posterior temporal slow waves were found on some occasions in all patients with bleeding from aneurysms of the middle cerebral artery and vertebrobasilar systems and in well over half the patients with aneurysms of the anterior and posterior communicating arteries. Such a feature is thus of little value in differentiating between bleeding sites. On the other hand, a slow wave focus in the Sylvian region, observed in 60 per cent of the patients with middle cerebral artery aneurysms, occurred in only one other case in the whole series and was thus of great localizing value.

The long-term EEG sequelae of subarachnoid haemorrhage are also similar to those seen after head injuries. In Walton's (1953) series of 312 cases, there were 120 survivors. Fifteen (12·5 per cent) developed epilepsy and in most of these the EEGs showed localized abnormalities. These were usually *delta* foci with sharp wave discharges (*Figure 7.9*), though occasionally only the slow activity persisted. In late cases without epilepsy, the EEG is often found to be normal even though there are neurological deficits, but in a few cases *delta* foci and even focal sharp wave discharges remain.

CEREBRAL FAT EMBOLISM

Serial EEG studies of 6 patients with cerebral fat embolism carried out by Müller and Klingler (1965) showed that the typical EEG abnormality was widespread, high voltage, polyrhythmic *theta* and *delta* activity, often best seen in the frontal and temporal areas, with disappearance of the normal rhythms. These findings correlate with the clouding of consciousness which is present. In one patient slow rhythmic patterns occurred not dissimilar from those seen in some cases of subacute spongiform encephalopathy. In patients who recovered, the EEGs returned to normal in a few weeks or months. Scherzer's (1967) findings were identical.

REFERENCES

Bergamasco, B., Bergamini, L., Doriguzzi, T. and Fabiani, D. (1968). 'EEG Sleep Patterns as a Prognostic Criterion in Post-traumatic Coma'. *Electroenceph. clin. Neurophysiol.* **24,** 374

Birchfield, R. I., Wilson, W. P. and Heyman, A. (1959). 'An Evaluation of Electroencephalography in Cerebral Infarction and Ischemia Due to Arteriosclerosis'. *Neurology* **9,** 859

Blonstein, J. L. (1961). 'EEGs of Boxers'. *Br. med. J.* **1,** 1174

Boonstra, S. and Notermans, S. L. H. (1967). 'The EEG in 17 Cases of Lesions of the Brain-stem, Established Post Mortem'. *Electroenceph. clin. Neurophysiol.* **23,** 496

Bruens, J. H., Gastaut, H. and Giove, G. (1960). 'Electroencephalographic Study of the Signs of Chronic Vascular Insufficiency of the Sylvian Region in Aged People'. *Electroenceph. clin. Neurophysiol.* **12,** 283

Chase, T. N., Moretti, L. and Prensky, A. L. (1968). 'Clinical and Electroencephalographic Manifestations of Vascular Lesions of the Pons'. *Neurology* **18,** 357

Chatrian, G. E., White Jr., L. E. and Daly, D. (1963). 'Electroencephalographic Patterns Resembling those of Sleep in Certain Comatose States after Injuries to the Head'. *Electroenceph. clin. Neurophysiol.* **15,** 272

— Shaw, C.-M. and Leffman, H. (1964). 'The Significance of Periodic Lateralized Epileptiform Discharges in EEG: An Electrographic, Clinical and Pathological Study'. *Electroenceph. clin. Neurophysiol.* **17,** 177

Cohn, R. (1949). *Clinical Electroencephalography.* p. 173. New York; McGraw-Hill

Corsellis, J. A. N. and Brierley, J. B. (1959). 'Observations on the Pathology of Insidious Dementia Following Head Injury'. *J. ment. Sci.* **105,** 714

Dawson, R. E., Webster, J. E. and Gurdjian, E. S. (1951). 'Serial Electroencephalography in Acute Head Injuries'. *J. Neurosurg.* **8,** 613

Dott, N. M. (1960). 'Brain, Movement and Time'. *Br. med. J.* **2,** 12

Dow, R. S., Ulett, G. and Raaf, J. (1944). 'Electroencephalographic Studies Immediately Following Head Injury'. *Am. J. Psychiat.* **101,** 174

Drift, J. H. A. Van der (1957). *The Significance of Electroencephalography for the Diagnosis and Localization of Cerebral Tumours.* Leiden; Stenfert Kroese

— (1961). 'Ischemic Cerebral Lesions'. *Angiology* **12,** 401

Evans, J. (1966). 'Transient Loss of Memory, an Organic Mental Syndrome'. *Brain* **89,** 539

Fisher, C. M. and Adams, R. D. (1964). 'Transient Global Amnesia'. *Acta neurol. scand.* **40,** Suppl. 9

Green, R. L. and Wilson, W. P. (1961). 'Asymmetries of Beta Activity in Epilepsy, Brain Tumour and Cerebrovascular Disease'. *Electroenceph. clin. Neurophysiol.* **13,** 75

Grünthal, E. and Remy, M. (1952). 'Über die Wirkung des Thalamusausfalles auf das EEG beim Menschen'. *Mschr. Psychiat. Neurol.* **124,** 263

Gurdjian, E. S., Webster, J. E. and Lissner, H. R. (1955). 'Mechanism of Brain Concussion, Contusion and Laceration'. *Electroenceph. clin. Neurophysiol.* **7,** 495

Hass, W. K. and Goldensohn, E. S. (1959). 'Clinical and Electroencephalographic Considerations in the Diagnosis of Carotid Artery Occlusion'. *Neurology* **9,** 575

Ingvar, D. H. (1967). 'The Pathophysiology of Occlusive Cerebrovascular Disorders'. *Acta neurol. scand.* **43,** Suppl. 31. p. 93

Jaffe, R. and Bender, M. B. (1966). 'EEG Studies in the Syndrome of Isolated Episodes of Confusion with Amnesia: "Transient Global Amnesia" '. *J. Neurol. Neurosurg. Psychiat.* **29,** 472

Jasper, H., Kershman, J. and Elvidge, A. (1945). 'Electroencephalography in Head Injury'. *Res. Publ. Ass. nerv. ment. Dis.* **24,** 388

Kaufman, I. C. and Walker, A. E. (1949). 'The Electroencephalogram after Head Injury'. *J. nerv. ment. Dis.* **109,** 383

Larsson, L. E., Melin, K. A., Nordström-Öhrberg, G., Silfverskiöld, B. P. and Öhrberg, K. (1954). 'Acute Head Injuries in Boxers; Clinical and Electroencephalographic Studies'. *Acta psychiat. neurol. scand.* Suppl. **95**

Lavy, S., Carmon, A. and Schwartz, A. (1964). 'Depression of Electrical Cortical Activity in Acute Cerebrovascular Accidents'. *Confinia neurol.* **24,** 349

Lindsley, D. B., Bowden, J. W. and Magoun, H. W. (1949). 'Effect upon the EEG of Acute Injury to the Brain Stem Activating System'. *Electroenceph. clin. Neurophysiol.* **1,** 475

Loeb, C., Rosadini, G. and Poggio, G. F. (1959). 'Electroencephalograms During Coma. Normal and Borderline Records in 5 Patients'. *Neurology* **9,** 610

Lou, H. (1968). 'Repeated Episodes of Transient Global Amnesia'. *Acta neurol. scand.* **44,** 612

Lundervold, A., Hauge, T. and Löken, A. C. (1956). 'Unusual EEG in Unconscious Patient With Brain Stem Atrophy'. *Electroenceph. clin. Neurophysiol.* **8,** 665

Margerison, J. H., Binnie, C. D. and McCaul, I. R. (1970). 'Electroencephalographic Signs Employed in the Location of Ruptured Intracranial Arterial Aneurysms'. *Electroenceph. clin. Neurophysiol.* **28,** 296

Marshall, W. H. (1959). 'Spreading Cortical Depression of Leão'. *Physiol. Rev.* **39,** 239

Meyer, J. S., Leiderman, H. and Denny-Brown, D. (1956). 'Electroencephalographic Study of Insufficiency of the Basilar and Carotid Arteries in Man'. *Neurology* **6,** 455

Müller, H. R. and Klingler, M. (1965). 'The Electroencephalogram in Cerebral Fat Embolism'. *Electroenceph. clin. Neurophysiol.* **18,** 278

Nesarajah, M. S., Seneviratne, K. N. and Watson, R. S. (1961). 'Electroencephalographic Changes in Ceylonese Boxers'. *Br. med. J.,* **1,** 866

Neubuerger, K. T., Sinton, D. W. and Denst, J. (1959). 'Cerebral Atrophy Associated With Boxing'. *Archs Neurol. Psychiat.* **81,** 403

Niedermeyer, E. (1963). 'The Electroencephalogram and Vertebrobasilar Artery Insufficiency'. *Neurology* **13,** 412

Otomo, E. (1966). 'Beta Wave Activity in the Electroencephalogram in Cases of Coma due to Acute Brain-Stem Lesions'. *J. Neurol. Neurosurg. Psychiat.* **29,** 383

Paillas, J. E., Bonnal, J., Gastaut, Y. and Barre, R. (1961). 'Electro-clinical Effects of Carotid Compression in Cases with Cerebral Circulatory Disturbances'. In *Cerebral Anoxia and the Electroencephalogram.* Ed. by H. Gastaut and J. S. Meyer. Springfield; Thomas

Pampus, F. and Grote, W. (1956). 'Elektrenkephalographische und klinische Befunde bei Boxern und ihre Bedeutung für die Pathophysiologie der traumatischen Hirnshadigung'. *Arch. Psychiat. NervKrankh.* **194,** 152

Phillips, B. M. (1964). 'Temporal-lobe Changes Associated with the Syndromes of Basilar-vertebral Insufficiency: An Electroencephalographic Study'. *Br. med. J.* **2,** 1104

Radermecker, J. (1967). 'Severe Acute Necrosis of the Pons with Long Survival: Electro-clinical Symptoms and Absence of Cerebral Lesions'. *Electroenceph. clin. Neurophysiol.* **23,** 281

Roger, J., Naquet, R., Gastaut, H., Lechner, H., Fernandez-Guardiola, A. and Bostem, F. (1961). 'Electroencephalographic and Electrocardiographic Manifestations Provoked by Carotid Compression in Cerebral Circulatory Insufficiences'. In *Cerebral Anoxia and the Electroencephalogram.* Ed. by H. Gastaut and J. S. Meyer. Springfield; Thomas

Roseman, E., Bloor, B. M. and Schmidt, R. P. (1951). 'The Electroencephalogram in Intracranial Aneurysms'. *Neurology* **1,** 25

Scherzer, E. (1967). 'EEG-Veränderungen bei zerebraler Fettemboli'. *Psychiatria Neurol.* **153,** 337

Solomon, S. (1966). 'Evaluation of Carotid Artery Compression in Cerebrovascular Disease; An Electroencephalographic-Clinical Correlation'. *Archs Neurol.* **14,** 165

Tharp, B. R. (1969). 'The Electroencephalogram in Transient Global Amnesia'. *Electroenceph. clin. Neurophysiol.* **26,** 96

Titeca, J. (1965). 'Contribution of EEG to the Study of Hemiplegias of Vascular Origin'. *J. belge Méd. phys. Rhum.* **11,** 89

Torres, F. and Shapiro, S. K. (1961). 'Electroencephalograms in Whiplash Injury'. *Archs Neurol.* **5,** 28

Ulett, G. A. (1955). 'Clinical and Experimental Studies of Mild Head Injuries'. *Electroenceph. clin. Neurophysiol.* **7,** 496

Walker, A. E., Kollros, J. J. and Case, T. J. (1944). 'The Physiological Basis of Concussion'. *J. Neurosurg.* **1,** 103

Walton, J. N. (1953). 'The Electroencephalographic Sequelae of Spontaneous Subarachnoid Haemorrhage'. *Electroenceph. clin. Neurophysiol.* **5,** 41

Whelan, J. L., Webster, J. E. and Gurdjian, E. S. (1955). 'Serial Electroencephalography in Recent Head Injuries with Attention to Photic Stimulation'. *Electroenceph. clin. Neurophysiol.* **7,** 495

Williams, D. (1941). 'The Electroencephalogram in Chronic Post-traumatic States'. *J. Neurol. Psychiat.* **4,** 131

— and Denny-Brown, D. (1941). 'Cerebral Electrical Changes in Experimental Concussion'. *Brain* **64,** 223

CHAPTER 8

INFECTIVE AND NON-INFECTIVE ENCEPHALOPATHIES

DELIRIUM AND COMA

Many of the conditions described in this chapter—the deliria, the meningoencephalitides and the encephalopathies, for instance—not only give rise to similar EEG abnormalities but share the important clinical feature of clouding of consciousness. In the absence of this phenomenon, the EEG is seldom affected to any marked degree, though it must be confessed that our clinical methods of judging slight degrees of impaired consciousness are crude and insensitive and that in many contexts we use the EEG itself as an indication of its level.

In delirium and in coma, clouding of consciousness is the cardinal symptom. No clear distinction other than that dictated by convention, can be drawn between the two states. When the degree of obnubilation is insufficient to preclude speech and observable behaviour, we use the term delirium; when these phenomena are abolished, we used the word coma. Both terms are purely descriptive and lack any nosological authority.

Many references have been made in earlier chapters to conditions in which clouding of consciousness occurs, notably raised intracranial pressure, 'concussion' and apoplexy. The common feature shared by most if not all of these cases in which structural lesions are present, is impairment of function of the reticular activating system of the midbrain and diencephalon, due most commonly to stretching and partial occlusion of the perforating arteries which supply this region.

In delirium too it is probable that direct involvement of these same anatomical regions occurs but as the areas projecting to and from the reticular formation are also likely to be affected it becomes difficult to apportion responsibility for the clinical and EEG changes.

Although in the meningoencephalitides changes in intracranial pressure or vascular abnormalities may play some part, in the deliria associated with such conditions as pneumonia or typhoid fever, or with renal or hepatic failure, it is difficult to conceive the intermediate mechanism as being other than metabolic in nature.

A direct relationship between the basic frequency of the EEG and the metabolic rate has long been recognized. Fever, for instance, may give rise to an increase in the *alpha* frequency. The level of tissue oxygen in the brain can be measured by electropolarography, and using this method Meyer, Fang and Denny-Brown (1954) showed in monkeys and cats that a fall of cerebral oxygen availability produced by vascular occlusion, is followed within a few seconds by EEG changes. These EEG abnormalities appear as a rule when the partial pressure of oxygen falls to 100 mmHg ($\equiv$ 12,000 ft A.S.L.) and becomes progressively more marked as it is reduced still further. Engel, Webb and Ferris (1945) showed that in the same individual, hypoxia, hypoglycaemia and alcohol, when causing comparable amounts of slow activity in the EEG also gave rise to similar effects on awareness, memory, attention and comprehension. A point stressed by these authors is that in the assessment of the EEGs of these patients the absolute frequency of the dominant rhythm is less important than the degree of slowing. A rhythm at 8–9 Hz may be significantly abnormal if it has replaced an *alpha* rhythm of higher frequency (*Figure 8.1*). This may explain why in some patients with clouding of consciousness the EEG appears to be normal, and emphasizes the need for obtaining serial recordings. Evidence that the frequency pattern of the EEG reflects the rate of oxygen utilization of the brain and in turn the rate of the cerebral blood flow has been reviewed by Ingvar (1967). The variability of the efficiency of cerebral homeostatic mechanisms in different individuals is likely to be of importance in accounting for the wide variations in the EEGs of individuals exposed to identical changes in their *milieu*.

In milder degrees of delirium the casual observer may be unaware of any change and the patient may experience no more than some difficulty in thinking and in recollection. In such cases the EEG

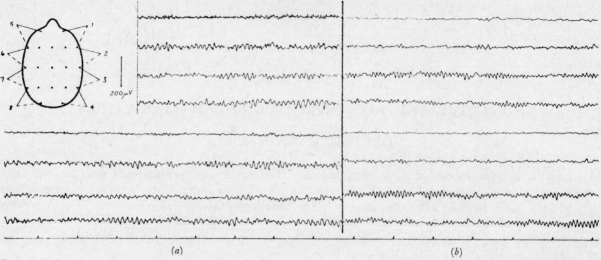

Figure 8.1—Pernicious anaemia with subacute combined degeneration of the cord. Man aged 64 years. (a) Before treatment. EEG: Alpha rhythm at 8 Hz extending into temporal regions. (b) 6 weeks after commencement of treatment with vitamin B_{12}. EEG: Alpha rhythm at 11 Hz confined to posterior half of head

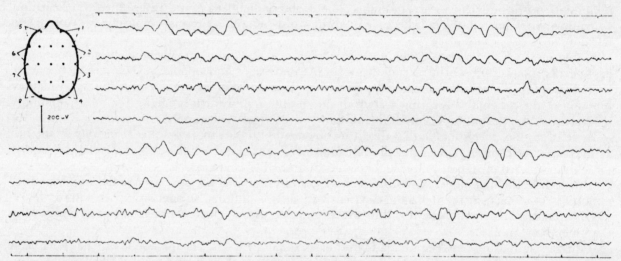

Figure 8.2—Severe delirium associated with bronchopneumonia. Woman aged 60 years. EEG: Bilaterally synchronous frontally predominant 2 Hz runs

may appear to be normal but as in Engel's cases of experimental delirium, there may be significant slowing of the basic rhythms insufficient in degree to transgress the arbitrary limits of normality. When confusion is evident the EEG becomes *theta* or even *delta* dominant though some *alpha* activity often persists. The *theta* activity commonly has the same distribution and reactivity as the *alpha* rhythm. In more advanced cases *delta* activity is clearly dominant, particularly in the frontal regions (*Figure 8.2*), and may be intermixed with faster frequencies; the reactivity of the EEG is usually slight or absent, but this is not always the case (*see Figure 8.16*). In coma, when the patient shows only a minimal response to stimuli, the most prominent activity is at 1–3 Hz and it may be bilaterally synchronous or more random in its distribution. Runs of such *delta* activity may alternate with periods of faster rhythms, or recur repetitively against a background of much lower voltage (*see* page 147). In deeper coma when the patient is quite unresponsive, the amplitude of the EEG diminishes and in the final stages when life can be maintained only by artificial respiration, the EEG becomes flat and featureless (Fischgold and Mathis, 1959). Whilst the EEG remains reactive to afferent stimulation, sleep and arousal patterns may occur, but in the deeper levels of coma such variations cease with certain rare exceptions (*see* page 130). In general, the prognosis is better when the EEG shows some periodicity and remains responsive to afferent stimuli.

Although frequently present, a direct and invariable relationship between the level of consciousness and the degree of EEG abnormality as emphasized by Engel and Romano (1959) is perhaps an over-simplification. These authors admit that in delirium tremens (alcoholic encephalopathy) records showing low to moderate voltage fast activity are more frequent than those with diffuse slow activity. Loeb (1958) in particular has stressed that although many records conform to the sequence of changes described, there is a significant number of exceptions. He points out that in the course of some cerebral lesions there may be little change in the EEG should consciousness become impaired and he feels that no one pattern should be regarded as characteristic of coma.

In addition to providing evidence of the depth of coma the EEG may be of some diagnostic help. It may indicate the presence of a space-occupying lesion, epileptogenic or otherwise, or it may suggest that the patient is suffering from barbiturate poisoning or from hepatic disease (Silverman, 1963).

SENSORY DEPRIVATION

The interest aroused by the similarity between the effects of sensory or perceptual deprivation and delirium is heightened by the fact that EEG changes of a comparable kind occur in both conditions. Heron (1961) found that the *alpha* rhythm slowed progressively during sensory deprivation. Sometimes 4–5 Hz activity appeared; the abnormalities persisted for several hours after a 96-hour period of isolation. His observations were confirmed by Zubeck, Welch and Saunders (1963) who found that after two weeks of sensory deprivation the slowing of the *alpha* rhythm was of the order of 2–3 Hz bringing the mean *alpha* frequency in one subject down to a little over 7 Hz. After a week, although considerable improvement had occurred, the mean frequency was still lower than that before deprivation. Smith, Thakurdas and Lawes (1961) reported even more marked changes in schizophrenic subjects and commented that without exception all records showed widespread slowing.

Infective Encephalopathies

ACUTE MENINGITIS

The EEG abnormalities associated with acute meningitis take the form of diffuse slow activity. In benign lymphocytic choriomeningitis, the clinical course of which is usually mild, such abnormalities as appear are slight and there may be only a moderate generalized excess of *theta* activity.

Purulent Meningitis

In purulent forms of meningitis the slow activity as a rule is prominent and falls within the *delta* range. In the cases described by Turrell and Roseman (1955) it was most marked over the posterior regions of the hemispheres. Children show more severe changes than adults (*Figure 8.3*). The abnormalities are likely to be related to circulatory disturbances involving the cerebral cortex and basal structures. The appearance of papilloedema is usually accompanied by an increase in the abnormality of the EEG. As Van der Drift (1957) remarks: 'the EEG findings resemble closely those seen with posterior fossa tumours'. With clinical improvement, the *delta* activity quickly diminishes in amount, being replaced by faster rhythms until finally the normal pattern is re-established. The rate of improvement of the EEG is particularly rapid in meningococcal meningitis. Should a cerebral abscess develop in the course of a purulent meningitis the EEG may provide valuable evidence both of its presence and of its location. Failure of the EEG to improve after two weeks of adequate treatment suggests either an error in diagnosis or that some complication has ensued.

Tuberculous Meningitis

Similar EEG abnormalities occur in tuberculous meningitis and show an approximate correlation with the clinical state of the patient, particularly with the level of consciousness. The bilateral slow

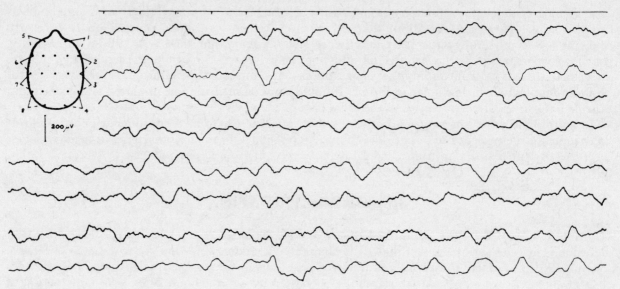

Figure 8.3—Acute streptococal meningitis—post-operative. Boy aged 7 years. Febrile with clouding of consciousness. EEG: Widespread random 1–2 Hz activity

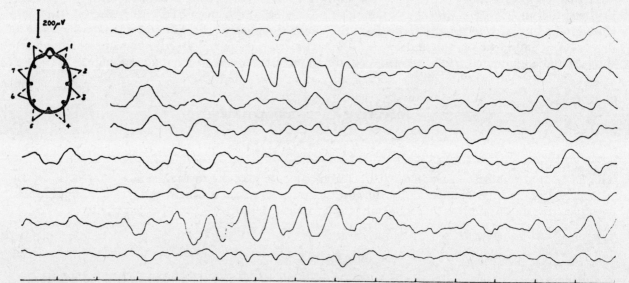

Figure 8.4—Tuberculous meningitis. Girl aged 4 years. Febrile with clouding of consciousness. EEG: Bilaterally synchronous 1–1·5 Hz runs superimposed upon random delta background

activity is often sinusoidal and regular and its amplitude moderate or high. The frequency may be as low as 0·5 Hz but is usually between 2–4·5 Hz. The slower activity is seen more often in children (*Figure 8.4*). Although the slow activity is usually distributed generally over the hemispheres, it is frequently more evident posteriorly. In addition, slow wave foci may be present and indicate incipient or frank focal lesions. Exacerbations of the meningitis, particularly when associated with hydrocephalus and raised intracranial pressure, are accompanied by a corresponding augmentation of the EEG abnormalities. The EEG may serve a useful function in judging the progress and duration of the treatment (Turrell *et al.*, 1953; Chaptal *et al.*, 1951).

NEUROSYPHILIS

The clinical manifestations of neurosyphilis are protean and there is considerable variation in the distribution of lesions in the nervous system and in their rate of development. It is only to be expected that the EEG findings vary widely in frequency and severity in different subgroups of this disease. The overall frequency of EEG abnormalities in unselected cases of active neurosyphilis is about 54 per cent (Arentsen and Voldby, 1952). As one might expect, their incidence is lower in cases in which the lesions are limited to the spinal cord. In tabes dorsalis the EEG abnormalities are slight in degree and occur with a frequency only a little above that of a normal group of subjects. In general paralysis, on the other hand, the incidence of EEG changes is 60–70 per cent and many cases show moderate to severe degrees of abnormality. In the presence of frank dementia, the incidence is even greater.

The EEG changes are fairly consistent throughout all groups and consist of a generalized excess of *theta* activity with some slowing of the basic *alpha* rhythm to the lower range of normality or even below it. In a few cases some 2–4 Hz activity is apparent. The changes are diffuse, although the slow activity may be more evident in the frontal and central areas. Asymmetry of the record is unusual and when present is relatively slight in degree.

The incidence of abnormalities in cases of neurosyphilis appears to fall off with increasing age and this is unrelated to the duration of the illness. Some improvement in the EEG abnormalities occurs in many cases following adequate treatment with penicillin.

ACUTE ENCEPHALITIS

In the encephalitides the degree of abnormality of the EEG corresponds approximately with the clinical state. Gloor, Kalabay and Giard (1968) believe that predominant involvement of the grey matter is associated with paroxysmal bilaterally synchronous slow activity. Involvement of subcortical grey matter is likely to be more important than involvement of the cortex. When white matter is involved, the characteristic EEG abnormality is diffuse polymorphous non-paroxysmal *delta* activity. Mixed cases show both.

In Group A encephalitides due to infections with neurotropic organisms, such as the encephalitis of mumps, St. Louis and equine encephalitis and acute anterior poliomyelitis, changes are relatively slight, the EEG showing some desynchronization with diffuse *theta* activity.

In acute anterior poliomyelitis these changes may progress so that the record becomes dominated by *delta* activity, but this phase lasts only a few days. There is no correlation between the EEG abnormality and the severity of paralysis (Garsche, 1951).

In the leucoencephalitides complicating infections with Group B (non-neurotropic) viruses, the EEG abnormalities are more marked. This group includes the encephalitides associated with measles, rubella, variola and the various post-vaccination states. The background rhythm virtually disappears

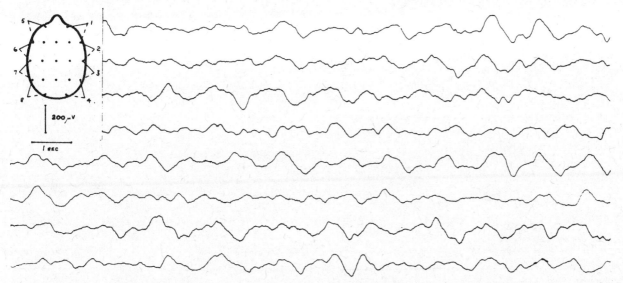

Figure 8.5—Measles encephalitis. Girl aged 2½ years. Rash appeared 4 days previously. Stuporose; occasional convulsions. EEG: Generalized asynchronous low frequency delta activity

and the record is made up of high voltage and often very slow *delta* activity (*Figure 8.5*). In most cases this subsides over a period of 2–4 weeks (Radermecker, 1955).

Doutlík and Janda (1963) point out that in some children the abnormalities persist much longer and frequently tend to become episodic. With the passage of time the episodes of slow activity tend either to disappear or to become asymmetrical and even focal. These latter cases are more likely to develop post-encephalitic epilepsy.

Sharp waves or sharp and slow wave complexes are rarely seen in the acute illness and when present are likely to be related to a pre-existing brain lesion (Pampiglione, Young and Ramsay, 1963).

A high incidence of EEG abnormalities in the febrile phase of rheumatic fever, even though there is no clinical evidence of involvement of the central nervous system, was noted by Lavy, Lavy and Brand (1964). In Sydenham's chorea (rheumatic encephalopathy) the majority of patients show a generalized excess of slow activity.

SUBACUTE VIRAL ENCEPHALOPATHIES

SUBACUTE SCLEROSING PANENCEPHALITIS

Subacute sclerosing panencephalitis is a disease of children and adolescents now recognized to be caused by the measles virus. Generally the onset is insidious and it progresses relentlessly, increasing global deterioration being punctuated by repetitive attacks of myoclonic epilepsy. As a rule a vegetative state is reached in a few months but on occasion the duration may be much longer and rarely the illness may run a remittent course (Cobb and Morgan-Hughes, 1968). It is associated with a characteristic EEG pattern which has been described by Radermecker (1949; 1956) and by Cobb and Hill (1950). The basic rhythm of the EEG becomes slower and more irregular, and high voltage (up to 1,400 μV) paroxysms appear consisting of a single diphasic slow wave or a brief run of slow activity at 1–3 Hz sometimes associated with one or more sharp waves. Occasionally the complexes appear against a background that is normal or relatively normal in appearance. The form and amplitude of the complex vary considerably from patient to patient and often in the same patient at different stages of the illness. Once established the paroxysms recur regularly though the repetition rate may vary throughout the illness. It is commonly between 6 and 16 times a minute but may be less frequent in the early phases of the illness. The duration of the individual paroxysms varied from 0·9 to 2·9 second in Cobb's (1966) series and the onset proved easier to define clearly than the termination. The paroxysms are bilaterally synchronous and as a rule generalized and symmetrical. Definite asymmetry is seen in some cases (*Figure 8.6*) and particularly in the earlier stages of the illness the complexes may be strictly unilateral; they are sometimes limited to the frontal or occipital regions. They persist but are less evident during sleep but once established are seldom influenced by any form

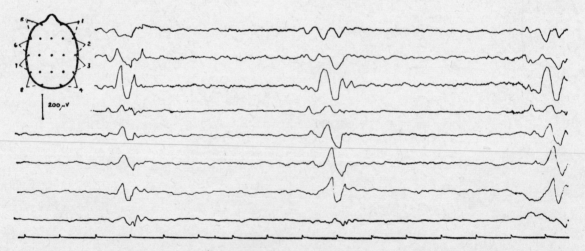

Figure 8.6—Subacute progressive encephalitis. Girl aged 7 years. Progressive organic deterioration, dyspraxia and dysphasia with generalized myoclonus for 4½ months. Died 5 months later. EEG: Periodic high voltage slow wave complexes occurring asynchronously on a low voltage background

of afferent stimulation. The background activity of the EEG consists of irregular *theta* or *delta* activity, sometimes increasing in amplitude immediately prior to the paroxysms. In occasional patients there may also be sporadic spikes or sharp waves. Later in the course of the illness the background activity is of remarkably low voltage. This flattening may initially be asymmetric, perhaps related to uneven progression of the disease. Myoclonic phenomena when present occur synchronously with the paroxysmal discharges and when both occur together they show a one to one relationship which Cobb (1964; 1966) regards as characteristic of the disease. Occasionally the complexes are accompanied by inhibitory phenomena so that at the time of each complex the child may fall. Cobb (1966) has pointed out that the constant form of the complexes in a particular patient on a particular occasion, their regularity and their constant relationship to myoclonic jerkings are features that are seldom mimicked precisely by any other disorder. Nevertheless, as Storm van Leeuwen (1964) amongst others has pointed out, the pattern falls a little short of being specific for the condition.

Subacute Spongiform Encephalopathy

Subacute spongiform encephalopathy was studied and defined by Jones and Nevin (1954). The condition affects, in the main, patients over 40 years of age, is never familial and ends fatally usually within 6 months after a relentless course characterized by visual symptoms, hypertonus, dysphasia, ataxia and progressive dementia. Myoclonus is often very prominent although not invariable, but major fits are relatively uncommon. Although not absolutely specific, the EEG findings are highly characteristic. In the early stages of the condition there may be a period in which generalized slow activity replaces the normal rhythms. The degree of EEG abnormality increases progressively and polyphasic complexes appear. These are of high voltage, are bilaterally synchronous and alternate with periods of lower voltage slow activity (*Figure 8.7*). The changes are not always symmetrical and

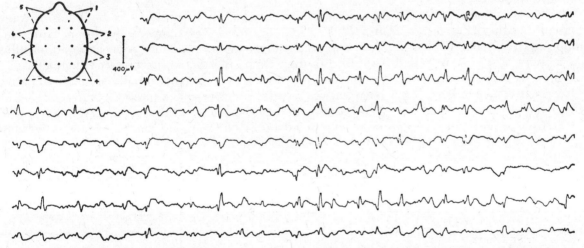

Figure 8.7—Subacute spongiform encephalopathy. Woman aged 70 years. Onset of illness 3 weeks previously; died 5 weeks later. Progressive rigidity and dementia. Frequent myoclonic jerkings of upper limbs and face. EEG: Bilateral high voltage polyphasic sharp waves occurring on a background of irregular slow activity

may be more obvious in any locality. The normal background rhythms become fragmentary and tend to disappear. The complexes in some patients show marked periodicity but in others occur with less regularity. They vary greatly in amplitude and form but include sharp and slow wave components. They are briefer (the duration being less than 200 ms), the sharp wave components are more prominent and the repetition rate faster than in the case of the complexes which occur in subacute sclerosing panencephalitis. As a rule they are easily inhibited by afferent stimuli. Myoclonic jerkings often accompany the complexes but are unrelated either to their amplitude or form. In the final stages of the illness the amplitude of the record diminishes; it becomes flat for long periods interrupted by brief bursts of slow or sharp and slow wave potentials (Nevin *et al.*, 1960).

Subacute spongiform encephalopathy has been transmitted to chimpanzees by combined intracerebral and intravenous inoculation of brain suspensions from biopsy or post-mortem material obtained from patients with the condition (Gibbs and Gajdusek, 1969).

PROGRESSIVE MULTIFOCAL LEUCOENCEPHALOPATHY

In the course of a number of chronic diseases, notably Hodgkin's disease, the leukemias, lympho-sarcoma, sarcoidosis and carcinomatosis, multiple areas of demyelination may occur in the white matter of the cerebral hemispheres, cerebellum, brainstem and spinal cord; these are likely to be viral in origin. The course of the resulting neurological disorder is subacute, death usually occurring within 6 months. The condition has been defined by Richardson (1961), and in those cases in which electroencephalography was carried out the records were always abnormal showing diffuse *theta* or *delta* activity with diminution or loss of the normal background rhythms. Asymmetry of the record was frequent and corresponded to the clinical picture. Unilateral sharp wave discharges were noted in a single case.

Farrell (1969) noted that focal *theta* or *delta* activity occurred in the early stages of the illness but later gave way to a generalized abnormality.

ACUTE NECROTIZING ENCEPHALITIS

Acute necrotizing encephalitis is now recognized to be caused by the herpes simplex virus. In 3 cases described by Millar and Coey (1959) localized single slow or sharp waves of regular periodicity occurred against a background of diffuse slow activity, the *alpha* rhythm having disappeared. In the cases described by Adams and Jennett (1967) 3 cases showed sharp wave foci. In 2, these were located at the vertex and in one of these they were 'frequent and repetitive'. A fourth case showed 'recurring slow wave complexes'.

The above authors described these various EEG findings at different stages of the illness. It is now apparent that the characteristic feature of the EEG changes is their temporal evolution. Upton and Gumpert (1970) have pointed out that 'triphasic complexes' occur against a background of diffuse slow activity between the second and fifteenth days of the illness and are not seen thereafter. The complexes are usually focal in the frontal or frontotemporal regions and initially are often unilateral (*Figure 8.8a*). Their bilateral occurrence carries a worse prognosis. The intervals between the complexes lengthen to a maximum of 3–3·5 seconds and then shorten over the course of a few days (*Figure 8.8b, c*). Concurrently they become more widespread and it is at this point that they may extend to the

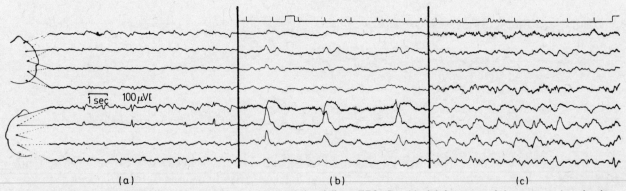

Figure 8.8—Herpes simplex encephalitis. Man aged 60 years. (a) *seventh day of illness. EEG: Repetitive left frontotemporal sharp waves on irregular slow-wave background.* (b) *ninth day of illness. EEG: repetitive slow-wave complexes in both frontotemporal regions, more marked on left.* (c) *twelfth day of illness. EEG: generalized increase in slow activity with repetitive sharp and slow-wave complexes predominantly in left frontotemporal region. (After Upton and Gumpert 1970)*

opposite hemisphere. The shortening of the intervals between the complexes is associated with clinical deterioration while the development of a hemiplegia is often accompanied by attenuation of the electrical activity over the affected temporal lobe. If the complexes occur bilaterally there is likely to be necrosis of both temporal lobes—a feature which may well be confirmed at autopsy or, should the patient survive, show itself in the form of a severe Korsakov syndrome. There is usually a lapse of 3–5 days between the stage at which the inter-complex intervals lengthen and the development of a low-voltage pattern.

The application of these criteria has allowed the diagnosis of herpes simplex encephalitis to be made in patients who were subsequently proved by brain biopsy to have the disease. This is of clinical importance because treatment with idoxuridine (5-iodo-2'-deoxyuridine) combined with a reduction of intracranial tension has improved the prognosis in many cases (Duffy, 1969). Even the exhibition of steroids at an early stage of the illness may be helpful in reducing pressure necrosis of the temporal lobes.

Periodic EEG Patterns

EEG patterns in which bursts of high voltage slow activity, sharp waves, or both, recur more or less regularly against a background of low amplitude slow activity are relatively uncommon. Two examples, the one associated with subacute sclerosing panencephalitis and the other with subacute spongiform encephalopathy, have just been described. The phenomenon described as 'burst suppression' which is characteristically seen in deep anaesthesia but also after cardiac arrest (Pampiglione, 1962), head injury (Zappoli, 1959), anoxic states and Wernicke's encephalopathy is another example (*Figure 8.9*). Periodic phenomena have been reported after attacks of grand mal (Cobb and Hill, 1950), in cases of acute encephalitis due to herpes simplex or infective mononucleosis and in cases of

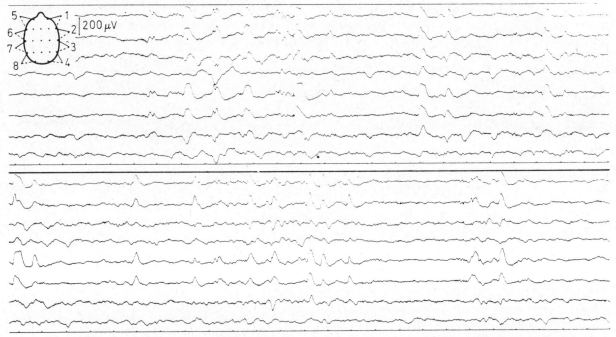

Figure 8.9—Burst suppression. Boy aged 11 years. Cardiac arrest following dental anaesthesia 30 hours previously. Deeply unconscious. EEG: Single and grouped slow delta complexes occurring bilaterally on background of lower voltage polymorphic slow activity

myoclonus epilepsy (Lesse, Hoefer and Austin, 1958), in some cases of hepatic coma (Foley, Watson and Adams, 1950), in subdural haematoma (Watson, Flynn and Sullivan, 1958), and in cerebral lipidosis. Periodicity therefore has no claim to specificity.

The mechanism underlying periodic EEG phenomena is by no means clear but a number of suggestions have been made. Zappoli (1959) believes that they occur when diffuse damage to cerebral white matter and brainstem structures leads to relative isolation of the cerebral cortex which is then free to produce 'periodic bioelectric phenomena'. A similar view was expressed by Fischer-Williams (1963) in regard to burst suppression. Others including Lombroso (1968) consider that the initial electrical event occurs in the reticular formation of the pons or midbrain and that this view is supported by observations of the time course of the events, particularly the fact that an ocular jerk may precede the myoclonic jerk and this in turn the periodic EEG discharge. Gloor, Kalabay and Giard (1968) postulate that the pathological state of the brain may be associated firstly with a readiness for neuronal discharges to generalize irrespective of their origin and secondly with a prolonged post-discharge refractory state. The normal afferent inflow might then be associated with repetitive synchronous discharges, their repetition rate depending on the duration of the refractory period.

Non-Infective Encephalopathies

SPHINGOLIPIDOSES

Ganglioside Lipidosis (*Infantile Amaurotic Family Idiocy; Tay Sachs' Disease*)

Schneck (1965) studied 14 cases of Tay Sachs' disease. In 4 cases the EEGs were recorded before the age of 10 months when vision was still intact; all were normal. Cases examined during the second year of life, which had become blind, had various neurological deficits and had developed epilepsy often with myoclonic attacks; all had abnormal EEGs showing high voltage *delta* activity with focal and generalized single and multiple spike potentials. In occasional patients symmetrical sharp and slow wave complexes occurred with a periodicity reminiscent of subacute sclerosing panencephalitis. It was this variety of EEG that was stressed in the earlier paper of Cobb, Martin and Pampiglione (1952). They described a number of cases of infantile and juvenile amaurotic family idiocy, although these conditions are likely to be genetically distinct. They emphasized that generalized high-voltage triphasic waves generally including a sharp wave component occurred against a background of irregular 1·5–6 Hz activity (*Figure 8.10*). In a minority of cases these complexes were accompanied by myoclonic

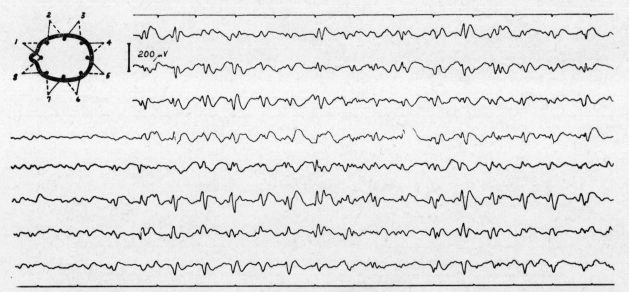

Figure 8.10—Amaurotic family idiocy (cerebral lipidosis). Boy aged 18 months. Development normal until 5 months. Occasional grand mal with progressive deterioration. Bilateral 'cherry red spots' at both maculae. EEG: Episodes of generalized repetitive sharp and slow wave complexes

jerkings. In some cases the EEG showed only bilateral paroxysmal *delta* activity. After the age of 3 years the EEG tends to show fewer epileptiform discharges and a general decrease in amplitude.

In a single case of late infantile amaurotic family idiocy (Bielschowsky type) the EEG at the age of 3 years showed high voltage 1–3 Hz activity with bioccipital asynchronous spikes (Klinken-Rasmussen and Dyggve, 1965).

Juvenile Amaurotic Family Idiocy (*Spielmeyer-Vogt's Disease; Batten-Mayou Disease*)

In the juvenile form of amaurotic family idiocy which generally begins between the ages of 5 and

8 years and runs its course in 10 to 15 years, the EEG also shows progressive abnormalities. In developing cases there may be generalized slow activity occurring continuously or in bursts. In the absence of epilepsy there may be no epileptiform features (Harlem, 1960) but often sporadic spikes are present. Photic stimulation at low flash rates often evokes large single or polyphasic spikes (Carels, 1960). In established cases the EEGs show widespread spike and wave complexes against a background of *theta* and *delta* activity (*Figure 8.11*). The sporadic and inconstantly focal spikes may persist. In the

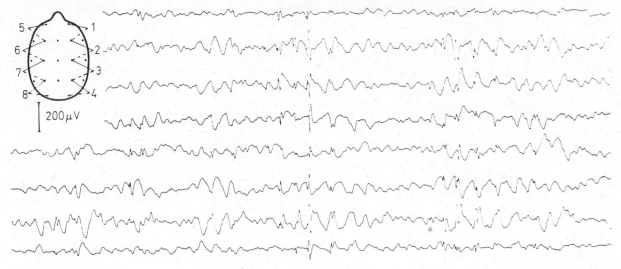

Figure 8.11—Spielmeyer-Vogt's disease. Girl aged 6 years. Frequent major seizures, severe mental subnormality and blindness. EEG: Bilateral irregular spike and wave discharges superimposed on polymorphic slow activity

later stages the background activity becomes slower, more irregular and the spike and wave complexes become less prominent. The periodicity sometimes seen in infantile amaurotic family idiocy has not been reported (Ellingson and Schain, 1969).

Cerebroside Lipidosis *(Gaucher's Disease)*

Literature concerning the EEG effects of Gaucher's disease is remarkably scanty. A pair of identical twins investigated by Espinas and Faris (1969) both had normal EEGs.

Sphinogomyelin Lipidosis *(Niemann-Pick's Disease)*

The EEG in Niemann-Pick's disease may sometimes show non-specific abnormalities (Schettler and Kahlke, 1967).

Sulphatide Lipidosis *(Metachromatic Leucodystrophy; Scholtz' Leucodystrophy)*

Cases of metachromatic leucodystrophy are characterized by demyelination with diffuse cerebral sclerosis. In.children the relatively rapid progress of the condition and the early appearance of a wide variety of neurological features contrasts with the much slower evolution of the adult form in which, for a considerable period, the clinical features may mimic functional psychoses, particularly schizophrenia. EEG examination, unfortunately, is unlikely to be helpful. The appearance of abnormalities is relatively delayed and often in the presence of neurological abnormalities the EEG may remain normal (Jervis, 1960) or show mild non-specific abnormalities (Pampiglione, 1961). Faster activity at 12–20 Hz over both the anterior and posterior regions usually becomes prominent later in the course of the disease superimposed upon slower rhythms (Pampiglione, 1968). Eventually the EEG may become dominated by high-amplitude irregular slow activity sometimes with multifocal sharp waves. Periodic phenomena do not occur so that the EEG may help in differentiating the condition from subacute sclerosing panencephalitis (Hagberg, Sourander and Svennerholm, 1962).

Krabbe's disease is included in this group by some authors although distinguished by others. Pampiglione (1968) noted that the EEGs showed earlier and more profound changes than in meta-chromatic leucodystrophy; his 3 cases all showed irregular slow activity with sharp waves and occasional spikes.

ENCEPHALOPATHIES DUE TO HEAVY METAL POISONING

The encephalopathy occurring in acute lead poisoning or after the administration of organic arsenical compounds is an acute illness in which clouding of consciousness and raised intracranial pressure are prominent features. In milder examples the only abnormal feature of the EEG may be the presence of random *theta* activity but in more florid cases the EEG is dominated by high amplitude generalized *delta* activity (Roseman, 1950).

HYPERTENSIVE ENCEPHALOPATHY

An elevated blood pressure in itself does not give rise to EEG abnormalities. During an attack of hypertensive encephalopathy when clouding of consciousness is apparent, the EEG is diffusely abnormal, consisting largely of *delta* activity. Between the attacks some generalized abnormalities may persist but are often slight unless raised intracranial pressure or severe renal impairment is present. In many cases EEG abnormalities due to cerebral infarction are likely to occur.

ACUTE PORPHYRIA

Relatively few records obtained from cases of acute porphyria have been published. In 8 personal cases there was a close correlation between the EEG abnormalities and the degree of clouding of consciousness. When the clinical picture consisted only of abdominal symptoms and peripheral neuritis, the EEG was within normal limits or at most showed a moderate excess of random *theta* activity. As delirious features appeared, the EEG became more and more abnormal and in severe cases, consisted largely of mixed *theta* and *delta* activity with high amplitude runs at 2 Hz, as in *Figure 8.12* (Kiloh and Nevin, 1950). The EEG abnormalities may persist for days or weeks after the delirium

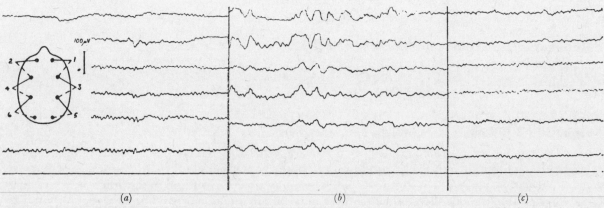

(a) (b) (c)

Figure 8.12—Acute porphyria. Man aged 32 years. (a) *10 days after onset. Abdominal pain; early peripheral neuropathy. EEG: Slight slowing of basic rhythms.* (b) *18 days after onset. Severe peripheral neuropathy with extensor plantar responses; confused and disorientated. EEG: Frontally predominant runs of 2 Hz activity.* (c) *2 months after onset. Residual but recovering peripheral neuropathy; mental state normal. EEG: Low voltage normal record*

has subsided. Similar EEG findings have been reported by Goldberg (1959). Dow (1961) has pointed out that the EEG changes are sometimes asymmetrical and that the slow activity may be paroxysmal. Spikes or sharp waves are not infrequently seen and though usually bilaterally synchronous, they may occasionally be unilateral. Epileptic attacks may form part of the clinical picture.

Barbiturates are often responsible for relapses in porphyric subjects and their exhibition, either for EEG purposes or for controlling fits, is inadvisable.

SYSTEMIC LUPUS ERYTHEMATOSUS

The EEG is frequently abnormal in systemic erythematosus, both in the acute and chronic stages of the condition. This perhaps is not surprising in view of the frequency of cerebral angiitis, fits and neurological complications in this condition. The EEG abnormality takes the form of an excess of *theta* or *delta* activity which may occur in runs, is sometimes asymmetrical and may even be lateralized or focal (Russell *et al.*, 1951; Lewis, Sinton and Knott, 1954; Larson, 1961).

RENAL DISEASE AND URAEMIA

In renal disease the EEG remains unchanged, even though there may be an increase in the blood urea, until clinical signs of renal failure become obvious. This is true both of acute glomerulonephritis (Hughes, Hill and Davis, 1950) and of chronic renal destruction whatever the aetiology.

In uraemia the same progression of EEG abnormalities occurs as in other encephalopathies with the same broad correlation with clouding of consciousness. *Theta* activity appears and the normal basic rhythms become disorganized and finally disappear. Reactivity of the EEG to afferent stimulation diminishes and the record becomes dominated by generalized *delta* activity (*Figure 8.13*). Not un-

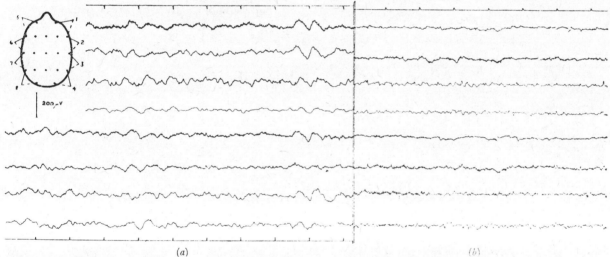

(a)　　　　　　　　　　　　　　　　　　　　　　　(b)

Figure 8.13—Renal failure treated by haemodialysis. Man aged 57 years. (a) Before dialysis. Clouding of consciousness. Plasma-urea level 250 mg per 100 ml. EEG: Runs of bilateral frontally predominant delta *activity occurring on a background of irregular* theta *activity. (b) 30 hours after dialysis. Consciousness clear. Plasma-urea level 50 mg per 100 ml. EEG: Low voltage posteriorly predominant mixed* alpha *and* theta *frequencies*

commonly, this is frontally predominant and may take on a markedly paroxysmal appearance. Although fits occur frequently in uraemia, interictal epileptiform discharges are infrequent although they have been reported by Klinger (1954). The nature of the disturbance of cerebral metabolism in uraemia is very complex and no single factor can be identified as the cause of the EEG abnormalities. These show no consistent relation to the level of the blood urea. Hypertension with cerebral oedema and vascular changes are present in many cases. Dehydration, cellular oedema, acidosis, hypocalcaemia, hyperkalaemia and an increased plasma magnesium may all contribute both to the clinical state and to the EEG changes.

Cadilhac and Ribstein (1961) note that about 20 per cent of infants with nephrotic syndromes show excessive occipital slow activity in the absence of renal failure or neurological symptoms. This abnormality appears to be unrelated to disturbances of the serum lipid and protein levels or to the presence of peripheral oedema. It is suggested that the slow activity may be related to cerebral oedema, to hypoxia secondary to hypovolaemia, to circulatory slowing or to hypocalcaemia. The abnormalities disappear as the patient improves.

Kennedy *et al.* (1963) have described the occurrence of marked EEG changes during haemodialysis of patients in renal failure. Five out of 13 of their patients had normal EEGs prior to dialysis, though all had plasma-urea levels in excess of 200 mg per 100 ml. Two hours after the commencement of dialysis all had markedly abnormal records, the commonest feature being the presence of intermittent or continuous high voltage *delta* activity. In 5 of 6 patients given intravenous hypertonic fructose, the degree of abnormality was reduced within a few minutes—an effect which lasted for periods of 10–15 minutes. Although raised intracranial pressure may be associated with these abnormalities, it is unlikely to be their sole cause as Kennedy *et al.* suggest. Jacob *et al.* (1965) believe that cerebral oedema is a more likely explanation. When the EEG is abnormal prior to dialysis, it is usually much less so 24 hours afterwards (*Figure 8.13*).

HEPATIC ENCEPHALOPATHY (PORTAL SYSTEMIC ENCEPHALOPATHY)

Patients with liver disease do not often show EEG abnormalities until the impairment of liver function is sufficient to give rise to clouding of consciousness. In the early phase of hepatic encephalopathy, the EEG shows progressive slowing and disorganization of the *alpha* rhythm which becomes mixed with random diffuse *theta* activity, often most marked in the temporal regions. As clouding of consciousness becomes more evident, the *theta* activity becomes dominant and its frequency falls. Runs of 4–7 Hz activity are best seen in the frontotemporal areas and as coma ensues, bilaterally synchronous 2 Hz activity begins to appear, particularly in the frontal regions (*Figure 8.14*). Later this *delta* activity dominates the EEG and suggests a grave prognosis. Further progression of the liver failure is associated with

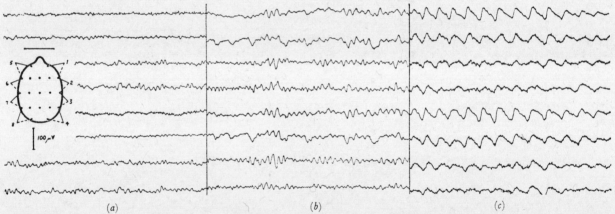

(a) (b) (c)

Figure 8.14—Hepatic encephalopathy (portal systemic encephalopathy). Man aged 33 years. (a) Mental state normal. Blood ammonia 200 μg 100 ml. EEG: Occasional slowing of alpha rhythm below 8 Hz with random theta components posteriorly. (b) Some clouding of consciousness. Blood ammonia 280 μ/100 ml. EEG: Widespread theta activity at 5–6 Hz (eye movement artefacts in channels 2 and 6). (c) Patient frankly delirious. Blood ammonia 500 μ/100 ml. EEG: High voltage rhythmical delta activity at 2 Hz, frontally predominant

diminishing amplitude of this *delta* activity, which becomes arrhythmic and finally disappears, so that prior to death the EEG shows a generalized absence of activity of any kind (Parsons-Smith *et al.*, 1957).

In a proportion of cases a more striking abnormality appears, taking the form of repetitive complexes. These were first described by Foley, Watson and Adams (1950) as 'blunt spike-wave' activity (*Figure 8.15*). In the patients described by Bickford and Butt (1955) such activity—which these authors called 'triphasic waves'—occurred in 11 out of 12 cases. In most clinics they are not seen as commonly but in part this may be due to lack of perseverance for their appearance may be ephemeral and repeated EEG examinations may be required to identify them. The triphasic complexes are usually best seen when the patient is stuporous though still responsive to painful stimuli but may occur earlier in association with clouding of consciousness. They are usually best seen in the frontal and frontotemporal regions reaching the occipital areas with lower amplitude after a delay of 25–140 ms. Occasionally the amplitude is highest in the occipital areas.

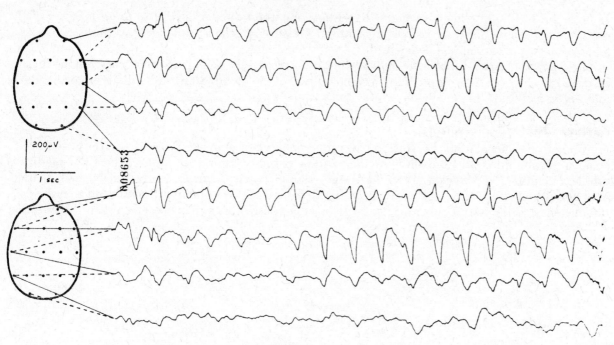

Figure 8.15—Hepatic coma. Man aged 47 years. EEG: Bilateral anteriorly predominant triphasic delta *waves at 2 Hz*

Commonly each complex consists of two electronegative waves separated by a positive wave of higher amplitude. One or more of the components may have a sharp or spike-like configuration and the general outline may vary considerably from patient to patient. As Silverman (1962) has pointed out, the term 'triphasic wave' is not always appropriate, for in an appreciable number of patients the discharge may be monophasic, biphasic or polyphasic. In some patients the discharge resembles spike and wave activity and in others the periodic discharge of subacute progressive encephalitis or cerebral lipidosis.

The relationship between the blood ammonia level and the EEG changes is far from being a precise and invariable one; many other metabolic abnormalities occur in liver failure which might play some part in determining the EEG abnormalities. EEG changes can be expected when the blood ammonia level reaches 200–400 μg per 100 ml (Friedlander, 1956). Feeding methionine, ammonium salts or a high protein diet to patients with hepatic encephalopathy leads to the absorption of larger amounts of nitrogenous compounds from the bowel; it aggravates the degree of clouding of consciousness and the EEG abnormalities. So too does the administration of morphine. Laidlaw and Read (1961) have used morphine in a dosage of 8 mg as a provocative test in mild cases of hepatic encephalopathy. A reduction in the nitrogen content of the gut, achieved by giving a low protein diet or by sterilizing the bowel contents with antibiotics, such as neomycin or by the administration of lactulose, has the opposite effect and may lead to improvement in the clinical state and the EEG.

ANOXIA

Anoxia produced by breathing gas mixtures low in oxygen content or by exposure in decompression chambers to atmospheres corresponding to altitudes of 12,000 feet or more, gives rise to progressive changes in the EEG which parallel the diminished awareness and impairment of consciousness of the subject. Initially and briefly the amplitude of the *alpha* rhythm may be increased but soon it diminishes in amount and frequency, becoming intermixed with random *theta* activity. Later, *delta* activity appears and eventually becomes the dominant rhythm. It may occur in bursts showing periodicity (burst suppression).

The EEG changes due to anoxia resulting from cardiac and respiratory disease are similar (Davidson and Jefferson, 1959). Hypercapnia and acidosis which often coexist in such cases may also contribute

153

to both the EEG and clinical changes. Retention of carbon dioxide gives rise to an increase in the cerebral blood flow and to a rise of intracranial pressure which, if prolonged, as in cases of severe emphysema, may cause papilloedema.

The EEG abnormalities and the clinical condition show only an approximate correlation; there is an even less close relationship with the oxygen tension of the blood. Some individuals are particularly tolerant to anoxia.

Carbon Monoxide Poisoning

Although the mechanisms at work in carbon monoxide poisoning sufficiently severe to give rise to coma are quite different from those of subacute or chronic respiratory failure, the EEG picture is similar (Lennox and Peterson, 1958; Bokonjić, 1963) (*Figure 8.16*). The generalized high voltage slow activity present is frequently maximal in the frontal or frontotemporal areas and may be continuous or occur in runs. It may persist for days after consciousness has been regained, the duration

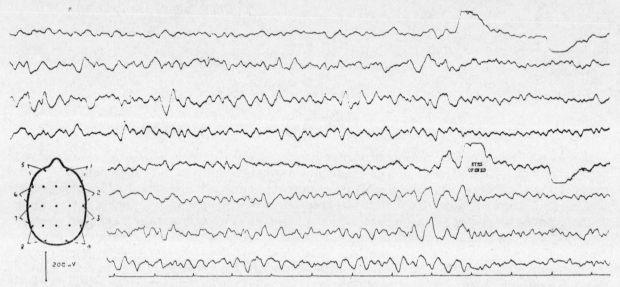

Figure 8.16—Carbon monoxide poisoning 36 hours previously. Woman aged 27 years. Suicidal attempt with coal gas. Drowsy and delirious but responding to commands. EEG: Bilateral posteriorly predominant delta and theta activity, the slower components responding to eye opening

varying with the length of the period of coma. The abnormalities may show some asymmetry, probably due to pre-existing relative vascular insufficiency. In such cases there may be focal damage to the brain. Neurological sequelae and severe sustained EEG abnormalities are more common in older patients. Although the EEG abnormalities improve and disappear within a week or two in most cases, some may persist indefinitely even though the patient may have recovered clinically. Conversely, on occasion the EEG may return to normal although the patient remains demented (Fischgold, Ajuriaguerra and de la Vigne, 1945). Treatment in a hyperbaric chamber with oxygen at 3 atmospheres for one hour may lead to rapid and remarkable changes in the EEG. In less severe cases in which some *alpha* activity persists, this increases in amount and voltage. In those who are mildly comatose and whose EEGs are composed of *theta* and *delta* activity, *alpha* activity appears and the slow activity diminishes in amplitude while increasing in frequency. In the deeply comatose patients, treatment has no effect on the EEG even though the patients may recover subsequently (Sluijter, 1967).

Congenital Heart Disease

Patients with congenital heart disease show a high incidence of EEG abnormalities particularly in cyanotic cases. A general excess of slow activity is usual but foci of slow waves may occur and epileptiform discharges are common (Shev and Robinson, 1961). In the children described by Kalyanaraman *et al.* (1968) 10 of 27 with cyanotic heart disease and 5 of 23 with acyanotic heart disease showed EEGs with epileptiform features. Of the total 50 patients, 21 experienced epileptic attacks. Ten of 12 patients with cyanotic heart disease studied by Kohner *et al.* (1967) had abnormal records showing various combinations of diffuse slow activity, focal *delta* activity and sharp waves. The early postoperative records were even more abnormal in 8 cases. This has been the general experience (Pampiglione, 1965) and is attributed to metabolic disturbances due to the operation. More surprising perhaps is that 3 months after operation, in spite of the relief of cyanosis, only 3 of the patients showed improvement in their EEGs and in 4 the EEGs had deteriorated further. Fowler, Kavan and Walter (1962) had previously noted that in 20 of 33 similar patients with abnormal EEGs these remained unchanged 1 to 2 years after operation. The immediate cause of the EEG abnormality is thought to be long-standing cerebral hypoxia and the persistence of the abnormality suggests that in some cases at any rate structural cerebral lesions occur.

Cardiac Surgery

A great deal has been learned about the effects of cerebral anoxia as the result of open-heart surgery; this is because the cerebral blood flow is controlled during such procedures, EEG monitoring is often carried out and unforeseen events occur not infrequently. When the cerebral circulation is cut off, the fast activity in the EEG associated with light anaesthesia disappears and is replaced by rhythms initially at about 3–4 Hz slowing to 0·5–1 Hz. Parallel with this slowing the amplitude falls progressively and the trace eventually becomes apotential (Storm van Leeuwen *et al.*, 1961). Sometimes the EEG becomes periodic, brief periods of very low potential separating bursts of slow activity and spikes (burst suppression). A similar sequence of changes including apotentiality can be seen in syncope (*see* page 104) and in Stokes–Adams attacks (Regis, Toga and Righini, 1961). Tonic seizures may occur during the apotential periods. Thies-Puppel and Wieners (1961) found that when the cerebral circulation was interrupted in the course of cardiac surgery it took 12–60 seconds for the EEG to become flat. Harden and Pampiglione (1966) showed that the time was also dependent on the degree of hypothermia; with a body temperature of 28–30°C. the average was 109 seconds. Hypothermia alone does not produce EEG changes unless the body temperature falls below 30°C. Slow activity initially of high amplitude appears, but as the temperature falls the amplitude of the record diminishes and at about 20°C repetitive complexes appear against a relatively flat background similar to burst suppression. Two patients with parkinsonism, one with a rectal temperature of 32·8°C and the other an axillary temperature of 35·9°C described by Gubbay and Barwick (1966) showed periodic features that the authors regarded as identical with those seen commonly in subacute spongiform encephalopathy.

Cardiac Arrest

Cardiac arrest and respiratory failure are common medical emergencies and if the consequent cerebral anoxia is not relieved in 4 to 8 minutes in these normothermic patients, irreversible cerebral damage occurs. By the time EEGs can be obtained the records are generally either of very low amplitude *delta* activity or are quite flat. Of 26 patients studied by Hockaday *et al.* (1965) showing such EEGs, irrespective of whether these were obtained early or late in the illness, all but one died without recovering consciousness. Several patients showed generalized spike and slow wave or polyspike and slow wave activity associated with myoclonic jerks. These epileptiform discharges were sometimes periodic and occurred even in cases with otherwise flat records. The authors regard the finding of a completely apotential EEG in these circumstances to have a very poor, if not hopeless, prognosis. Deterioration in the appearance of the EEG after a lapse of a few days also proved to have a very poor prognosis. Prior (1969) found sustained apotential EEGs in 25 out of 96 patients with cardiorespiratory arrest. All died and post-mortem examination in 9 who survived at least one day revealed extensive anoxic brain damage. In a further 26 patients burst suppression was found; 24 of these died but the other 2 recovered completely. Bickford, Dawson and Takeshita (1965) also noted that in similar patients there was no hope of recovery if the EEG was found to be apotential and that in patients showing burst suppression who survived, little more than a vegetative existence could be anticipated. Pampiglione and Harden (1968) obtained EEGs from 120 children suffering spontaneous cardiac arrest. Of those that had apotential EEGs for periods of 24 hours or longer none survived. Nor did any of those who showed burst suppression. Even patients whose records consisted of generalized slow activity without improvement in the first 24 hours fared badly, many dying within a week, the others suffering varying degrees of intellectual and neurological disability.

Death

The interpretation of the very low potential EEG has achieved importance because with modern clinical technology it has become increasingly difficult to declare with confidence that a patient is dead. Clearly from what has been said such an EEG indicates a grave state of affairs. Clearly too, the nature of the underlying condition must influence the prognosis both directly and indirectly. Certainly an apotential EEG in the course of barbiturate coma does not have such a poor prognosis as when associated with cardiac arrest. Thus Bird and Plum (1968) describe a patient in barbiturate coma for 5 days whose EEG was apotential for at least 23 hours yet recovered. Fischgold and Mathis (1959) stressed that in severe anoxic states a flat EEG might last for hours or even days without signifying brain death. Indeed Lindgren, Petersén and Zwetnow (1968) have described a patient who attempted suicide by hanging whose EEG remained apotential for 4 weeks following which some increasing 5–6 Hz activity at 20–30 μV appeared. The patient was still alive 18 months later although admittedly leading a vegetative existence. Bental and Leibowitz (1961) described a patient with a clinical diagnosis of 'encephalitis' whose EEG also remained apotential for 4 weeks who showed complete EEG and clinical recovery.

Lorentz (1969), too, insists that an apotential EEG is not an absolute indication of brain death but adds that if it is associated with a delay of circulation time after cerebral angiography exceeding 15 seconds 'such an EEG is incompatible with life'.

Schwab (Schwab *et al.*, 1963) has been closely concerned with the establishment of the criteria of brain death. Rosoff and Schwab (1968) listed these: a continuously apotential EEG at a sensitivity of 100–50 μV/cm for a minimum period of 30 minutes; an absence of clinical and EEG response to noise or pinching; an absence of reflexes, spontaneous breathing or muscle activity; and an absence of hypothermia or anaesthesia. If these criteria are all satisfied and provided that after a lapse of 24 to 72 hours the same negative responses are obtained, one can state 'there is no chance of brain activity recovering'. It should be noted that the EEG interpreter can only discuss 'brain death'. It is not possible to diagnose 'death' by the EEG alone—certainly not until an adequate definition is available!

WATER BALANCE—ELECTROLYTE DISTURBANCES

Disturbances of water balance occur in many conditions, both medical and surgical, particularly when vomiting and diarrhoea are prominent. They make their contribution to both clinical and EEG changes in severe renal disease, states of malnutrition and of profound weakness, and in such endocrine disorders as Addison's disease.

Hydration

As far as the EEG is concerned, dehydration is very much better tolerated than water intoxication. Dehydration without gross electrolyte disturbances leads to little change in the EEG, though there may be some general reduction in its amplitude and some admixture of *theta* activity. Water intoxication, on the other hand, gives rise to an encephalopathy with headache, vomiting, impaired consciousness, muscle cramps and even fits. The EEG shows high voltage generalized *delta* activity, often irregular in form and occurring in runs. Overhydration produced by drinking large quantities of water aided by an injection of pitressin was used by McQuarrie and Peeler (1931) to provoke fits in suspected epileptics.

Acidosis

Acidosis due for instance to the retention of sulphates and phosphates, as may occur with diminished glomerular function, is well tolerated and has little effect upon the EEG. Slight degrees of acidosis produced by the inhalation of 10 per cent carbon dioxide tend to cause some reduction in the amplitude of the EEG and an increase in the amount of fast activity. In such clinical conditions as diabetic coma, uraemia and toxic states, in which both acidosis and EEG abnormalities are prominent, the other biochemical disturbances are likely to be of much greater importance.

Alkalosis

Alkalosis is much more potent in its effects although it is not the elevation in arterial pH that is directly responsible for the EEG changes (Wyke, 1963). Clinically, alkalosis may occur in many conditions, particularly those in which vomiting is prominent. The plasma pH and alkali reserve are increased and there may be some hypokalaemia. Its effects on the nervous system may be marked and include clouding of consciousness and muscle spasms. The EEG shows high voltage runs of generalized rhythmic *delta* against a background of faster activity. In very severe cases, the *delta* activity becomes arrhythmic and of lower amplitude.

Plasma Cation Disturbances

As far as disturbances in the level of the more common cations in the plasma are concerned, the position is complicated by the fact that clinically, such disturbances are generally accompanied by abnormalities of water balance and of the acid base equilibrium. The evidence available suggests that variations in the plasma sodium level have very little direct effect upon the EEG. Changes in the potassium level, too, have little effect and such increases in its plasma concentration as produce marked dysfunction of the cardiovascular system have little or no effect on the EEG. In attacks of family periodic paralysis, when the plasma potassium may fall to 1·8 mEq/litre, the EEG often remains normal, although sometimes a little diffuse *theta* activity occurs (Saunders, 1954).

VITAMIN DEFICIENCIES

Acute Thiamin Deficiency

From an EEG point of view, the only vitamin deficiencies of importance are those of the B group. Acute thiamin deficiency gives rise to the clinical picture of Wernicke's encephalopathy, in which punctate haemorrhages occur mainly in the region of the upper midbrain and diencephalon. Clouding of consciousness of various degrees is present. In the milder cases the EEG shows a general slowing of the *alpha* rhythm, giving place to a *theta* dominant record which remains reactive to sensory stimulation. In more advanced cases, the EEG is made up of moderate amplitude generalized *delta* which is bilaterally synchronous and as a rule symmetrical (Frantzen, 1966). There is a reasonable correlation between the clinical state and the EEG abnormalities. In moribund patients generalized sharp and slow wave complexes, lasting for 1–2 seconds, separated by flat stretches of record similar to the EEGs in severe anoxic states have been described (Fournet and Lanternier, 1956).

Pellagra and Nicotinic Acid Encephalopathy

Twenty-two of 29 pellagrins studied by Srikantia *et al.* (1968) showed EEGs containing excess of diffuse *theta* and sometimes *delta* activity. Only 6 showed obvious psychiatric symptoms. The EEG abnormalities were aggravated by the administration of either L-leucine or quinolinic acid. EEG abnormalities whether spontaneous or induced disappeared following treatment in all cases, the time taken varying from 10 to 42 days.

In cases of nicotinic acid encephalopathy with clouding of consciousness, depression, catatonia and extrapyramidal disturbances EEG changes are to be expected. In the case described by Vallat *et al.* (1962) runs of generalized slow activity were present which were somewhat asymmetrical and most evident in the temporal areas. Rapid improvement both of the EEG and the clinical features occurred following parenteral vitamin therapy.

Deficiency of Vitamin B$_{12}$

Vitamin B$_{12}$ (cyanocobalamin) deficiency may give rise to pernicious anaemia, subacute combined degeneration of the cord and psychiatric abnormalities including depressive states, paranoid reactions and both acute and chronic organic reactions. It is not surprising that EEG abnormalities are particularly common. Of a group of 80 untreated cases studied by Walton *et al.* (1954), two-thirds had abnormal EEGs. Seven patients showed mild organic reactions and in all of these the EEGs were abnormal.

The abnormalities in vitamin B_{12} deficiency consist of slowing and disorganization of the *alpha* rhythm, which disappears altogether in the more advanced cases. Many show diffuse *theta* activity which may dominate the record, and in some this *theta* activity is intermixed with generalized *delta* activity which may be continuous or occur in runs. In occasional patients, the slow activity is asymmetrical and it may be focal. Temporal lobe sharp waves without any history of epilepsy have also been noted in a few patients. The most common type of abnormal record is one showing a generalized excess of *theta* activity. The response of the EEG to the administration of vitamin B_{12} is even more dramatic than the clinical improvement and in the great majority the EEG returns to normal, improvement beginning within 7 days and being complete within a few weeks (*Figure 8.17*). As would be predicted by

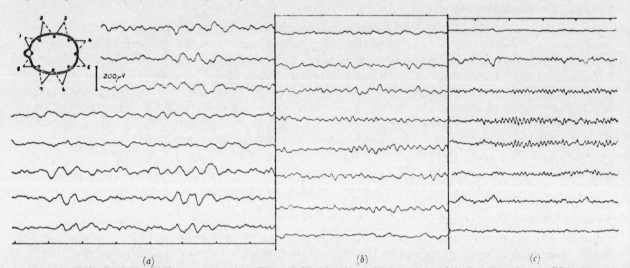

(a) (b) (c)

Figure 8.17—Pernicious anaemia. Woman aged 65 years. (a) Untreated. Hb 8·0g/100 ml. Moderate degree of clouding of consciousness. EEG: Bilateral frontally predominant 2 Hz delta runs. (b). 1 week after treatment with 300 µg cyanocobalamin. Hb. 9·6 g per 100 ml. Slight degree of clouding of consciousness. EEG: Dominant posterior rhythm at 5–6 Hz. (c) After 2 months treatment with 100 µg cyanocobalamin every 2 weeks. Hb 14·6 g/100ml. Mental state normal. EEG: Dominant posterior rhythm at 9–10 Hz

Engel *et al.* (1945), some of the pre-treatment EEGs classified as normal show a significant increase in the frequency of the *alpha* rhythm during the course of treatment (*see Figure 8.1*). The EEG abnormalities show no correlation with the degree of anaemia present and studies of patients with idiopathic hypochromic anaemia, with anaemia due to chronic blood loss or with haemolytic anaemia, show that quite low haemoglobin values may have little or no effect upon the EEG. Nor is there any parallel with the intensity of the neurological signs. Some correlation is seen with intellectual deterioration and clouding of consciousness, but the EEG changes are frequently present in patients in whom neither of these phenomena can be detected.

Pyridoxine Deficiency

In infants, pyridoxine deficiency has been reported due to feeding with a dried milk preparation lacking this vitamin. Fits occur and the EEG may show generalized spike and slow wave discharges or hypsarrhythmic patterns (Coursin, 1954). The symptoms and the EEG abnormalities respond dramatically to the administration of pyridoxine. Pyridoxine dependency, an inborn error of metabolism, gives rise to fits and similar EEG abnormalities in infants (Bejsovec *et al.*, 1967).

ENDOCRINE DISORDERS

HYPERTHYROIDISM

In hyperthyroidism, comparison of the EEG with premorbid recordings often shows an increase in the frequency of the *alpha* rhythm, the degree of change showing some relationship to the increase in the basal metabolic rate. The amount of *alpha* activity is often diminished and there is an increase in fast activity (15–30 Hz) in the central regions. A little sporadic *theta* activity may also be present and in a few patients may be prominent (Wilson and Johnson, 1964). The abnormalities generally disappear within three months of adequate surgical treatment (Vague *et al.*, 1961).

HYPOTHYROIDISM

In myxoedema the EEG tends to be of low voltage and the *alpha* rhythm is slow and poorly sustained. Variable amounts of random *theta* and *delta* activity may be present. There is little or no response to hyperventilation. In many cases the record can be declared abnormal only if one is able to compare it with a premorbid recording or with one obtained after recovery. In myxoedema coma with marked hypothermia (Nieman, 1959) the EEG is almost featureless, although a little very low amplitude slow activity may be evident. Hypothermia appears to be at least a contributory factor to the general decrease in amplitude of the trace, and artificially induced hypothermia has similar effects upon the EEG (Scott, 1955) (*see* page 155). The EEG changes together with the clinical state respond to the administration of thyroid extract or L-triiodothyronine.

Lansing and Trunnell (1963) withdrew treatment for periods of 4–6 weeks from 28 patients previously demonstrated to have little or no functioning thyroid tissue. At the end of this time there was a decrease in the mean *alpha* frequency from 10·3 to 9·5 Hz and the persistence and amplitude of the response to photic stimulation at 11–30 f/s were significantly reduced, the maximal effect being at 13 f/s. Re-establishment of therapy reversed these changes.

Cretins diagnosed before the age of 6 months show an unusually regular *theta* rhythm which is remarkably constant in its amplitude and frequency. The record may be of low voltage but this is by no means always the case. Adequate treatment for a few weeks leads to the appearance of a normal EEG pattern in most cases but if the patient remains retarded, presumably because of the presence of cerebral dysgenesis, the EEG may show paroxysmal activity, often with spikes or sharp waves (Nieman, 1961).

ADDISON'S DISEASE

In mild cases of Addison's disease, the EEG usually remains unaffected but may show a moderate excess of generalized *theta* activity. In more advanced cases and during crises the record may be made up entirely of generalized *theta* and *delta* activity, the latter often of high voltage. The biochemical disturbance in Addison's disease is complex and no consistent correlation between the severity of the EEG changes has been established with the blood sugar level or with the sodium, potassium or chloride plasma levels. In occasional cases the abnormalities may disappear if the blood sugar is raised to normal but in others this procedure is without effect. The administration of cortisone leads to a dramatic improvement in the EEG. DOCA has less predictable effects; improvement often follows its administration but sometimes the EEG may deteriorate, even though the clinical state improves (Dreyfus-Brisac and Mises, 1953).

ADRENAL HYPERCORTICISM

As a rule, EEG changes with tumours or hyperplasia of the suprarenal cortex are slight or non-existent, but cases have been described in which excessive amounts of *theta* and of fast activity have been found (Austt, Torrents and Fournier, 1950; Rohmer, Wackenheim and Kurtz, 1959).

DIABETES AND HYPERINSULINISM

Diabetic Coma

In a compensated diabetic the EEG shows no abnormality directly attributable to the absence of functioning islet tissue, but in incipient or frank diabetic coma abnormalities appear. The *alpha* rhythm becomes disorganized and is replaced by generalized *theta* or *delta* activity, usually of moderate amplitude. In the unconscious patient the record is *delta* dominant. Changes in water balance and ionic concentrations and the presence of abnormal metabolites are the significant factors. The hyperglycaemia is of no importance. The EEG often fails to return to normal until several days after effective treatment has been given (Cadilhac, Ribstein and Jean, 1959).

Hypoglycaemia

There is a considerable individual variation in sensitivity to the effects of hypoglycaemia, both as regards the clinical state and the EEG abnormalities, although the same person usually shows consistent responses to repeated lowering of the blood sugar level. The EEG findings are similar whether the hypoglycaemia is due to an islet cell tumour or is induced by an injection of insulin.

One of the earliest EEG changes in hypoglycaemia is an increased sensitivity to overbreathing, bursts of bilaterally synchronous slow activity appearing earlier and more readily than in the same individual with a normal blood sugar. The resting record may show slowing of the *alpha* rhythm and later generalized *theta* activity appears. Such changes are likely when the blood glucose has fallen to 50 mg/100 ml. As the blood sugar level continues to fall, runs of bilaterally synchronous *delta* activity, often more evident in the frontal regions, appear against this abnormal background and as the coma deepens the *delta* activity becomes more and more prominent. Particularly in those cases of islet cell tumour that present with behavioural abnormalities the EEG provides valuable diagnostic help.

Hypoglycaemia is associated with a diminished cerebral oxygen consumption and this may well be an important factor in producing the EEG abnormalities. Electrolyte disturbances and cerebral oedema may also play their part. Although occasional records obtained during hypoglycaemia may show spike or spike and slow wave discharges, even those cases in which fits occur generally show none of these features. It must be remembered that hypoglycaemia is a well recognized and potent activating agent. Not uncommonly, the slow activity shows some asymmetry and occasionally a well marked focal abnormality may be seen. This may be related to vascular factors and corresponding signs of a neurological lesion may also be present.

In the great majority of cases the abnormalities in the EEG disappear rapidly when the blood sugar is restored to normal (*Figure 8.18*). Occasionally a focal abnormality may persist, implying that local

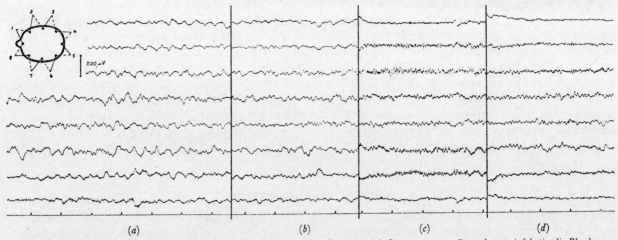

Figure 8.18—Spontaneous hypoglycaemia. Woman aged 38 years with an islet cell tumour. (a) Stuporose; responding only to painful stimuli. Blood sugar 20 mg/100 ml. (b) Following intravenous injection of 2 g glucose. (c) 30 seconds later. Total 4 glucose given. (d) 30 seconds later. Total 6 g glucose given. EEGs: Dominant generalized delta activity gives way progressively to a 9 Hz alpha rhythm and a little theta activity posteriorly

structural changes have occurred. After a particularly prolonged or very deep coma, it may be several days before the abnormalities disappear completely. After so-called irreversible coma the abnormalities persist long after the blood sugar level is normal and in the more severe cases, when degenerative changes have occurred in the cerebral cortex with secondary gliosis, the EEG may remain of low voltage with an irregular background of mixed frequencies, showing little organized *alpha* rhythm and dominated by irregular *delta* activity (Cadilhac, Ribstein and Jean, 1959).

Hypopituitarism

In hypopituitarism the EEG changes are similar to those seen in Addison's disease. In the more severe cases the EEG is made up of generalized *theta* and *delta* activity, the latter occurring in bilaterally synchronous runs which may be accentuated by overbreathing. The abnormalities may be aggravated

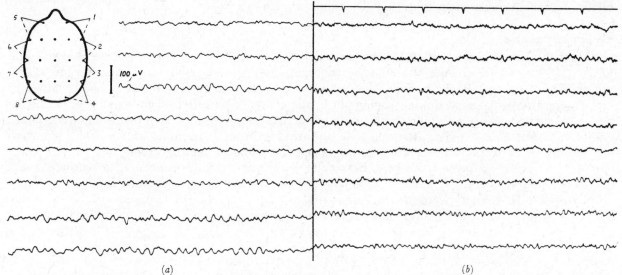

(a)   *(b)*

Figure 8.19—Hypopituitarism. Man aged 51 years. (a) *Mentally slow, retarded and apathetic. EEG: Dominant rhythm at 4–5 Hz.* (b) *Following the administration of ACTH. Mental state normal. EEG: Dominant components at 8–9 Hz*

by the administration of thyroid extract or DOCA, but they disappear if cortisone or ACTH is given (Hughes and Summers, 1956) (*Figure 8.19*). The administration of glucose generally has little effect.

Diabetes Insipidus

Diabetes insipidus in the absence of a tumour or other structural lesion does not give rise to EEG abnormalities.

Pituitary Tumours

Pituitary tumours in the absence of endocrine changes cause no EEG abnormality unless they erode out of the pituitary fossa and invade the floor of the third ventricle or, rarely, the cerebral hemispheres. Hyperplasia of acidophil cells, associated clinically with the syndrome of acromegaly, gives rise to no consistent EEG change, although in some cases slowing of the *alpha* rhythm and an admixture of slower activity is evident (Rohmer, Wackenheim and Kurtz, 1959).

Hypoparathyroidism

In mild cases of hypoparathyroidism, the only clinical feature of which is the occurrence of occasional attacks of tetany, the EEG may show some diminution in the *alpha* rhythm and the addition of diffuse *theta* activity which is most marked in the central regions. Runs of higher amplitude *theta* activity also appear and a very marked response to overbreathing occurs. In severe cases, particularly those in which there are convulsions, the *alpha* rhythm disappears more or less completely and the trace is polymorphic, being made up of a mixture of *theta* and *delta* frequencies often of high amplitude. Superimposed on this background there may be bilaterally synchronous paroxysms of high voltage rhythmical *delta* activity together with isolated sharp waves. The abnormalities are aggravated by overbreathing. Treatment by intravenous calcium salts, large doses of vitamin D, AT10 or Para-thor-mone leads to rapid improvement in the EEG (Rohmer, Wackenheim and Kurtz, 1959; Glaser and Levy, 1960).

Pseudohypoparathyroidism

In pseudohypoparathyroidism, although hyperphosphataemia and hypocalcaemia are accompanied by tetany and often by fits, the parathyroids are normal or hyperplastic and the electrolyte disturbances are unaffected by the administration of Para-thor-mone. The EEG shows a diminution of *alpha* activity and is made up largely of 4–7 Hz and fast activity. Paroxysms of atypical spike and slow wave activity, sporadic spikes or irregular mixtures of spikes and slow waves occur and are commonly bilaterally synchronous and generalized (Dickson *et al.*, 1960).

Hypercalcaemia

Relatively little has been published on the effects of hypercalcaemia on the EEG. Lehrer and Levitt (1960), and Beare and Millar (1951) refer to cases secondary to excessive consumption of vitamin D or calciferol in which diffuse slow activity becomes prominent in the EEG, while Edwards and Daum (1959) reported similar findings in a single case of parathyroid tumour. Wilson (1965) refers to a further case of parathyroid adenoma whose EEG showed slowing of the dominant rhythm with some diffuse *theta* activity; after operation the EEG returned to normal. Moure (1967) reported 8 cases, 1 with a parathyroid tumour and the others with tumours elsewhere usually associated with widespread bone metastases. It is likely that at the times the EEGs were recorded all showed some degree of clouding of consciousness. In each case diffuse slow activity was present; brief runs of high amplitude 2–4 Hz activity were present often with a marked frontal predominance. In 2 cases the *delta* activity took a triphasic form similar to the discharges sometimes seen in hepatic encephalopathy.

MULTIPLE SCLEROSIS

The incidence of abnormal EEGs in cases of multiple sclerosis is about 50 per cent (Funkhouser and Nagler, 1959). Abnormalities are more frequent in cases in relapse than those in remission. Commonly one finds bilateral 5–7 Hz activity often most prominent frontally but *delta* dominant records may occur particularly in cases with acute and widespread lesions. Ashworth and Emery (1963) suggest that the incidence of abnormality is greater when there is clinical evidence of brainstem involvement.

Gibbs and Becka (1968) found localized areas of attenuation most commonly in the occipital areas in 13 of 123 patients but in others slow wave foci occurred. Of 74 patients described by Fuglsang-Frederiksen and Thygesen (1951) three-quarters showed abnormal EEGs. Serial recordings indicated migratory foci in 47 per cent which appeared to be related to the clinical course of the disease. In some patients it is impossible to relate the EEG foci to the clinical signs.

Improvement in the EEG may occur although the clinical signs persist, but sometimes the reverse situation may be encountered (Macrae and Aird, 1954).

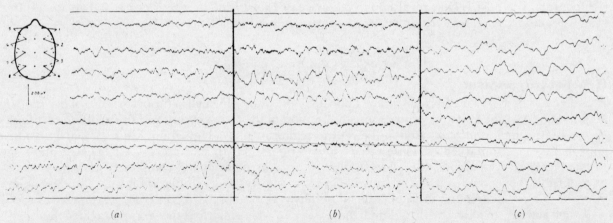

Figure 8.20—Schilder's disease. Boy aged 9 years. Progressive deterioration of intellectual capacity over previous two years. Ataxic with fluctuating confusion. Failure of speech and vision. (a) EEG: Bilateral parieto-occipital irregular slow activity spreading into right central region. (b) Two weeks later. EEG: Higher-voltage slow activity with slight right-sided preponderance. (c) Six weeks later. EEG: Generalized asynchronous lower frequency delta *activity;* theta *components more evident on the left side. Death occurred 10 weeks later*

In some of the small proportion of cases of multiple sclerosis that develop epilepsy, bilateral or localized spikes may occur (Ashworth and Emery, 1963), but as Gibbs and Becka (1968) emphasize, sharp wave and other epileptiform discharges are not a feature of the EEG in multiple sclerosis.

Generalized irregular slow activity (Cobb, Martin and Pampiglione, 1952) or high voltage slow activity with spikes (Gibbs and Gibbs, 1941) may occur in Schilder's disease (*Figure 8.20*).

NEUROMYELITIS OPTICA (DEVIC'S DISEASE)

Reilly and Wilson (1969) found that 6 of 9 cases of neuromyelitis optica had abnormal EEGs. The records showed diffuse *theta* and *delta* activity and it appears that such abnormalities occur more frequently than in multiple sclerosis. The abnormalities become more common a few weeks after the onset of the illness than at the time of the initial visual loss.

MUSCULAR DYSTROPHY

Barwick, Osselton and Walton (1965) were unable to confirm suggestions made in earlier studies that there was any increase in incidence of EEG abnormalities in muscular dystrophy. In patients with dystrophia myotonica, however, the incidence of abnormalities was 61 per cent. Lundervold, Refsum and Jacobsen (1969) found abnormalities in 23 out of 49 patients; the abnormalities consisted of slowing of the *alpha* rhythm with diffuse and occasionally paroxysmal slow activity which they believed to be related to cerebral and metabolic abnormalities including cerebral atrophy that are commonly found in such patients. In myasthenia gravis too, a relatively high incidence of abnormalities has been found by Hokkanen and Toivakka (1969), 34 of 92 cases showing excessive amounts of slow activity, sometimes diffuse and in others, paroxysmal.

PARKINSON'S DISEASE

A number of EEG studies on patients with parkinsonism have shown that although in the majority the EEG remains normal the incidence of abnormalities is greater than that in a normal population. Unfortunately, although parkinsonism can result from a variety of pathological states no aetiological distinctions are drawn as a rule in these studies. Sixty-four per cent of the 223 patients described by Yeager, Alberts and Delattre (1966) had normal EEGs. In the remainder, diffuse slow activity was evident, generally of *theta* frequency but sometimes in the *delta* range. In a few cases focal slow activity was evident but showed no consistent localization in different patients. The findings of Sirakov and Mezan (1963) and Ganglberger (1961) were similar.

Following unilateral stereotactic lesions in the globus pallidus or ventral lateral nucleus of the thalamus the EEG became abnormal in 49 per cent of those with normal preoperative records. The postoperative records were generally obtained about 3 months after operation. The most common abnormalities noted were diffuse slow activity, focal slow activity—generally ipsilateral to the lesion—or both. Paroxysmal slow activity and even bursts of spikes or sharp waves were seen occasionally. Some amplitude asymmetry of the slow activity was present in some cases, the higher amplitude being evident on the side of the lesion. Whether the globus pallidus or the ventral lateral nucleus of the thalamus was the site of the lesion made no difference.

HEPATO-LENTICULAR DEGENERATION (WILSON'S DISEASE)

Heller and Kooi (1962) collating 80 cases from the literature found that EEG abnormalities had been reported in 43. These usually took the form of generalized slow activity or bursts of slow waves. In 28 patients described by Hansotia, Harris and Kennedy (1969), 14 showed similar abnormalities. One case of epilepsy had multifocal and generalized spikes. Improvement of both the EEG and clinical

163

findings has been observed on a number of occasions after treatment with BAL or penicillamine. A rough correlation exists between the EEG abnormality and the severity of the overall clinical picture. Not surprisingly the most severe abnormalities are seen in patients with advanced liver disease.

REFERENCES

Adams, J. H. and Jennett, W. B. (1967). 'Acute Necrotizing Encephalitis: A Problem in Diagnosis'. *J. Neurol. Neurosurg. Psychiat.* **30,** 248

Arentsen, K. and Voldby, H. (1952). 'Electroencephalographic Changes in Neurosyphilis'. *Electroenceph. clin. Neurophysiol.* **4,** 331

Ashworth, B. and Emery, V. (1963). 'Cerebral Dysrhythmia in Disseminated Sclerosis'. *Brain* **86,** 173

Austt, E. G., Torrents, E. and Fournier, J. C. M. (1950). 'The Electroencephalogram in Cushing's Syndrome'. *Electroenceph. clin. Neurophysiol.* **2,** 103

Barwick, D. D., Osselton, J. W. and Walton, J. N. (1965). 'Electroencephalographic Studies in Hereditary Myopathy'. *J. Neurol. Neurosurg. Psychiat.* **28,** 109

Beare, J. M. and Millar, J. H. (1951). 'Epileptiform Fits during Calciferol Therapy'. *Lancet* **1,** 884

Bejsovec, M., Kulenda, Z. and Ponca, E. (1967). 'Familial Intrauterine Convulsions in Pyridoxine Dependency.' *Archs Dis. Childh.* **42,** 301

Bental, E. and Leibowitz, U. (1961). 'Flat Electroencephalograms during 28 days in a Case of "Encephalitis".' *Electroenceph. clin. Neurophysiol.* **13,** 457

Bickford, R. G. and Butt, H. R. (1955). 'Hepatic Coma: The Electroencephalographic Pattern'. *J. clin. Invest.* **34,** 790

— Dawson, B. and Takeshita, H. (1965). 'EEG Evidence of Neurologic Death'. *Electroenceph. clin. Neurophysiol.* **18,** 513

Bird, T. D. and Plum, F. (1968). 'Recovery from Barbiturate Overdose Coma with a Prolonged Isoelectric Electroencephalogram'. *Neurology* **18,** 456

Bokonjić, N. (1963). 'Stagnant Anoxia and Carbon Monoxide Poisoning: A Clinical and Electroencephalographic Study in Humans' *Electroenceph. clin. Neurophysiol.* Suppl. 21, 47

Cadilhac, J. and Ribstein, M. (1961). 'The EEG in Metabolic Disorders'. *Wld. Neurol.* **2,** 296

— — and Jean, R. (1959). 'EEG et troubles métaboliques'. *Revue neurol.* **100,** 270

Carels, G. (1960). 'Etude physiopathologique d'un syndrome myoclonique chez deux enfants atteints d'une forme infantile tardive de l'idiotie amaurotique'. *Acta neurol. psychiat. belg.* **60,** 435

Chaptal, J., Passouant, P., Brunel, D., Latour, H., Jean, R. and Cadilhac, J. (1951). 'Le trace de monorhythmie sinusoïdale lente à prédominance postérieure au cours de la méningite tuberculeuse de l'enfant. Intérêt diagnostique et prognostique'. *Bull. Soc. méd. Hôp. Paris* **67,** 1409

Cobb, W. A. (1964). 'Subacute Progressive Encephalitis'. *Electroenceph. clin. Neurophysiol.* **17,** 604

— (1966). 'The Periodic Events of Subacute Sclerosing Leucoencephalitis'. *Electroenceph. clin. Neurophysiol.* **21,** 278

— and Hill, D. (1950). 'Electroencephalogram in Subacute Progressive Encephalitis'. *Brain* **73,** 392

— Martin, F. and Pampiglione, G. (1952). 'Cerebral Lipidosis: an Electroencephalographic Study'. *Brain* **75,** 343

— and Morgan-Hughes, J. A. (1968). 'Non-Fatal Subacute Sclerosing Leucoencephalitis'. *J. Neurol. Neurosurg. Psychiat.* **31,** 115

Coursin, D. B. (1954). 'The Relationship of Vitamin B-6 to Convulsive Seizures'. *Electroenceph. clin. Neurophysiol.* **6,** 695

Davidson, L. A. G. and Jefferson, J. M. (1959). 'Electroencephalographic Studies in Respiratory Failure'. *Br. med. J.* **2,** 396

Diamond, E. F. and Tentler, R. (1962). 'The Electroencephalogram in Rheumatic Fever'. *J. Am. med. Ass.* **182,** 685

Dickson, L. G., Morita, Y., Cowsert, E. J., Graves, J. and Meyer, J. S. (1960). 'Neurological, Electroencephalographic and Heredo-familial Aspects of Pseudohypoparathyroidism and Pseudo-pseudohypoparathyroidism'. *J. Neurol. Neurosurg. Psychiat.* **23,** 33

Doutlik, S. and Janda, V. (1963). 'Episodic EEG Activity in Exanthematic Parainfectious Encephalitis'. *Confin. neurol.* **22,** 81

Dow, R. S. (1961). 'The Electroencephalographic Findings in Acute Intermittent Porphyria'. *Electroenceph. clin. Neurophysiol.* **13,** 425

Dreyfus-Brisac, C. and Mises, R. (1953). 'Etude EEG de 28 addisoniens'. *Electroenceph. clin. Neurophysiol.* **5,** 133

Drift, J. H. A. Van der (1957). *The Significance of Electroencephalography for the Diagnosis and Localization of Cerebral Tumours.* Leiden; Stenfert Kroese

Duffy, G. J. (1969). 'Herpes Simplex Encephalitis: Neurosurgical Implications and Treatment'. *J. Neurol. Neurosurg. Psychiat.* **32,** 634

Edwards, G. A. and Daum, S. M. (1959). 'Increased Spinal Fluid Protein in Hyperparathyroidism and other Hypercalcemic States'. *Archs intern. Med.* **104,** 29

Ellingson, R. J. and Schain, R. J. (1969). 'EEG Patterns in Juvenile Cerebral Lipidosis'. *Electroenceph. clin. Neurophysiol.* **27,** 191

Engel, G. L. and Romano, J. (1959). 'Delirium, a Syndrome of Cerebral Insufficiency'. *J. chron. Dis.* **9,** 260

— Webb, J. P. and Ferris, E. B. (1945). 'Quantitative Electroencephalographic Studies of Anoxia in Humans. Comparison with Acute Alcoholic Intoxication and Hypoglycaemia'. *J. clin. Invest.* **24,** 691

Espinas, O. E. and Faris, A. A. (1969). 'Acute Infantile Gaucher's Disease in Identical Twins'. *Neurology* **19,** 133

Farrell, D. F. (1969). 'The EEG in Progressive Multifocal Leukoencephalopathy'. *Electroenceph. clin. Neurophysiol.* **26,** 200

Fischer-Williams, M. (1963). 'Burst-Suppression Activity as an Indication of Undercut Cortex'. *Electroenceph. clin. Neurophysiol.* **15,** 723

Fischgold, H. and Mathis, P. (1959). *Obnubilations, Comas et Stupeurs:* Etudes Electroencéphalographiques. *Electroenceph. clin. Neurophysiol.* Suppl. 11

— Ajuriaguerra, J. and Vigne, R. de la (1945). 'L'électroencéphalogramme dans l'intoxication oxycarbonnée'. *C. r. Soc. Biol.* **139,** 401

REFERENCES

Foley, J. M., Watson, C. M. and Adams, R. D. (1950). 'Significance of the Electroencephalographic Changes in Hepatic Coma'. *Trans. Am. neurol. Ass.* **75,** 161

Fournet, A. and Lanternier, Mlle. (1956). 'Constatations électroencéphalographiques dans 17 cas d'encéphalopathie de Gayet-Wernicke'. *Revue neurol.* **94,** 644

Fowler, W. M., Kavan, E. M. and Walter, R. D. (1962). 'Open-Heart Surgery: Neurological Findings and Electroencephalographic Patterns, Before, During and After Open-Heart Surgery'. *Am. J. Dis. Child.* **104,** 131

Frantzen, E. (1966). 'Wernicke's Encephalopathy'. *Acta neurol. scand.* **42,** 426

Friedlander, W. J. (1956). 'Electroencephalographic Changes in Hyperammonemia'. *Electroenceph. clin. Neurophysiol.* **8,** 513

Fuglsang-Frederiksen, V. and Thygesen, P. (1951). 'The Electroencephalogram in Multiple Sclerosis: Analysis of a Series Submitted to Continuous Examination and Discussions'. *Arch. Neurol. Psychiat.* **66,** 504

Funkhouser, J. B. and Nagler, B. (1959). 'The Electroencephalogram in Multiple Sclerosis'. *Dis. nerv. Syst.* **20,** 41

Ganglberger, J. A. (1961). 'The EEG in Parkinsonism and its Alteration by Stereotaxically Produced Lesions in Pallidum or Thalamus'. *Electroenceph. clin. Neurophysiol.* **13,** 828

Garsche, R. (1951). 'Über die hirnelektrischen Veränderungen bei der Kindlichen Poliomyelitis. Eine klinishe und elektro-encephalographische Studie der Epidemic das Jahres 1950'. *Arch. Psychiat. Nervenkr.* **187,** 363

Gibbs, C. J. and Gajdusek, D. C. (1969). 'Infection as the Etiology of Spongiform Encephalopathy (Creutzfeldt–Jakob Disease)'. *Science* **165,** 1023

Gibbs, F. A. and Gibbs, E. L. (1941). *Atlas of Electroencephalography.* p. 159. Cambridge, Mass.; Cummings

— and Becka, D. (1968). 'Reappraisal of the Electroencephalogram in Multiple Sclerosis'. *Dis. nerv. Syst.* **29,** 589

Glaser, G. H. and Levy, L. L. (1960). 'Seizures and Idiopathic Hypoparathyroidism: A Clinical-Electroencephalographic Study'. *Epilepsia* **1,** 454

Gloor, P., Kalabay, O. and Giard, N. (1968). 'The Electroencephalogram in Diffuse Encephalopathies: Electroencephalographic Correlates of Grey and White Matter Lesions'. *Brain* **91,** 779

Goldberg, A. (1959). 'Acute Intermittent Porphyria. A Study of 50 Cases'. *Q. Jl. Med.* **28,** 183

Gubbay, S. S. and Barwick, D. D. (1966). 'Two Cases of Hypothermia in Parkinson's Disease with Unusual EEG Findings'. *J. Neurol. Neurosurg. Psychiat.* **29,** 459

Hagberg, B., Sourander, P. and Svennerholm, L. (1962). 'Sulfatide Lipidosis in Childhood'. *Am. J. Dis. Child.* **104,** 644

Hansotia, P., Harris, R., and Kennedy, J. (1969). 'EEG Changes in Wilson's Disease'. *Electroenceph. clin. Neurophysiol.* **27,** 335

Harden, A. and Pampiglione, G. (1966). 'EEG Studies in Children with Circulatory Arrest during Hypothermia'. *Electroenceph. clin. Neurophysiol.* **21,** 202

Harlem, O. K. (1960). 'Juvenile Cerebroretinal Degeneration (Spielmeyer-Vogt)'. *Am. J. Dis. Child.* **100,** 918

Heller, G. L. and Kooi, K. A. (1962). 'The Electroencephalogram in Hepato-lenticular Degeneration (Wilson's Disease)'. *Electroenceph. clin. Neurophysiol.* **14,** 520

Heron, W. (1961). 'Cognitive and Physiological Effects of Perceptual Isolation'. In *Sensory Deprivation,* p. 6. Ed. by P. Solomon *et al.* Cambridge, Mass.; Harvard University Press

Hockaday, J. M., Potts, F., Epstein, E., Bonazzi, A. and Schwab, R. S. (1965). 'Electroencephalographic Changes in Acute Cerebral Anoxia from Cardiac or Respiratory Arrest'. *Electroenceph. clin. Neurophysiol.* **18,** 575

Hokkanen, E. and Toivakka, E. (1969). 'Electroencephalographic Findings in Myasthenia Gravis'. *Acta neurol. scand.* **45,** 556

Hughes, J. G., Hill, F. S. and Davis, B. C. (1950). 'Electroencephalographic Findings in Acute Nephritis'. *J. Pediat.* **36,** 451

Hughes, R. R. and Summers, V. K. (1956). 'Changes in the Electroencephalogram Associated with Hypopituitarism due to Post-partum Necrosis'. *Electroenceph. clin. Neurophysiol.* **8,** 87

Ingvar, D. H. (1967). 'Cerebral Metabolism, Cerebral Blood Flow and EEG'. In *Recent Advances in Clinical Neurophysiology.* Ed. by L. Widen. *Electroenceph. clin. Neurophysiol.* Suppl. 25, 102

Jacob, J. C., Gloor, P., Elwan, O. H., Dossetor, J. B. and Pateras, V. R. (1965). 'Electroencephalographic Changes in Chronic Renal Failure'. *Neurology* **15,** 419

Jervis, G. A. (1960). 'Infantile Metachromatic Leucodystrophy (Greenfield's Disease)'. *J. Neuropath. exp. Neurol.* **19,** 323

Jones, D. P. and Nevin, S. (1954). 'Rapidly Progressive Cerebral Degeneration (Subacute Vascular Encephalopathy) with Mental Disorder, Focal Disturbances and Myoclonic Epilepsy'. *J. Neurol. Neurosurg. Psychiat.* **17,** 148

Kalyanaraman, K., Niedermeyer, E., Rowe, R. and Wolf, K. (1968). 'The Electroencephalogram in Congenital Heart Disease'. *Archs Neurol.* **18,** 98

Kennedy, A. C., Linton, A. L., Luke, R. G. and Renfrew, S. (1963). 'Electroencephalographic Changes during Haemodialysis'. *Lancet* **1,** 408

Kiloh, L. G. and Nevin, S. (1950). 'Acute Porphyria with Severe Neurological Changes'. *Proc. R. Soc. Med.* **43,** 948

Klinger, M. (1954). 'EEG Observations in Uraemia'. *Electroenceph. clin. Neurophysiol.* **6,** 519

Klinken-Rasmussen, L. and Dyggve, H. V. (1965). 'A Case of Late Infantile Amaurotic Idiocy of the Myoclonus Type'. *Acta neurol. scand.* **41,** 172

Kohner, E. M., Allen, E. M., Saunders, K. B., Emery, V. M. and Pallis, C. (1967). 'Electroencephalogram and Retinal Vessels in Congenital Cyanotic Heart Disease before and after Surgery'. *Br. med. J.* **4,** 207

Laidlaw, J. and Read, A. E. (1961). 'The Electroencephalographic Diagnosis of Manifest and Latent "Delirium" with Particular Reference to that Complicating Hepatic Cirrhosis'. *J. Neurol. Neurosurg. Psychiat.* **24,** 58

Lansing, R. W. and Trunnell, J. B. (1963). 'Electroencephalographic Changes Accompanying Thyroid Deficiency in Man'. *J. clin. Endocr.* **23,** 470

Larson, D. L. (1961). *Systemic Lupus Erythematosus,* pp. 41, 57 and 103. Boston; Little, Brown

Lavy, S., Lavy, R. and Brand, A. (1964). 'Neurological and Electroencephalographic Abnormalities in Rheumatic Fever'. *Acta neurol. scand.* **40,** 76

Lehrer, G. M. and Levitt, M. F. (1960). 'Neuropsychiatric Presentation of Hypercalcemia'. *J. Mt. Sinai Hosp.* **27,** 10

Lennox, M. A. and Peterson, P. B. (1958). 'Electroencephalographic Findings in Acute Carbon Monoxide Poisoning'. *Electroenceph. clin. Neurophysiol.* **10,** 63

Lesse, S., Hoefer, P. F. A. and Austin, J. H. (1958). 'The Electroencephalogram in Diffuse Encephalopathies'. *Arch. Neurol. Psychiat.* **79,** 359

165

Lewis, B. I., Sinton, D. W. and Knott, J. R. (1954). 'Central Nervous System Involvement in Disorders of Collagen'. *Archs intern. Med.* **93,** 315

Lindgren, S., Petersén, I. and Zwetnow, N. (1968). 'Prediction of Death in Serious Brain Damage'. *Acta chir. scand.* **134,** 405

Loeb, C. (1958). 'Electroencephalographic Changes During the State of Coma'. *Electroenceph. clin. Neurophysiol.* **10,** 589

Lombroso, C. T. (1968). 'Remarks on the EEG and Movement Disorder in S.S.P.E.'. *Neurology* **18,** January Suppl. 69

Lorenz, R. (1969). 'Concerning Electrical Death of the Brain'. *Electroenceph. clin. Neurophysiol.* **26,** 449

Lundervold, A., Refsum, S. and Jacobsen, W. (1969). 'The EEG in Dystrophia Myotonica'. *Europ. Neurol.* **2,** 279

McQuarrie, I. and Peeler, D. B. (1931). 'The Effects of Sustained Pituitary Antidiuresis and Forced Water Drinking in Epileptic Children. A Diagnostic and Etiologic Study'. *J. clin. Invest.* **10,** 915

Macrae, D. and Aird, R. B. (1954). 'The Electroencephalogram in Multiple Sclerosis'. *Electroenceph. clin. Neurophysiol.* **6,** 699

Meyer, J. S., Fang, H. C. and Denny-Brown, D. (1954). Polarographic Study of Cerebral Collateral Circulation'. *Archs Neurol. Psychiat.* **72,** 296

Millar, J. H. D. and Coey, A. (1959). 'The EEG in Necrotizing Encephalitis'. *Electroenceph. clin. Neurophysiol.* **11,** 582

Moure, J. M. B. (1967). 'The Electroencephalogram in Hypercalcemia'. *Archs Neurol.* **17,** 34

Nevin, S., McMenemey, W. H., Behrman, S. and Jones, D. P. (1960). 'Subacute Spongiform Encephalopathy—A Subacute Form of Encephalopathy Attributable to Vascular Dysfunction (Spongiform Cerebral Atrophy)'. *Brain* **83,** 519

Nieman, E. A. (1959). 'The Electroencephalogram in Myxoedema Coma. Clinical and Electroencephalographic Study of Three Cases'. *Br. med. J.* **1,** 1204

— (1961). 'The Electroencephalogram in Congenital Hypothyroidism: A Study of 10 Cases'. *J. Neurol. Neurosurg. Psychiat.* **24,** 50

Pampiglione, G. (1961). 'EEG in Inborn Errors of Metabolism'. *Excerpta med. Int. Congress Series* **39,** 2

— (1962). 'Electroencephalographic Studies after Cardiorespiratory Arrest'. *Proc. R. Soc. Med.* **55,** 653

— (1965). 'Electroencephalographic and Metabolic Changes after Surgical Operations'. *Lancet* **2,** 263

— (1968). 'Some Inborn Metabolic Disorders Affecting Cerebral Electrogenesis'. In *Some Recent Advances in Inborn Errors of Metabolism,* p. 80. Ed. by K. S. Holt and V. P. Coffey. Edinburgh; Livingstone

— and Harden, A. (1968). 'Prognostic Value of Neurophysiological Studies in the First Hours Following Resuscitation: A Review of 120 Children after Cardiac Arrest'. *Electroenceph. clin. Neurophysiol.* **25,** 91

— Young, S. E. J. and Ramsay, A. M. (1963). 'Neurological and Electroencephalographic Problems of the Rubella Epidemic of 1962'. *Br. med. J.* **2,** 1300

Parsons-Smith, B. G., Summerskill, W. H. J., Dawson, A. M. and Sherlock, S. (1957). 'The Electroencephalograph in Liver Disease'. *Lancet* **2,** 867

Prior, P. F. (1969). 'EEG Findings in Dying and Resuscitated Adult Patients'. *Electroenceph. clin. Neurophysiol.* **27,** 333

Radermecker, J. (1949). 'Aspects électroencéphalographiques dans cas d'encéphalite subaiguë'. *Acta neurol. belg.* **49,** 222

— (1955). 'The EEG in the Encephalitides and Related Cerebral Disorders'. *Electroenceph. clin. Neurophysiol.* **7,** 448

— (1956). 'Systématiques et électroencéphalographie des encéphalities et encéphalopathies'. *Electroenceph. clin. Neurophysiol.* Suppl. **5**

Regis, H., Toga, M. and Righini, C. (1961). 'Clinical, Electroencephalographic and Pathological Study of a Case of Adams-Stokes Syndrome'. In *Cerebral Anoxia and the Electroencephalogram,* p. 295. Ed. by H. Gastaut and J. S. Meyer. Springfield; Thomas

Reilly, E. L. and Wilson, W. P. (1969). 'EEG Findings in Devic's Disease'. *Electroenceph. clin. Neurophysiol.* **27,** 549

Richardson, E. P. (1961). 'Progressive Multifocal Leukoencephalopathy'. *New Engl. J. Med.* **265,** 815

Rohmer, F., Wackenheim, A. and Kurtz, D. (1959). 'L'EEG dans les syndromes endocriniens hypophysaires, thyroïdiens, surrenaux et dans le tétanie de l'adulte'. *Revue neurol.* **100,** 297

Roseman, E. (1950). 'Electroencephalographic Studies of the Encephalopathies I. Arsenical "Haemorrhagic Encephalopathy" '. *Archs Neurol. Psychiat.* **64,** 448

Rosoff, S. D. and Schwab, R. S. (1968). 'The EEG in Establishing Death'. *Electroenceph. clin. Neurophysiol.* **24,** 283

Russell, P. W., Haserick, J. R. and Zucker, E. M. (1951). 'Epilepsy in Systemic Lupus Erythematosus: Analysis of 100 Cases'. *J. Am. med. Ass.* **171,** 1055

Saunders, M. G. (1954). 'Electroencephalographic Findings in a Case of Familial Periodic Paralysis with Hypopotassaemia'. *Electroenceph. clin. Neurophysiol.* **6,** 499

Schettler, G. and Kahlke, W. (1967). 'Niemann–Pick Disease'. In *Lipids & Lipidoses,* p. 291. Ed. by G. Schettler. New York; Springer

Schneck, L. (1965). 'The Early Electroencephalographic and Seizure Characteristics of Tay–Sachs' Disease'. *Acta neurol. scand.* **41,** 163

Schwab, R. S., Potts, F. and Bonazzi, A. (1963). 'EEG as an Aid in Determining Death in the Presence of Cardiac Activity (Ethical, Legal and Medical Aspects)'. *Electroenceph. clin. Neurophysiol.* **15,** 147

Scott, J. W. (1955). 'The EEG During Hypothermia'. *Electroenceph. clin. Neurophysiol.* **7,** 466

Shev, E. S. and Robinson, S. J. (1961). 'Electroencephalographic Findings Associated with Congenital Heart Disease'. In *Cerebral Anoxia and the Electroencephalogram.* Ed. by H. Gastaut and J. S. Meyer. Springfield; Thomas

Silverman, D. (1962). 'Some Observations on the EEG in Hepatic Coma'. *Electroenceph. clin. Neurophysiol.* **14,** 53

— (1963). 'Retrospective Study of the EEG in Coma'. *Electroenceph. clin. Neurophysiol.* **15,** 486

Sirakov, A. A. and Mezan, I. S. (1963). 'EEG Findings in Parkinsonism'. *Electroenceph. clin. Neurophysiol.* **15,** 321

Sluijter, M. E. (1967). 'The Treatment of Carbon Monoxide Poisoning by Administration of Oxygen at High Atmospheric Pressure'. *Prog. Brain Res.* **24,** 123

Smith, S., Thakurdas, H. and Lawes, T. G. G. (1961). 'Perceptual Isolation and Schizophrenia'. *J. ment. Sci.* **107,** 839

Srikantia, S. G., Veeraraghava Reddy, M. and Krishnaswamy, K. (1968). 'Electroencephalographic Patterns in Pellagra'. *Electroenceph. clin. Neurophysiol.* **25,** 386

Storm van Leeuwen, W. (1964). 'Electroencephalographical and Neurophysiological Aspects of Subacute Sclerosing Leucoencephalitis.' *Folia psychiat. neurol, neurochir. neerl.* **67,** 312

— Mechelse, K., Kok, L. and Zierfuss, E. (1961). 'EEG during Heart Operations with Artificial Circulation'. In *Cerebral Anoxia and the Electroencephalogram,* p. 268. Ed. by H. Gastaut and J. S. Meyer. Springfield; Thomas

REFERENCES

Turrell, R. C. and Roseman, E. (1955). 'Electroencephalographic Studies of the Encephalopathies IV. Serial Studies of Meningococcic Meningitis'. *Archs Neurol. Psychiat.* **73,** 141

— Shaw, W., Schmidt, R. P., Levy, L. L. and Roseman, E. (1953). 'Electroencephalographic Studies of the Encephalopathies II. Serial Studies in Tuberculous Meningitis'. *Electroenceph. clin. Neurophysiol.* **5,** 53

Upton, A. and Gumpert, J. (1970). 'Electroencephalography in the Diagnosis of Herpes-simplex Encephalitis'. *Lancet* **1,** 650

Vague, J., Gastaut, H., Codaccioni, J. L., Roger, A. and Miller, G. (1961). 'L'électroencéphalogramme des hyperthyroides'. In *Advances in Thyroid Research*, p. 253. Ed. by R. Pitt-Rivers. Oxford; Pergamon

Vallat, J. N., Lepetit, J. M., Demarti, D. and Boutet, P. (1962). 'Accidents neurologiques de la pellagre. A propos d'une observation électro-clinique'. *Presse méd.* **70,** 625

Walton, J. N., Kiloh, L. G., Osselton, J. W. and Farrall, J. (1954). 'The Electroencephalogram in Pernicious Anaemia and Subacute Combined Degeneration of the Cord'. *Electroenceph. clin. Neurophysiol.* **6,** 45

Watson, C. W., Flynn, R. E. and Sullivan, J. F. (1958). 'A Distinctive Electroencephalographic Change Associated with Subdural Haematoma Resembling Changes which Occur with Hepatic Encephalopathy'. *Electroenceph. clin. Neurophysiol.* **10,** 780

Wilson, W. P. (1965). 'The Electroencephalogram in Endocrine Disorders'. In *Applications of Electroencephalography in Psychiatry*, p. 102. Ed. by W. P. Wilson. Durham, N. Carolina; Duke University Press

— and Johnson, J. E. (1964). 'Thyroid Hormone and Brain Function. I: The EEG in Hyperthyroidism with Observations on the Effect of Age, Sex and Reserpine in the Production of Abnormalities'. *Electroenceph. clin. Neurophysiol.* **16,** 321

Wyke, B. (1963). *Brain Function and Metabolic Diseases*. London; Butterworths

Yeager, C. L., Alberts, W. W. and Delattre, L. D. (1966). 'Effects of Stereotaxic Surgery upon Electroencephalographic Status of Parkinsonian Patients'. *Neurology* **16,** 904

Zappoli, R. (1959). 'Transient Electroencephalographic Pattern Characteristic of Subacute Leucoencephalitis in a Case of Acute Head Injury'. *Electroenceph. clin. Neurophysiol.* **11,** 571

Zubek, J. P., Welch, G. and Saunders, M. G. (1963). 'Electroencephalographic Changes during and after 14 Days of Perceptual Deprivation'. *Science* **139,** 490

CHAPTER 9

PSYCHIATRY

INTRODUCTION

It must be admitted that from clinical, nosological and prognostic points of view, the value of the EEG in psychiatry is limited. Nevertheless, many interesting observations have been made in this field and although their significance is often far from clear, they represent a challenge to investigators and heuristically may prove to be of importance.

There are many difficulties facing electroencephalographers concerned with psychiatric problems. A number of conditions, notably the neuroses, the behaviour disorders and subnormality, show only quantitative differences from normality and there is more than a hint of artifice about the distinctions we are forced to make on practical grounds. Furthermore—and this is particularly true of the three categories mentioned—any one patient may show the features of two or more clinical syndromes and it is clear that systems of rigid diagnostic classification that have proved their value in neurology and other medical disciplines are more difficult to apply to psychiatric cases. Even in the psychoses the establishment of correlates between EEG patterns and clinical groups is hindered by the great variations in diagnostic criteria employed in different centres. The concept of schizophrenia, in particular, is a source of constant disagreement. A further difficulty arises from the absence of adequate methods of quantification which can be applied to psychiatric symptoms. Attempts to grade or rank the complaints of patients are for the most part purely subjective estimates.

Even if the EEG data have proved difficult to evaluate it must be admitted that they have not been well handled. In so many studies groups of patients differing widely in age, diagnosis and duration of illness have been examined and no attempt has been made to match them with controls. Often insufficient allowance has been made for the effects of variations in the emotional state, for the effects of fatigue and of drowsiness and for changes in physiological variables such as the blood sugar. Differences in interpretation hinder the comparison of results from different centres and it is not always realized how subjective interpretation may be. Publications of single exceptional cases though of interest, tend to exert a disproportionate influence and even in more elaborate studies, statistical evaluation of results is sometimes omitted.

The conventional method of detecting brain potentials by means of electrodes on the scalp is relatively crude and it would show undue optimism to expect characteristic and helpful EEG patterns in psychiatric conditions, in many of which the cerebral dysfunction is of an extremely subtle kind.

PERSONALITY

As Hill (1950) points out, the pattern of the adult EEG is as characteristic as a finger-print, although it should be added that one must make due allowance for the effect of ageing and for any untoward cerebral insults that may occur. The striking similarities between the EEGs of identical twins suggest that the EEG pattern of the individual is dependent on genetic factors (Lennox, Gibbs and Gibbs, 1942).

Many attempts have been made to relate the pattern of the EEG, particularly the *alpha* index, to personality traits. Short and Walter (1954) suggest that M type subjects are predominantly visual thinkers, that P types are essentially verbal thinkers, while R types employ mixed imagery (*see* page 54). A more precise measurement of the *alpha* changes during the solution of visual and verbal problems by Stewart and Smith (1959) has failed to show any significant differences between the performances of

M, P and R subjects, though they did find that the solution of visual problems caused a greater reduction in *alpha* amplitude than those of a verbal or abstract nature. This trend was the same for all three groups of subjects.

An attempt to correlate EEG patterns with personality structure as revealed by psychoanalysis was made by Saul, Davis and Davis (1949) who found that individuals classed as 'passive', that is who were inclined to be dependent and were reluctant to accept responsibility, almost all had high amplitude *alpha* rhythms of the P or R types with little activity at other frequencies. A contrasting group comprised those classed as 'active', in other words those who tended to be independent, competitive and inherently aggressive. This group consisted mainly of women with either marked masculine trends or unusually strong maternal drives; a large proportion of them had low amplitude M type records. A further type of EEG pattern in which there was a considerable amount of fast activity often associated with an irregular *alpha* rhythm, was claimed to correlate with 'frustration'. This pattern too was more frequent in women. It is of interest that these findings, which appear to anticipate those obtained by Gastaut, Dongier and Dongier (1960), provided the first evidence that certain EEG patterns occur more often in one sex than the other. Some of these observations must be accepted with reserve as the subjects were undergoing analysis because of personality difficulties and cannot be regarded as representative of the population as a whole.

The association of a high *alpha* index with passivity was also noted by Palmer and Rock (1953). Individuals with these features showed ready acceptance of authority, immature attitudes and were unduly submissive. This study too is not entirely satisfactory. Gastaut, Dongier and Dongier (1960) have made similar claims in regard to patients undergoing prolonged psychotherapy.

Attempts made to relate EEG patterns to intelligence have likewise produced indecisive results. A suggestion by Walter (1953) that there might be a relationship with the EEG frequency-pattern variation has not been confirmed (Ellingson *et al.*, 1957).

Apprehension or unexpected sensory stimulation leads to a reduction in the amount of *alpha* rhythm and an increase in fast activity. The changes are comparable to the activation response described in animals by Magoun and are similar to those occurring spontaneously in anxiety states. There may also be an increase in *alpha* frequency. Hughes and Hendrix (1968) using telemetric recording found that during periods of anxiety and anticipation the *alpha* rhythm of a football player rose from 9–9·5 Hz to 13 Hz. Induced anger or frustration may lead to the appearance of *theta* activity in the temporal areas, especially in children.

DISORDERS OF BEHAVIOUR AND OF PERSONALITY

Many studies have been made of the EEGs of children and adults with disturbances of behaviour or personality abnormalities. There is general agreement that a substantial proportion of their records show evidence of 'immaturity'—that is the EEG pattern is of a type that would be accepted as normal in a younger age group. The use of the word 'immaturity' implies that there has been a lag in development of the appropriate chronological EEG features and carries the further suggestion that in time the pattern might eventually become normal. This undoubtedly is true of a large proportion of cases and evidence has been advanced by Knott *et al.* (1953), particularly the high incidence of morphologically similar records in the parents of these individuals, that the defect is dependent upon genetic determinants. Nevertheless, abnormalities of an indistinguishable kind may follow a variety of lesions both in children and in adults and in some cases the so-called 'immaturity' may be an expression of a birth injury or later cerebral trauma, of a past attack of encephalitis or meningitis, or may be associated with epilepsy. Such illnesses are also well-recognized antecedents of disturbed behaviour and perhaps the grossest of all psychopaths are those suffering from the sequelae of encephalitis lethargica. Another possibility is that in some cases the 'immaturity' may be a psychosomatic effect; psychological influences giving rise to autonomic or endocrine disturbances might cause changes in the biochemical *milieu* of the brain which in turn would be reflected both in the EEG and in abnormal patterns of behaviour (Ellingson, 1954–55). The evidence suggests that although structural lesions, and possibly these psychosomatic effects, are important in some cases, in the majority the EEG abnormalities are associated with delayed maturation and that genetic determinants may play some part.

Behaviour Disorders in Children

An incidence of 50–60 per cent of abnormal EEGs is found in children with behaviour disorders as compared with 10–15 per cent in normal children. The excess of slow activity may be diffuse but is often predominant in—or in older children confined to—the temporal regions. It may be of *theta* or *delta* frequency depending on the age of the child and degree of 'immaturity'. Asymmetry of the slow activity is common and it is often more obvious on the left side, as one might expect from the fact that during normal maturation *theta* activity tends to persist longer in the left temporal region. The amplitude of the slow activity usually fluctuates widely during the recording and may do so in such a way

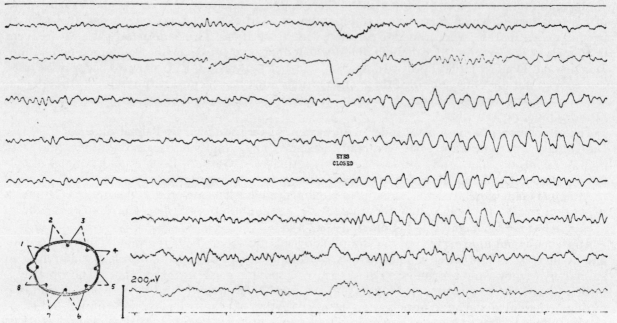

Figure 9.1—Immaturity. Boy aged 7 years with nocturnal enuresis. EEG: Posterior 3 Hz delta rhythm following eye closure

as to impart a paroxysmal quality to the record (*Figure 9.1*). Occipital slow activity is also present to excess in many immature records (Cohn, 1958).

There is no relationship between the degree or type of abnormality and the particular form of the behaviour disorder. Cases of nocturnal enuresis, school phobia, anxiety reactions, antisocial behaviour —the whole range of childhood disorders—show a similar incidence of abnormalities. It is interesting that behaviour disorders occur more commonly in boys than in girls and that maturation of the EEG is usually later in the former (Rey, Pond and Evans, 1949).

Nocturnal Enuresis

Nocturnal enuresis occurs both in children and in young adults. Several authors, including Spear and Turton (1953), have reported a high incidence of epileptiform discharges in such cases but this is not the general experience and must be discounted. The 8 boys studied by Pierce *et al.* (1961) were all enuretic during deep sleep. Ditman and Blinn (1954–55) carried out prolonged EEG recordings on patients with nocturnal enuresis, the great majority of whom were over the age of 17 years. Although the number of children investigated was too small to draw any firm conclusions, the EEG findings tended to confirm the belief that enuretics fall into two groups, those who micturate during deep sleep and those who micturate when their EEGs show a 'waking pattern'. The former state is more common in children, the latter in adolescents and young adults. Indeed, of the 22 cases over the age of 17 years, all but one showed a 'waking *alpha* dominant pattern' when micturition occurred. The subjects often remained unresponsive to stimuli and none was aware of wetting the bed. Schiff (1965) noted that in 3 enuretic soldiers aged 17, 19 and 26 years the EEGs before, during and after enuretic episodes showed low voltage fast activity without REM. In view of this finding and the fact that when Ditman and Blinn published their observations, the variations of the EEG during sleep were not well understood, it seems probable that these patients micturated in a state of dissociation.

SOMNAMBULISM

All night recordings by Kales *et al.* (1966a & b) and Gastaut (1966) showed that episodes of somnambulism occur during slow wave sleep (stages 3 and 4) and never in the REM periods. Somnambulism can sometimes be induced when subjects are raised to their feet in the slow wave period but a similar manoeuvre in the REM phase leads to awakening. As compared with normal children the somnambulistic subjects showed sudden high voltage bursts of *delta* activity during slow wave sleep, which the authors regard as evidence of 'immaturity'. Generally, the sleepwalking episode began with one of these bursts. In the longer episodes the slow wave activity was replaced by low voltage fast activity. Nightmares are generally associated with REM sleep.

KLEINE–LEVIN SYNDROME (PERIODIC HYPERSOMNIA)

The aetiology of the Kleine–Levin syndrome, which is characterized by hypersomnia lasting for periods of several days often accompanied by compulsive overeating, remains unknown, although it is believed that the diencephalon is implicated. Two of Critchley's (1962) patients had abnormal EEGs during the attacks but the changes were slight and non-specific; they were less obvious than might have been expected at a comparable stage of normal sleep. In the patient described by Elian and Bornstein (1969) the EEG was normal when the patient was well but showed bursts of high amplitude slow activity against a normal or *theta* dominant background during an attack even though the patient was kept awake while the recording was in progress. Thacore, Ahmed and Oswald's (1969) patient could not be fully aroused from his sleepy state; his EEG showed diffuse *theta* and *delta* activity with frequent high amplitude bursts of *delta* activity. The appearances were not those of sleep and in particular, spindles were never seen.

PERSONALITY DISORDERS AND PSYCHOPATHY

Terminological differences and varying diagnostic criteria make it difficult to compare the work on personality disorders and psychopathy carried out at different centres. Schneider's (1958) approach provides a more logical and useful classification but Henderson's (1939) concepts are perforce followed in this section, as it is in the main the grosser psychopaths, in particular those showing aggressive behaviour, who have been most extensively studied. A large proportion of patients presenting with personality disturbances give a history of disordered behaviour in childhood.

One of the largest and most detailed investigations was carried out by Hill (1952). In 194 non-epileptic psychopaths, the majority of whom showed aggressive behaviour, Hill found that one or more of three varieties of abnormality might occur, all indicative of a maturational defect of cerebral organization.

The commonest finding was an excess of bilateral rhythmical *theta* activity with an amplitude equal to or greater than that of the *alpha* rhythm (*Figure 9.2*). It predominated in the temporal and central areas and showed no blocking response to visual stimulation but was accentuated, often grossly so, on overbreathing. In the majority an *alpha* rhythm was present, but in some it was poorly developed or absent. The incidence of this type of record, which is similar to that already described in children with behaviour disorders, was 22 per cent as compared with 11·7 per cent in a control group.

In 3·2 per cent of Hill's cases *alpha* variants were present as compared with 1 per cent of the controls, the *alpha* rhythm being associated with subharmonic components. Higher harmonics of the *alpha* frequency were often present but were not correlated with abnormal behaviour.

The most interesting abnormality was the occurrence, in 14 per cent of cases, of foci of 3–5 Hz activity in the posterior temporal regions (*Figure 9.3*), this phenomenon occurring in only 2 per cent of the controls. This focal slow activity tended to be episodic and its amplitude was often greater than that of the *alpha* rhythm. It was frequently bilateral and symmetrical but was sometimes unilateral. Right-sided foci were rather more common than left. In two-thirds of cases, the slow activity showed

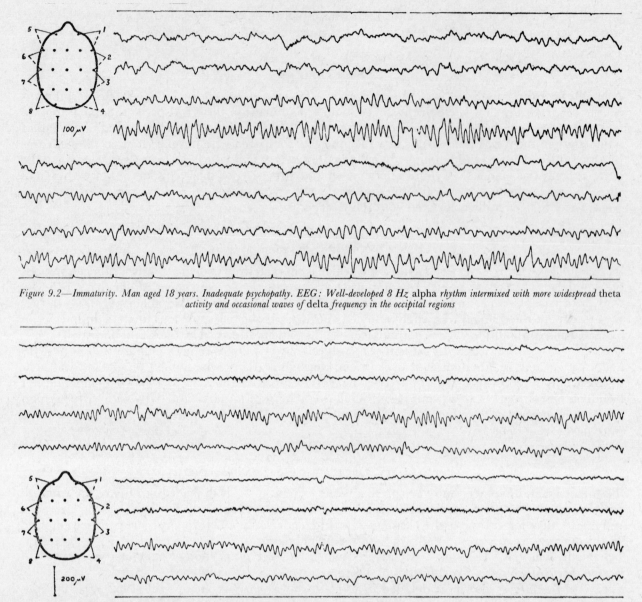

Figure 9.2—Immaturity. Man aged 18 years. Inadequate psychopathy. EEG: Well-developed 8 Hz alpha rhythm intermixed with more widespread theta activity and occasional waves of delta frequency in the occipital regions

Figure 9.3—Posterior temporal delta foci in psychopath. Man aged 21 years. EEG: Well-developed 8–9 Hz alpha rhythm associated with irregular delta activity confined to and sometimes focal in the posterior temporal regions. Both alpha and delta components slightly more marked on the right side

blocking to visual stimuli and it also tended to block on photic stimulation. It was usually accentuated by overbreathing. The bilateral occipital slow activity described by Cohn and Nardini (1958–59) was associated with aggressive behaviour in 75 per cent of cases and also showed blocking to visual stimuli. It is almost certainly the same phenomenon as that described by Hill, and in view of the electrode placements used it is difficult to see why its distribution is not described as posterior temporal.

These maturational defects are usually intermixed with a normal *alpha* rhythm and do not give the impression of replacing it as often occurs with the diffuse slow activity resulting, for instance, from a head injury or from the presence of a posterior fossa tumour. The response of these maturational abnormalities to physiological stimuli is also more marked than that of slow activity due to acquired lesions. All the abnormalities described tend to diminish and even to disappear with increasing age and it is well recognized that there is often a parallel improvement in behaviour.

Although in Hill's series, paroxysmal disturbances—including spike and slow wave discharges, poly-spikes and temporal lobe spikes—occurred in a few cases, their incidence was low and not significantly different from that in the control group.

In many epileptics, particularly those with attacks of a temporal lobe origin, the interseizure behaviour has all the hallmarks of psychopathy. In these cases, similar maturational defects are often evident, combined with frank epileptiform features. Removal of the abnormal temporal lobe in such a case may lead not only to cessation of the fits but to an improvement in the EEG and in behaviour. Nuffield (1961) demonstrated that there were clear behavioural differences between those epileptic children with temporal lobe foci and those with centrencephalic discharges. The former showed high scores for aggression and low scores for neuroticism, whilst the reverse was found in the latter. It is of great theoretical interest that both maturational defects and structural lesions of the temporal lobe should be associated with such similar forms of abnormal behaviour. The incidence and severity of maturational defects, particularly the posterior temporal slow wave foci, are greatest in those psychopaths showing aggressive behaviour. This was particularly evident in the series reported by Williams (1969). After excluding those with epilepsy, mental subnormality or a history of major head injury he compared prisoners who were habitually aggressive with others who had committed single, major violent crimes. The incidence of EEG abnormalities was 57 per cent in the former as compared with 12 per cent in the latter group. In the habitually aggressive group the abnormalities were almost always seen over the anterior part of the brain, the temporal lobes being affected in all.

Alcoholism

Whether or not one accepts alcoholism as a 'disease', from an EEG point of view it seems that the complications are more important than the underlying disorder, although the latter might be expected to be associated with an incidence of non-specific EEG abnormalities higher than that found in the general population. In the absence of prospective studies some care is needed in the interpretation of published figures but those provided by Arentsen and Sindrup (1963) would seem to support this view. In patients with established dependence on alcohol but no other drugs, and whose EEGs were obtained 8 days after withdrawal, the percentages of abnormal records in those classified as normal, neurotic or psychopathic were 21, 26 and 38 per cent respectively. The incidence in the dependent group as a whole was higher in those classified as social drinkers—30 per cent compared with 13 per cent. It seems most probable that these are pre-existing abnormalities and in the absence of complications it does not seem that chronic alcoholism as such gives rise to EEG abnormalities (Greenblatt, Levin and di Cori, 1944).

There were only 8 cases in the Arentsen and Sindrup series with complications such as delirium tremens and 5 of these had abnormal records.

In states of acute intoxication, although many EEGs remain within normal limits, an excess of fast activity, most prominent in the central areas, is frequently seen to be mixed with low amplitude *theta* activity. There may be some reduction in the amount of *alpha* activity. Sobriety is associated with a return of the EEG to normal. The changes in delirium tremens are similar (Funkhouser, 1953; Bennett, Doi and Mowery, 1956). In Wernicke's encephalopathy, bilateral high amplitude *delta* activity is likely (*see* page 157).

Fast activity is frequently prominent in alcoholics with Korsakow states or chronic alcoholic deterioration (alcoholic dementia) but diffuse slow activity with some delta components is equally prominent.

Chromosomal Abnormalities

Cases with XYY chromosome constitution have in large part been identified from prison and mental hospital populations and in these, at any rate, personality abnormalities and criminality, often with aggressive components, are common. It is not surprising perhaps that amongst these the frequency of abnormal EEG patterns is higher than in a normal population. Of 28 such cases assembled from their own case material and the literature by Nielsen and Tsuboi (1969), 12 had abnormal EEGs.

In a psychiatrically biased material, Mellbin (1966) found that all 4 of his patients with Turner's syndrome had abnormal EEGs, 1 showing an excess of slow activity, the other 3 having epileptiform discharges; 2 of the latter patients suffered from epilepsy. In 45 patients with Klinefelter's syndrome, largely culled from mental hospitals and institutions for the mentally subnormal, a slow dominant rhythm or excessive slow activity occurred in 33 (73 per cent) (Hambert and Torsten, 1964). When patients were obtained from medical or neurological clinics by Nielsen and Pedersen (1969) (*see also* Nielsen, 1969) abnormalities were found in only 7 of the 25 cases; 5 of these patients were epileptics. The patients described by Pasquelini, Vidal and Bur (1957) were all supporting themselves in the community—all had normal EEGs.

Criminals

The incidence of EEG abnormalities in criminals is high (Table 9.1), the most frequent abnormality being the presence of 'immature' patterns.

Apart from the difference in incidence, there is nothing to distinguish the EEG abnormalities of psychopaths in prison from those who remain in the community. In other words, such differences as exist are of a quantitative nature. Stafford-Clark and Taylor (1949) carried out an interesting study of 64 individuals whose common link was that they had been charged with murder. In those who had committed motivated murder under considerable provocation, the incidence of abnormal EEGs was 17 per cent, scarcely higher than that in the general population. Those who murdered incidentally or accidentally during the course of committing some other felony showed an incidence of 25 per cent. Amongst explosive psychopaths who had committed murder without motive and without provocation —except in some cases the excitement of aggressive sexual acts—73 per cent showed abnormal EEGs, whilst the highest incidence of 86 per cent occurred in those obviously psychotic at the time they committed their crimes. The figures obtained by Sayed, Lewis and Brittain (1969) were comparable. Of 32 murderers confined to a state mental hospital, 14 were regarded as psychopaths and 50 per cent of these showed abnormal EEGs. The other 18 were all schizophrenics, except for 3 cases of psychotic depression; 78 per cent had abnormal EEGs. Why the incidence of abnormalities should be higher in these than in the functional psychoses in general is not known.

TABLE 9.1

RELATION OF PERSONALITY DISORDER TO INCIDENCE OF ABNORMAL EEGs
[From Stafford-Clark (1959). *Br. med. J.* 2, 1199.]

Category	Incidence of abnormal EEGs (per cent)	Authority
Flying personnel	5	Williams, 1941
RAMC personnel	10	Williams, 1941
Mixed controls	15	Hill and Watterson, 1942
Controls in prison	25	Stafford-Clark, Pond and Doust, 1951
Mixed psychoneurotics	26	Williams, 1941
Inadequate psychopaths	32	Hill and Watterson, 1942
Aggressive psychopaths	65	Hill and Watterson, 1942
Motiveless murderers	73	Stafford-Clark and Taylor, 1949
Aggressive psychopaths in prison	83	Stafford-Clark, Pond and Doust, 1951

A significant difference, as might be anticipated, has been demonstrated between individuals of relatively stable personality with single convictions and those with more obvious personality defects and multiple convictions. In the former, Levy (1952) found the incidence of abnormalities to be 17 per cent compared with 34 per cent in the recidivists.

Fourteen and Six per Second Positive spikes

Runs of 14 and 6 per second positive spikes in sleep EEGs were first described by Gibbs and Gibbs (1951), who claimed that there was an association between this activity and attacks of 'thalamic or hypothalamic epilepsy' in the waking state. They regard such attacks as one of the more common— although frequently unrecognized—forms of epilepsy occurring particularly in adolescents and young adults. The attacks might take the form of syncopal-like states, unrelated to posture but often followed by headache and drowsiness, of episodic pain, usually diagnosed as atypical migraine, neuralgia or sciatica, of paraesthesiae or of episodes of rage and aggressive behaviour including determined homicidal attacks. In the majority of cases they admit that no other form of epileptic attack occurs.

Gibbs and Gibbs (1963) have reviewed this EEG phenomenon. They identified 14 and 6 per second positive spikes in 5,165 of over 38,000 patients in whom sleep and waking records were made, an incidence, they feel, that makes this pattern by far the most common of all the 'paroxysmal cerebral

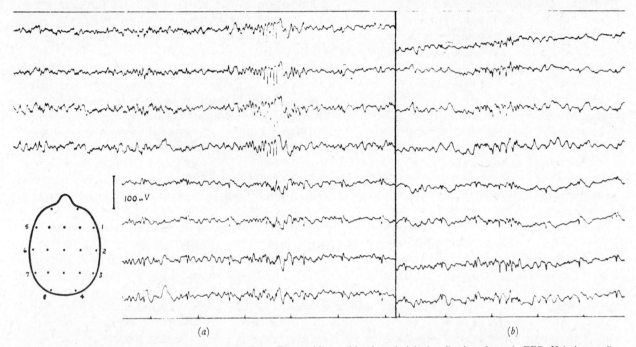

Figure 9.4—14 and 6 per second positive spikes. Boy aged 12 years. Foreceps delivery; delayed speech; behaviour disorder and enuresis. EEG: Unipolar recording during sleep. Channels 1–4 referred to left under-ear electrode; channels 5–8 referred to right under-ear electrode, contaminated by recurrent ECG artefact. (a) Right-sided burst of 14 per second positive spikes. (b) Predominantly right-sided run of 6 per second positive sharp waves

dysrhythmias'. Yet in other EEG laboratories such spikes are seldom identified. In all probability this reflects the recording methods in use. To demonstrate the phenomenon it is usually necessary to use a unipolar montage with wide spacing between the active and reference electrodes (*Figure 9.4*).

Fourteen- and six-per second spikes occur at all ages but are most common in children and young adults. In the series of patients described by Hughes, Gianturco and Stein (1961) the mean age was 15·5 years. Whereas in young children the spikes occur only in deep sleep, with increasing age they occur at progressively lighter stages of sleep so that in adults they may be seen in the waking state. The spikes are most evident in the occipital and temporal areas with a particular predilection for the posterior temporal regions. They are commonly bilateral and synchronous but runs may occur independently on either side and in a few cases the discharges may be persistently unilateral. Analysis of the waveform by Hughes (1965) showed that the precise repetition rate varied from patient to patient and in the same patient from time to time. The frequency of the slow form fell in the range 6·0 to 8·3 per second and the fast form from 12·0 to 19·5 per second, the mean frequencies being 7·1 and 15·2 per second respectively. The fast bursts tended to slow to about 14 per second before giving way to the slower form at about 7 per second which Hughes believes to be a subharmonic. The actual discharges are not accompanied by any clinical phenomena and in most cases the waking EEGs are normal.

The concept of thalamic and hypothalamic epilepsy and its association with the 14 and 6 per second phenomenon is not generally accepted, although Kellaway, Crawley and Kagawa (1960) have put forward a strong plea in its support. They describe a group of 459 children with a 'specific electroclinical syndrome' comprising episodic attacks of headache or abdominal pain or both, associated with other autonomic disturbances and the 14 and 6 per second EEG pattern during sleep. Those in whom recordings were obtained during an attack, showed high voltage slow activity in their EEGs. They claim that amelioration of the attacks is most likely to occur following treatment with phenytoin sodium (Dilantin) or acetazolamide (Diamox).

The literature concerned with the clinical correlates of the 14 and 6 per second phenomenon is confusing and indeed contradictory. Walter *et al.* (1960) classified a number of children into groups according to the EEG findings. Full studies of the children by observers who were ignorant of these failed to show any correlation between behavioural abnormalities and the 14 and 6 per second phenomenon. Refsum *et al.* (1960) found 14 and 6 per second spikes in just over 3 per cent of 3,272 patients drawn from a hospital population. When compared with the patients not showing this abnormality they were noted to suffer a significantly higher incidence of paroxysmal headache, attacks of dizziness, gastrointestinal disturbance, syncope, psychoneurosis and behaviour disturbance.

An interesting study of the clinical correlates of this phenomenon has been carried out by Schwade and Geiger (1960). The patients in the main were under 16 years of age and presented with destructive behaviour, outbursts of uncontrolled rage, violent motiveless and unprovoked acts including larceny, arson, aggressive sexual activity, and occasionally homicide. Emotional blunting and some degree of amnesia for the outbursts were characteristic. Of these patients 73 per cent showed 14 and 6 per second positive spikes, often confined to the temporal and occipital areas of one hemisphere. In a large control group 14 and 6 per second spikes were found in only 1·5 per cent and retrospectively it was discovered that most of these suffered from temper tantrums. These findings are very much in accord with the earlier observation of Grossman (1954) that 14 and 6 per second positive spikes occurred in the posterior regions of the head in aggressive psychopaths.

Long and Johnson (1968) noted 14 and 6 per second positive spikes in 30 of 119 male volunteers. No correlation could be established with scores on the Minnesota Multiphasic Personality Inventory (MMPI) or the Cornell Medical Inventory (CMI), with temper tantrums, altercations with authority or any features of their psychiatric histories. Lombroso *et al.* (1966) found 14 and 6 per second spikes in the sleep EEGs of 90 (58 per cent) of 155 boys aged 13 to 15 years. No significant correlation with any events in the boys' medical histories could be established. Small, Sharpley and Small (1968) found that in children admitted to a psychiatric hospital the presence of 14 and 6 per second spikes correlated with hyperkinesis and other evidence of brain damage, although this was not the case with adults. Pollack *et al.* (1969) could find no difference in the incidence of 14 and 6 per second spikes when they compared psychiatric patients with their siblings. They concluded that this EEG phenomenon is related to maturity of the EEG and has no special psychiatric significance.

The occurrence of 14 and 6 per second positive spikes must now be accepted as an authentic EEG phenomenon. Clinically there is a loose association with a wide range of psychoneurotic symptomatology and behavioural disturbance. It occurs in individuals whose EEGs show other minor abnormalities which are often subsumed under the term 'immaturity'. It is of interest that Hughes, Gianturco and Stein (1961) noted an association with posterior temporal slow activity, particularly on the right side (*see* page 171). Although their spatial distribution differs, 14 per second spikes bear some resemblance to sleep spindles in which the negative phase is rounded off and the positive phase sharpened, a waveform which may be considered as a 14 Hz fundamental plus even order harmonics. If, as has been claimed by Hughes (1960), it is really a 14 and 7 per second phenomenon, it would be possible to explain its waveform in terms of a combination of harmonics. If so, it is doubtful whether the use of the word 'spike' is appropriate; indeed Grossman (1963) has suggested that the term 'burst' should be substituted.

Six Per Second Spike and Wave Complexes

Although commonly described as 6 per cent spike and wave activity, Gibbs and Gibbs (1964) pointed out that the actual repetition rate may vary from 4 to 7 per second. The discharges are usually bilaterally synchronous and symmetrical, the slow wave component being more prominent than the spike. They are best seen during light sleep. The episodes are generally short, lasting under 1 second. Gibbs and Gibbs regard these discharges as epileptiform believing that their most common cause is trauma. Although various authors have attempted to confirm the epileptiform nature of 6 per second spike and wave complexes, no convincing case has been made out and several studies (Silverman, 1967; Small and Small, 1967; Thomas and Klass, 1968) have found no such association. In different series this EEG feature has been found in 0·4–1 per cent of control subjects. Although it is possible that those with these complexes are more likely to experience such symptoms as syncope or abdominal pain or to show personality disorders, the relationship at best is a vague one. Small (1968) however, made the rather surprising observation that 5 per cent of acutely ill hospitalized psychiatric patients showed these 6 per second spike and wave complexes and that their presence was a good prognostic sign.

Because he was able to induce the phenomenon in the EEGs of 10 of 34 subjects by the intravenous injection of 50 mg diphenhydramine, Tharp (1967) concluded that it was a 'normal physiologic cerebral discharge'.

The findings of Silverman (1967) are of considerable interest; after selecting 142 patients because they showed either 6 per second spike and wave complexes or 14 and 6 per second positive spikes, all but 36 showed both. Of the 36, 30 showed only 14 and 6 per second positive spikes and 6 the 6 per second spike and wave complexes. Such an association had been noted by previous authors but not considered to have significance. Silverman believes that the two phenomena are variants of one another and points out that if we accept 14 and 6 or 14 and 7 per second positive spikes as harmonically related frequencies, then if both the 14 and 6 (or 7) components occurred in the same complex the result would be a 6 per second spike and wave complex. He believes that we see these complexes more often in adults because the slower positive spikes are more common than the faster variety in older age groups.

PSYCHONEUROSES

ANXIETY STATES

Although it may be difficult in practice to distinguish between them, it should be remembered that there are two ways in which EEG abnormalities may be associated with anxiety. First, changes may occur in relation to the actual experience of this symptom in the same way that there may be changes in other physiological variables, such as the blood pressure and the pulse; and, secondly, there may be persistent abnormalities in those individuals who comprise the group we designate as chronic anxiety states.

The diminution of the *alpha* rhythm and the increase in fast activity, particularly in the central areas, which occur when anxiety is induced in normal subjects, has already been mentioned and has a precise parallel in patients with anxiety reactions. It is not surprising that when large groups of patients with anxiety states are surveyed, they show statistically a diminished per cent time *alpha* and more fast activity than normal controls, even though the records remain within the limits of normality. The scatter of the EEG phenomena in anxious patients is therefore wider than that of normal controls. The high incidence of 'flat' EEGs in neurotic patients noted by Adams (1959)—19 per cent as compared with 10 per cent of normals having EEGs with an amplitude not greater than 20 μV—is presumably an expression of the same phenomenon. Such patients often show a great deal more *alpha* activity towards the end of the recording as they relax, if they become a little drowsy, or at the commencement of overbreathing.

Maturational defects are common, particularly the presence of 4–7 Hz activity, sometimes limited to the temporal regions or, if generalized, of maximal amplitude in these areas; they may be expected in 20 per cent of cases as compared with 10 per cent of normals.

Ulett *et al.* (1953) found that anxiety-prone individuals tend with photic stimulation to show less driving than normals in the range 8–18 f/s but more in the 2–7 f/s and 20–30 f/s ranges. They also tend to show a response richer in harmonics, especially second harmonics of the 10–15 f/s and fourth harmonics of the 5–7 f/s stimuli (*Figure 9.5*). They are particularly liable to report strange or unpleasant experiences during photic stimulation, such as dizziness, anxiety, nausea, faintness, depersonalization and illusions.

Patients with severe prolonged anxiety respond predictably to repeated light stimuli with *alpha* blocking in the same way as normal subjects. Auditory stimuli give rise to a transient response in both anxious and non-anxious groups. Wells and Wolff (1960) showed that conditioned cerebral responses

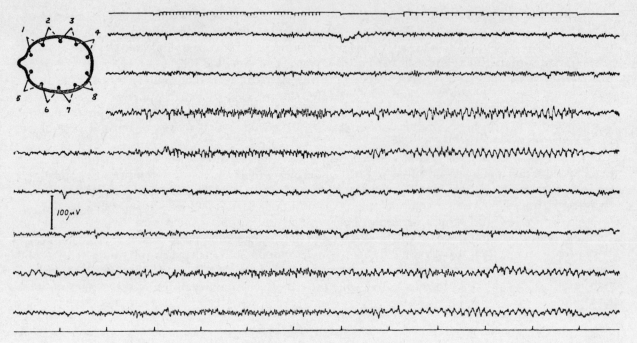

Figure 9.5—Chronic anxiety state—photic stimulation. Man aged 29 years. EEG: Initial stimulation at 14 f/s evokes second harmonic response. Subsequent stimulation at 8 f/s evokes fundamental plus second harmonic response

could be established when the sound was suitably paired with the visual stimulus. It proved much more difficult to establish such responses in anxious patients. The mean number of conditioned cerebral responses in controls given 50 paired stimulations was 10·9 (SD±3·25). In the patients with anxiety the mean number of responses was 4·8 (SD±3·28)—a highly significant difference.

The photo-metrazol threshold is unaffected in anxiety states. The question of the sedation threshold is considered on page 180.

HYSTERIA

A stable *alpha* rhythm has been described as characteristic of hysterical patients but the evidence is unsatisfactory. The incidence of maturational defects is high.

In hysterical blindness, normal blocking of the *alpha* rhythm occurs on eye opening. Similar blocking may occur if an 'anaesthetic' area is pricked with a pin, while evoked potentials can be demonstrated in the appropriate area of the cerebral cortex (*see* page 208).

Hypnosis has no effect in itself on the EEG rhythms. If a tense, anxious patient is hypnotized a good *alpha* rhythm may appear as the patient relaxes and if physiological sleep is induced by suggestion, a normal sleep pattern will develop. Blocking of the *alpha* rhythm may occur if a visual stimulus is suggested to the subject.

In anorexia nervosa Crisp, Fenton and Scotton (1968) found a high incidence of abnormalities. Thirteen of the 32 patients examined had normal records and these tended to be those with shorter illnesses. In the other 19 some showed a general excess of *theta* activity and others slowing of the dominant rhythm below 8 Hz, frequently with an unstable hyperventilation response. Four patients showed epileptiform activity but all had histories of epilepsy. The EEG abnormalities correlated with low serum sodium, potassium and chloride levels. There were 2 cases with severe hypothermia; 1, with a temperature of 31·6°C had a dominant rhythm at 7 Hz and the other, with a temperature of 34°C had a dominant rhythm at 5–6 Hz. The abnormalities appear therefore to be epiphenomena.

OBSESSIONAL STATES

Examination of the literature on EEG abnormalities in obsessional states suggests that these are

178

common. Closer scrutiny shows that in some series, that of Pacella, Polatin and Nagler (1944) for instance, both epileptics and schizophrenics are included. Other papers describe single atypical cases.

Rockwell and Simons (1947) distinguish between true obsessional neuroses and psychopaths with obsessive compulsive features. As compared with the latter, the incidence of abnormalities is low in the true obsessional states. The study of Ingram and McAdam (1960) indicates a low incidence of abnormalities. Amongst 22 cases, only 1 showed bursts of synchronous generalized *delta* activity and this patient was subject to outbursts of temper. In the remainder the EEGs were normal.

HEADACHES AND MIGRAINE

In patients with recurrent headaches unassociated with organic disease, EEG patterns of an immature kind are noted with much the same frequency as in chronically anxious patients. Perhaps this is not surprising for there is a considerable overlap between the two groups. When those patients with indubitable migraine are separated out, they too show a similar incidence and variety of abnormalities between attacks. In 459 patients described by Selby and Lance (1960) 30 per cent of the EEGs recorded when the patients were headache-free showed such abnormalities. Smyth and Winter (1961) found similar EEG changes in 43 per cent of 202 patients. They also demonstrated an association between migraine and a flicker response to flash rates above 20 per second. Hockaday and Whitty (1969) found that 61 per cent of 560 migrainous subjects had abnormal EEGs. Lateralized changes were common especially in cases that experienced lateralized non-visual auras. There was no correlation with duration of history or frequency of attacks and the changes were not regarded therefore as being secondary to the attacks themselves. This series is remarkable both for the number of patients with a personal or family history of epilepsy that amounted to 126 and for the number showing 'dysrhythmic' EEGs, 227 being so described. Weil (1952) described a small number of patients with severe but typical attacks of migraine in whom the slow activity present was of high voltage and had a paroxysmal quality. He proposed the term 'dysrhythmic migraine' for this group, but such a differentiation scarcely seems justifiable.

Engel *et al.* (1944) found that after periods in decompression chambers at simulated altitudes of 30,000 ft or more, some subjects developed attacks of migraine in association with decompression sickness. When a scotoma occurred it was accompanied by a focus of *delta* activity over the contra-lateral occipital lobe. Similar foci were observed during spontaneous migrainous auras by Smyth and Winter (1961) in 2 patients. In 1 the focal *delta* was abolished immediately after the inhalation of carbon dioxide. Camp and Wolff (1961) found that three types of *theta* or *delta* foci could be observed in patients with migraine. In the first the focus develops simultaneously and disappears promptly with resolution of the clinical symptoms; it is likely to be related to local ischaemia. The second variety persists for hours or days and may be related to localized oedema. The third type continues for a longer period and may be associated with lasting focal neurological signs; it usually indicates infarction. During the actual headaches Arellano (1951), using nasopharyngeal and tympanic electrodes, has noted 5–7 Hz activity in the basal areas.

AFFECTIVE DISORDERS

In the field of affective disorders EEG studies have mostly been carried out in manic-depressive psychosis and apart from Shagass' work on sedation thresholds, which is reviewed at the end of this section, there has been little interest shown in the EEG aspects of the neurotic forms of depression. Perris (1966) however, in the course of his very detailed study of the EEG in affective disorders found that 16 out of 39 patients with 'reactive depression' showed 'immature' records. They had a higher *alpha* index than patients with endogenous depression.

Many of the studies of EEG changes found in mania, endogenous depression and involutional depression suffer from the faults enumerated at the beginning of this chapter; a large proportion of them are unsatisfactory and their results inconclusive. Nevertheless, certain trends emerge which appear to have some validity.

179

Even though the majority of patients with manic-depressive illness have normal EEGs, the incidence of abnormalities—20–40 per cent—and the scatter of normal EEG attributes is greater than in the general population. Ten of Dalén's (1965) 35 cases of mania had abnormal records.

A proportion of cases show fast dominant records of the same type described in schizophrenia by Davis (1939–40) as 'choppy'. Their incidence in manic-depressive illness is similar to that seen in schizophrenia. As in this latter condition one suspects that in a proportion of these at any rate, the fast activity may have been barbiturate induced. Finley (1944) found that in some cases the fast activity diminished or disappeared during periods of clinical remission. Hurst, Mundy-Castle and Beerstecher (1954) claimed that in addition to an increase in the frequency, amplitude and amount of fast activity, the mean frequency and the amplitude of the *alpha* rhythm together with the per cent time *alpha* were lower in manic-depressive illness. The significance of these observations is diminished by the fact that the mean age of their cases was 55 years as compared with 22 years in the controls. Using photic stimulation these authors claimed that manic-depressives showed a response of higher amplitude in the range 4–20 f/s and of lower amplitude in the range 21–26 f/s, than the controls.

An observation made originally by Davis (1941) and confirmed by Hurst *et al.* is that the mean *alpha* frequency tends to be high in manic patients and relatively low in depressed patients, although surprisingly, in patients alternating between the two states, the *alpha* frequency does not shift with the changing phases of the illness. As compared with depressives, manic patients show a significantly greater incidence of second and third order harmonics and of responses at the flash frequency in the 14–26 f/s range during photic stimulation.

In a group of depressed patients, Margerison *et al.* (1962) showed that the degree of depression, as measured by reduced verbal output, was accompanied by a tendency towards sodium retention and a decrease in the amount of activity at 6·5–10·5 Hz in the EEG. On the other hand Anderson *et al.* (1964) claimed in a single patient that the amount of *alpha* activity was diminished in the manic as compared with the depressive phase of the illness.

An interesting case of manic-depressive illness is described by Hes (1960), in which a normal EEG with an *alpha* rhythm at 11 Hz occurred in the depressive phases, while in the periods of mania there were brief bursts of symmetrical, high voltage slow activity, of greatest amplitude in the frontal regions.

A study of 3 patients suffering from rapidly alternating periods of mania and depression by Harding *et al.* (1966) has confirmed that one must expect such variations in the EEGs of individual patients. Two of the patients showed a decrease of *alpha* activity in the manic phase with an increase in mean frequency, together with an increase in *beta* activity. In both it was possible to predict the mood of the patient from inspection of the EEG. In the other patient almost opposite results were obtained. These authors conclude that although the EEG does show changes related to the mood of the particular phase of the illness, no constant relationship exists between the type of EEG change, the mood and the biochemical variations.

The association of depression with temporal lobe epilepsy is well recognized. It may be an aural or prodromal phenomenon or occur episodically after temporal lobectomy. In the cases described by Weil (1954), periods of depression were associated with an increased incidence of temporal lobe spikes.

SEDATION THRESHOLD

In the procedure described by Shagass (1954) for establishing the sedation threshold, an intravenous injection of 0·5 mg/kg body weight of amylobarbitone sodium is repeated every 40 seconds until well past the point at which speech becomes slurred. The amount of 15–30 Hz activity recorded from the frontal areas is measured. Initially, Shagass did this visually with the aid of an additive ruler but later he employed a frequency analyser. If muscle artefact interferes with measurement of the frontal fast activity, more posterior electrode placements may be used. A dosage-response curve is plotted between the integrated dosage of sodium amytal and the integrated amount of fast activity. The curve tends to be S-shaped (*Figure 9.6*) and shows an inflection point corresponding roughly with the onset of slurred speech. Beyond this point the amount of fast activity produced by further increments of the drug is sharply diminished. The sedation threshold is defined as the amount of amylobarbitone sodium in mg/kg body weight required to reach this inflection point. Other workers attempting to repeat

180

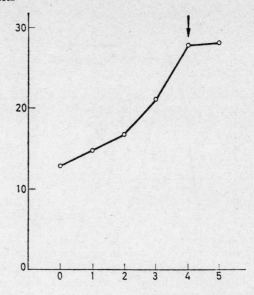

Figure 9.6—Sedation threshold. Normal subject. Ordinate: Mean amplitude of frontal fast activity in μV. Abscissa: Integrated amount of amylobarbitone sodium given intravenously in mg/kg body weight. Arrow denotes point of slurred speech

(From Shagass, C. (1954) 'The sedation threshold. A method for estimating tension in the psychiatric patients.' *Electroenceph. clin. Neurophysiol.* **6**, 221, by courtesy of the Editor)

Shagass' work have encountered considerable difficulty in defining an accurate inflection point, so much so that Ackner and Pampiglione (1959), amongst others, have disputed the validity of Shagass' results. Others, including Nymgaard (1959), have satisfied themselves that the technique is practicable though difficult and have obtained broad confirmation of the earlier work.

The sedation threshold shows no sex distinction and provided care is taken to exclude cases of depression and organic psychoses, there is no alteration with age. In non-psychotic subjects the threshold is correlated with manifest anxiety. Shagass and Jones (1958) found the threshold in non-patient controls to be 3·09 mg/kg compared with 2·79 mg/kg in conversion hysteria, 3·91 mg/kg in anxiety hysteria, 4·42 mg/kg in obsessive-compulsive states, 4·78 mg/kg in neurotic depression and 5·27 mg/kg in anxiety states. It must be emphasized that, although these results have been shown to be highly significant statistically, their standard deviation is too great to permit them much diagnostic significance in individual cases.

Marked differences were found between groups of cases of the major psychoses. In the organic psychoses the mean sedation threshold was 1·94 mg/kg, the lowest of any group, in endogenous depression it was 2·81 mg/kg, in mania 3·45 mg/kg, in 'acute' schizophrenia 2·66 mg/kg, and in chronic schizophrenia it was 4·27 mg/kg.

Perhaps the most interesting application of the sedation threshold is in the differentiation of neurotic or reactive depression from endogenous depression. In contrast to the high threshold found in neurotic depression, in endogenous depression it is low, regardless of the degree of agitation present. The overlap of test results in the two groups is relatively small and Shagass suggests that the procedure has considerable differentiating value when these two diagnoses are under consideration.

Shagass' findings have largely been confirmed in a study by Nymgaard (1959) who found that thiopentone sodium gave comparable results to amylobarbitone sodium and that the test-retest results showed the procedure to be reliable. Although recommending that the administration of other barbiturates and phenothiazine compounds should be discontinued for 10 days before carrying out the test, Nymgaard found that in fact the administration of chlorpromazine 100 mg three times a day, phenobarbitone 100 mg twice a day or amylobarbitone 200 mg three times a day produced little or no effect upon the result. She also found significant differences between groups of neurotic and endogenous depressives, although the overlap between them was rather greater than that noted by Shagass (*Figure 9.7*). Perris (1966), too, has found the technique reliable. He divided the patients with endogenous depression into bipolar and unipolar groups. The patients in the bipolar group were depressed at the time of examination but had all previously experienced at least one attack of mania, while those in the unipolar group had had at least three episodes of depression without ever suffering mania. Interestingly, those with unipolar depression (mean 5·0 mg/kg) were found to have sedation thresholds of the same order as those with neurotic depression (mean 5·2 mg/kg), while the bipolar patients had thresholds with a mean value of 2·2 mg/kg.

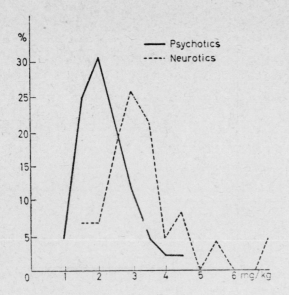

Figure 9.7—*Percentage distribution of sedation thresholds in mg/kg body weight for psychotic and neurotic depression groups. Mean sedation threshold for psychotics: 2·23 mg/kg. Mean sedation threshold for neurotics: 3·39 mg/kg*

(From Nymgaard, K. (1959). 'Studies on the sedation threshold.' *Arch. gen. Psychiat.* **1**, 530, by courtesy of the Editor)

Fenton, Hill and Scotton (1968) aware of the difficulties some workers have found in identifying an end-point have suggested that a different technique based upon the observation that in the fourth stage of thiopentone-induced sleep (Kiersey, Bickford and Faulconer, 1951) 'burst suppression' occurs; following the stage of generalized high amplitude slow activity, bursts of activity at various frequencies alternate with periods of electrical silence. They used a 2·5 per cent solution of thiopentone sodium and gave an initial dose of 4 mg/kg body weight over 15 seconds. After a 15 seconds interval further doses of 50 mg were given at 15 second intervals until burst suppression occurred. The end-point was indicated by the first period of electrical silence, lasting 1 second in all channels. The technique proved to be highly reliable but comparison of groups of orthopaedic and psychiatric patients showed no significant difference in their mean thresholds. On the other hand, in the case of depressed patients treated with ECT a significant decrease was demonstrated following treatment in those who recovered.

Although one might anticipate that a tense and anxious patient would have an increased tolerance to sedatives, the sedation threshold test is important, for it represents one of the first attempts to apply objective and quantitative methods to the study of psychiatric symptoms.

SCHIZOPHRENIA

There is no general agreement on the precise limits that should be placed on the concept of schizophrenia and it may well subsume a multiplicity of nosological entities. It is hardly surprising that the incidence and variety of EEG abnormalities reported vary so much in view of the differing diagnostic criteria used by the authors. From the multiplicity of findings published only two facts emerge clearly. First, there is no particular EEG pattern that can be regarded as characteristic of schizophrenia and second, that in the overall majority of cases the EEG is within normal limits; furthermore, in most of the others the abnormalities are relatively slight in degree. The variability of those EEG patterns classified as normal is striking (Hill, 1957). In regard to the amount of *alpha* rhythm, of low voltage fast and slow activity and in the response to physiological variables, they show a wider scatter about the mean than do normal controls.

The incidence of EEG abnormalities in schizophrenia varies from 20 per cent to 60 per cent of cases, according to the author, with a mean of 30 per cent (Ellingson, 1954–55). Abnormalities are more common in cases with a family history of the same disorder and a positive correlation exists with early onset, with severity of the symptoms and with long duration of the illness. In most series the incidence is highest in the catatonic group and lowest in paranoid schizophrenics.

Non-specific EEG abnormalities occur frequently in the siblings of schizophrenics. Chamberlain and Gordon-Russell (1952) found their incidence to be 44 per cent in patients, 6·5 per cent in their parents and 31 per cent in their siblings, as compared with 11·6 per cent in a group of controls.

A number of EEG variants may be found in schizophrenic patients and these are dealt with in turn. It must be remembered that more than one of these may be found in any one patient.

Alpha Variations

In many schizophrenics the *alpha* rhythm shows reduced responsiveness to visual, emotional and intellectual stimuli.

Fast Activity

Fast activity is found more frequently in the EEGs of schizophrenics than in a normal population (Finley, 1944). This accounts for the so-called 'choppy' activity described by Davis (1939–40) who applied the term to records deficient in *alpha* rhythm and dominated by low voltage irregular fast activity (*Figure 9.8*). The very high incidence of 61 per cent of such records in schizophrenia noted by

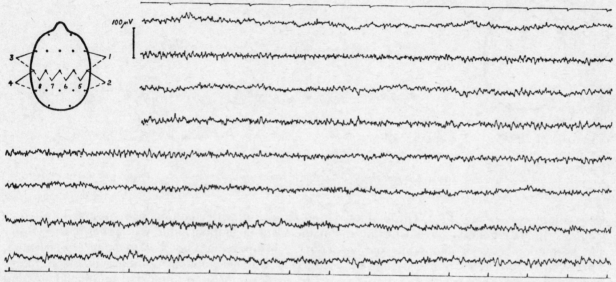

Figure 9.8—Schizophrenia. Man aged 42 years. EEG: 'Choppy' activity comprising mixed low voltage alpha, beta *and occasional* theta *components*

Davis (1942–43) has not been confirmed. Finley reported an incidence of about 30 per cent but Hill (1952) believes that the true incidence is under 20 per cent; he points out that such records could well occur as the result of emotional tension which causes blocking of the *alpha* rhythm and an increase of fast activity. Unrecognized contamination with muscle potentials would heighten the illusion of 'choppiness'. A more likely explanation of the high incidence in the earlier studies is that the fast activity was due to medication with barbiturates or paraldehyde. It is of interest that Small and Small (1965) do not refer to fast activity at all in their study of 88 acute schizophrenic patients and that Volavka, Matoušek and Roubíček (1966) in a study of schizophrenic patients deprived of all medication found, if anything, that they showed less *beta* activity than a control group.

'Epileptiform' Discharges

'Epileptiform' activity reminiscent of subcortical epilepsy is reported in the EEGs of 20–25 per cent of schizophrenics (Hill, 1957). Discharges of bilaterally synchronous slow wave activity, of spikes and slow waves and of polyspikes may be seen. It must be stressed that their amplitude is usually low and that they seldom present dramatically against the background rhythms (*Figure 9.9*). They also differ from the discharges seen in subcortical epilepsy in their distribution, usually being most evident in the post-central areas, and in their repetition frequency which tends to be over 4 per second. These fast spike and wave and polyspike discharges are very similar to the responses sometimes seen in normal individuals during photic stimulation. Personal experience has failed to show such a high incidence of sharp wave abnormalities and again one wonders to what extent different criteria of interpretation may be responsible and in how many the EEG abnormality can be explained as 6 per second spike

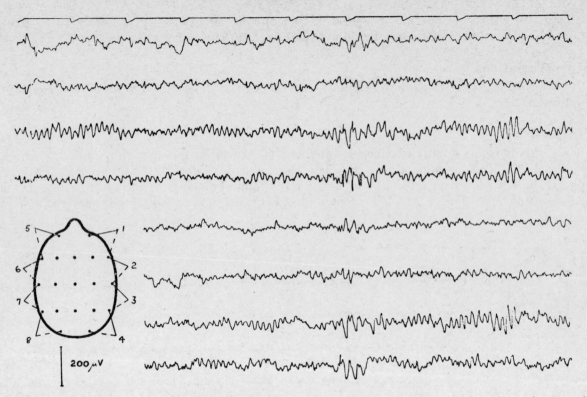

Figure 9.9—Catatonic schizophrenia. Man aged 36 years. EEG: Burst of theta *activity with low voltage spikes posteriorly standing out from symmetrical 9·5 Hz* alpha *rhythm and more widespread low voltage* theta *components*

wave complexes (*see* page 176). The loading of some case series with catatonic patients may be another factor, for there is general agreement that the incidence of such abnormalities is higher in this group. The distinction between 'idiopathic' and 'secondary' schizophrenia is not always made—or accepted. This is particularly relevant in regard to those epileptics who develop schizophrenic-like states. Slater and Beard (1963) have shown that there appears to be a causal connection between the epilepsy and the psychosis and that these patients cannot be regarded as schizophrenics who happen to have epilepsy. Another factor that has to be considered is medication with analeptic drugs such as the phenothiazines. Small and Small (1965) found epileptiform discharges in 18 per cent of 88 patients with acute schizophrenia and noted a significant correlation with medication.

Slow Activity

Although Hill (1957) believes that the proportion of EEGs showing a generalized excess of slow activity is no higher than in normal controls, other authors such as Volavka, Matoušek and Roubíček (1966) find a slightly increased incidence. In catatonic stupor the normal EEG rhythms tend to disappear and their place is taken by generalized low amplitude 2–6 Hz activity (*Figure 9.10*). In some cases the EEG abnormality only appears as clinical improvement begins. There may be considerable variation in the precise form of the abnormality in successive attacks.

Igert and Lairy (1962) after studying 62 female schizophrenics have suggested that a normal EEG indicates a poor prognosis and a continuing illness. Records showing the variations or abnormalities described above occurred in 54 per cent of their patients and these were more likely to show episodic illnesses and to respond better to treatment. Similarly, Small and Stern (1965) have found that a normal EEG with abundant *alpha* activity tends to be associated with a poor prognosis whereas patients with abnormal EEGs had a better prognosis.

Provocation Techniques

The photo-metrazol threshold is often low in schizophrenia and in the series described by Leffman and Perlo (1955) this was the case in 64 per cent of patients with overt symptoms. Among schizophrenics

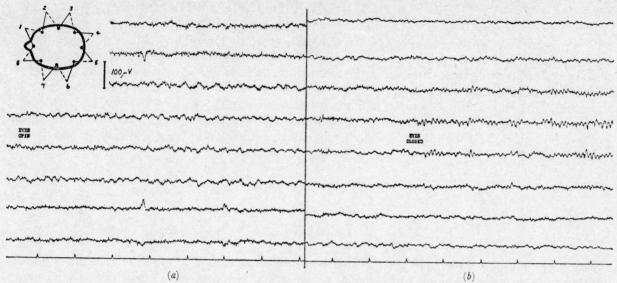

Figure 9.10—Catatonic schizophrenia. Man aged 17 years. (a) *In stupor, with eyes open. EEG: Low voltage 2–4 Hz activity posteriorly.* (b) *After recovery EEG: 11 Hz* alpha *rhythm following eye closure*

in remission 35 per cent had low thresholds. Sometimes the photo-metrazol threshold is zero; that is, the discharges appear on photic stimulation alone without the need for leptazol (Metrazol). Driver (1962) found that whereas a photoconvulsive response occurred in 75 per cent of a group of epileptics, it was also found in 40 per cent of schizophrenics. In depressed patients the response was seen in only 6 per cent of cases.

Chamberlain and Gordon-Russell (1953) claim that the photo-metrazol threshold is related, at least in part, to body build. Leptosomatic patients have significantly lower thresholds than those of pyknic habitus.

Variations in the photo-metrazol threshold may occur during the course of the illness, particularly in the catatonic cases. Hoenig and Leiberman (1953) noted that although in the stuporose phases the threshold was low, it fell to zero in the normal periods. Results such as these suggest a fluctuating sensitivity of the centrencephalic mechanisms related to the phases of the illness.

Caldwell and Domino (1967) have found that, during sleep, many chronic schizophrenic patients show little or no stage 4 and a reduction of stage 3 sleep. Feinberg *et al.* (1964) found in acutely ill patients that there was a significant decrease in REM sleep.

When simple visual analysis of the EEG proved to be clinically unhelpful a number of refinements, either in technique or record analysis, were evolved, their originators claiming that the results correlated with the clinical diagnosis. It must be pointed out that no adequate confirmation of any of these claims has been provided and even if this is achieved the nature of the tests and the level of correlation between the results and clinical status are such that they are unlikely to be of other than heuristic interest. Consequently, only brief reference is made to these studies. Goldman (1959) (*see also* Galbrecht, Caffey and Goldman, 1968) claimed that the rapid intravenous injection of thiopentone sodium gave rise to EEG features which were characteristic of schizophrenia and disappeared following the administration of chlorpromazine. Kennard, Rabinovitch and Fister (1955) suggested that the frequency spectra of the EEG in various scalp derivations differed between schizophrenic and normal subjects. Bruck (1964; 1967) investigated the average voltage values and the 'synchrony ratios' of EEGs in schizophrenics and controls. The 'synchrony ratio' is obtained by counting the total number of waves over 10μV in a chosen epoch of two EEG channels and relating to this the number of waves that proved to be synchronous. Goldstein *et al.* (1965) (*see also* Sugerman *et al.* 1964) have assessed the 'energy content' of the EEG in schizophrenics using an integrator which transforms the EEG into a series of electrical pulses, the number of which is a function of the amplitude of the EEG integrated over time.

185

AUTISM AND CHILDHOOD SCHIZOPHRENIA

The nosological relationship of cases diagnosed as early infantile autism and childhood schizophrenia to cases of adult schizophrenia is uncertain. Nor has the place of brain damage as an aetiological factor been satisfactorily evaluated, although the fact that 19 of the 102 patients discussed by White, DeMyer and DeMyer (1964) suffered seizures suggests that organic factors may have operated frequently in this series. Fifty-three of these patients had abnormal records and 45 showed focal spikes, paroxysmal spike and wave activity or both. Creak and Pampiglione (1969) found a variety of EEG abnormalities in 29 of 35 autistic and withdrawn children, but none of them could unequivocally be classified as brain damaged.

DEMENTIA

Some of the conditions which may give rise to dementia have already been considered—epilepsy, brain injury, space-occupying lesions, myxoedema, pernicious anaemia, disseminated sclerosis and neuro-syphilis—and the appropriate sections may be consulted. The main purpose of this section is to consider the senile and presenile dementias.

There is general agreement that in senility the frequency and abundance of the *alpha* rhythm are both reduced and that the amount of fast activity tends to be increased. There is no unanimity regarding the occurrence of *theta* activity. Obrist (1954) surveyed a group of 150 normal adults aged from 65 to 94 years and compared their EEGs with those of 1,000 young adults previously classified by Gibbs, Gibbs and Lennox (1943). His findings confirmed the shift that occurs in the frequency of the dominant rhythm with increasing age. In subjects aged 65–79 years, 18 per cent had EEGs with a dominant rhythm slower than 8·5 Hz, a few as slow as the *delta* range, while in those aged over 80 years the proportion rose to 30 per cent. In the young adults such EEGs occurred in 8·3 per cent. Unforfunately, cases known to have cerebrovascular disease were not excluded from the series. In the study by Mundy-Castle *et al.* (1954) every care was taken to exclude cases with organic lesions and it was concluded that normal senility is not associated with any increase in the amount of slow activity in the EEG. McAdam and McClatchey (1952) and Weiner and Schuster (1956) came to the same conclusion.

Many studies of the senile psychoses are invalidated by the assumption that any psychosis occurring in the senium is organic in nature irrespective of its symptomatology. Mundy-Castle *et al.* (1954) classified their cases into depressions, paranoid states and dementias and found, surprisingly, that the overall incidence of abnormal records of 54 per cent was little different in each of these three groups. The later study by Weiner and Schuster (1956) in which the incidence of abnormalities was 78 per cent, showed clearly that functional psychoses in old age without dementia were not generally associated with abnormal EEGs. This view receives support from Frey and Sjögren (1959) and from Lyketsos, Belinson and Gibbs (1953).

Senile Dementia

In senile dementia the most common abnormality is an accentuation of the usual senile EEG features, one result of which is that the remaining *alpha* rhythm may slow below 8 Hz. Diffuse *theta* and even diffuse *delta* activity, usually of low amplitude, may also be present so that the general appearance of the EEG is polyrhythmic (*Figure 9.11*). The reduction of the *alpha* index and the amount of slow activity show only a very approximate relation to the degree of dementia. In advanced cases no *alpha* or faster frequencies may be identifiable.

Why a substantial proportion of cases of senile—and of presenile—dementia should retain normal EEGs while others show such obvious abnormalities is mystifying. In a few cases the explanation may be that the premorbid EEGs were made up of faster rhythms and the slowing which occurs fails to transgress the lower limits of normality.

ARTERIOSCLEROTIC DEMENTIA

Arteriosclerotic dementia occurs on average a decade earlier than senile dementia. The frequency and

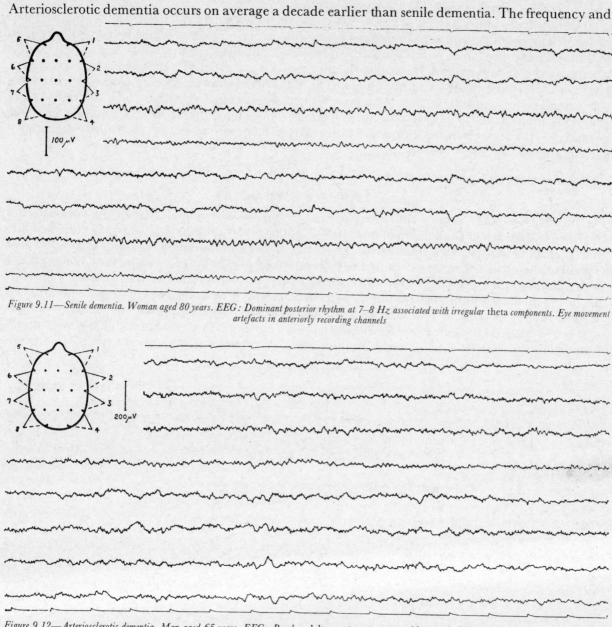

Figure 9.11—Senile dementia. Woman aged 80 years. EEG: Dominant posterior rhythm at 7–8 Hz associated with irregular theta components. Eye movement artefacts in anteriorly recording channels

Figure 9.12—Arteriosclerotic dementia. Man aged 65 years. EEG: Random delta components, more evident on the left side, occurring on a background of irregular theta and beta activity

variety of the EEG abnormalities are similar to those of senile dementia but tend to be rather more severe (*Figure 9.12*). In a substantial number of cases there are also focal abnormalities due to cerebral infarction.

Episodes of delirium occur frequently in cases of generalized cerebral arteriosclerosis and in these bifrontal sinusoidal *delta* activity commonly appears, which Van der Drift (1961) attributes to ischaemia of the anterior region of the diencephalon.

JAKOB-CREUTZFELDT'S SYNDROME

The literature concerned with dementia in the presenile period is confusing. Many cases have been described as examples of Jakob–Creutzfeldt's syndrome which it now seems in the light of Nevin's (1967) work were really cases of subacute spongiform encephalopathy. Thus, Lesse, Hoefer and Austin

(1958) and Abbott (1959) describe EEG findings in Jakob–Creutzfeldt's syndrome identical with those associated with subacute spongiform encephalopathy.

As the result of a critical review of the literature and the study of personal cases, Nevin concludes that in Jakob–Creutzfeldt's syndrome the lesions are multifocal, its onset on average is 10 years later than that of subacute spongiform encephalopathy, it may be familial and its mean duration is 19·6 months as compared with 5·26 months. Clinically, the progressive organic deterioration is associated sooner or later with increasing rigidity and myoclonus. The EEG never shows periodic complexes with sharp wave components and instead there is a progressive loss of normal rhythms which are replaced by generalized slow activity of low to medium voltage. In Gordon and Sim's (1967) 4 cases the EEG was normal in 1, the others showing diffuse 2–5 Hz activity of moderate amplitude; so-called 'spiking' was present in one case.

ALZHEIMER'S DISEASE

The incidence of EEG abnormalities in Alzheimer's disease is very high and in the various series described by Letemendia and Pampiglione (1958), Liddell (1958), Swain (1959), and Gordon and Sim (1967), all the cases had abnormal EEGs. The series of 48 cases described by Gordon and Sim is of particular interest as all cases were confirmed by cerebral biopsy. In the early stages the EEG may be of low amplitude with a reduction in the *alpha* activity. Later the background activity consists of generalized low to medium amplitude irregular *theta* frequencies with little or no *alpha* rhythm. Superimposed on this are runs of random *delta* activity, often of moderately high amplitude and sometimes most evident in the frontal regions (*Figure 9.13*). Nevin (1967) attributes this to ischaemic changes secondary to amyloid degeneration of small vessels in these areas. Asymmetry of the slow activity is not uncom-

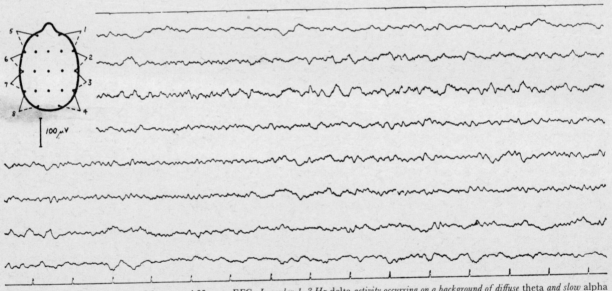

Figure 9.13—Alzheimer's disease. Woman aged 55 years. EEG: Irregular 1–3 Hz delta activity occurring on a background of diffuse theta and slow alpha frequency components

mon and occasional sharp waves are present in a few patients. Focal features are rarely seen. In cases subjected to photic stimulation by Letemendia and Pampiglione, all showed parieto-occipital responses to single flashes. Fast activity induced by barbiturates was scanty and limited to the region of the vertex. Sleep spindles, too, tended to be poorly developed and K-complexes were difficult or impossible to evoke. The slow activity present in the routine record tended to diminish when sleep was induced.

It has always seemed illogical that in correlative studies little relationship could be shown between duration and severity of illness and the degree of EEG abnormality. This is probably to be explained by the fact that most previous studies have been made on patients already well advanced in their illnesses, as in Letemendia and Pampiglione's cases in which no change was evident after a year. Gordon (1968) has reported serial EEGs obtained in 13 cases of presenile dementia. In 7 with

Alzheimer's disease progressive EEG changes were evident, except in 1 patient who already had a severely abnormal EEG when first seen. Nevin (1967) comments that in his 25 cases the degree of change correlated with the duration of illness and that by 3 years little *alpha* activity was evident.

The EEG changes in Alzheimer's disease are as a rule much more marked than those in senile dementia but the differences are in degree only.

PICK'S DISEASE

In Pick's disease the EEG is often normal (Gordon and Sim, 1967; Nevin, 1967). When abnormal, *alpha* activity can usually still be discerned and may remain prominent. Otherwise the changes are similar to those seen in Alzheimer's disease and senile dementia, although they tend to be less marked. Focal changes are not a feature of the EEG in Pick's disease and in Swain's (1959) 4 cases, for example, none could be detected.

SIMPLE PRESENILE DEMENTIA

Many cases of dementia occurring in the presenium lack distinctive features and are difficult to classify. They are doubtless of varied aetiology. EEG abnormalities are similar to those seen in senile dementia but are frequently mild and in many cases the EEGs may be within normal limits. Five of the 19 cases described by Gordon and Sim (1967) had normal records. In none of the others was the *alpha* rhythm completely lost.

HUNTINGTON'S CHOREA

In developed cases of Huntington's chorea the EEG is frequently abnormal. The *alpha* rhythm is poorly developed or absent and the record may be of very low voltage. In others, generalized low voltage fast activity is prominent and low to medium voltage random slow activity is often evident.

Patterson, Bagchi and Test (1947–48) claimed that nearly three-quarters of the offspring of cases of Huntington's chorea showed bilateral paroxysms of slow activity in the central areas, often associated with spikes. Their *alpha* rhythms were well developed and none of them gave a history of epilepsy. It is difficult to see what relationship these abnormalities have to those occurring in actual cases of Huntington's chorea and it is very doubtful indeed if they have any predictive value as to the development of the choreiform syndrome. This appears to be a unique study though the offspring of patients with Huntington's chorea do undoubtedly show a high incidence of non-specific abnormalities which can be correlated with their incidence of psychopathy. Twenty-three of the 26 offspring of patients with Huntington's chorea described by Patterson *et al.* have been re-examined by Chandler (1966). Their predictions based on the EEG findings were correct in 11 and incorrect in 12!

NORMAL PRESSURE HYDROCEPHALUS

Normal pressure hydrocephalus was described by Adams *et al.* (1965) (*see also* Adams, 1966). It presents with dementia and a gait disturbance, generally in the presenile period and is important because considerable improvement in the dementia can be achieved by introducing a ventriculo-atrial shunt. The EEG is almost always abnormal in some degree at the time of diagnosis although in milder cases the abnormality is limited to a small excess of generalized *theta* activity. In more severe cases diffuse *delta* activity may be prominent. Air encephalography is necessary for the diagnosis and not infrequently exacerbates both the clinical features and the EEG abnormalities. Some improvement in the EEG may occur in those cases which show clinical improvement after operation.

Considering the presenile and senile dementias as a group, it appears that the degree of EEG abnormality is more closely related to the rate of progress of the condition than to the degree of dementia. This view is held by Hill (1948), by Weiner and Schuster (1956) and is well demonstrated in the series of patients described by Lundervold, Engeset and Lönnum (1962).

The significance of the slow activity in these cases of dementia is in some doubt. Hill (1948) believes that it indicates 'active involvement of nerve cells' and therefore that it is directly associated with cortical degeneration. Alternatively, the slow activity might have its origin in subcortical centres, either in the upper brain stem or diencephalon. The fact that it is bilateral, sometimes synchronous and often frontally predominant may be cited in favour of this latter view.

PHYSICAL TREATMENTS

BILATERAL PREFRONTAL LEUCOTOMY

After a bilateral prefrontal leucotomy there is frequently a period when the EEG consists of generalized *delta* activity, sometimes of high voltage and often showing a frontal predominance. This is especially the case when the operation is followed by a drowsy, anergic state in which some degree of impairment of consciousness is evident. The generalized abnormality diminishes, leaving bifrontal, moderate or high amplitude *delta* activity which is sometimes asymmetrical and may occur in runs. *Theta* activity is intermixed with it and after several weeks becomes more prominent as the *delta* activity gradually disappears. In many cases the EEG returns approximately to its pre-operative state within three months, but in a few, particularly when post-operative epilepsy has ensued, low amplitude frontal *theta* or *delta* activity may persist indefinitely. Even in those cases experiencing fits, it is unusual to find spike or sharp wave discharges. There appears to be no correlation between the EEG changes and the other effects of the operation (Levin *et al.*, 1949–50), though sometimes, when a marked decrease of tension results, there may be an increase in the *alpha* index and a decrease of fast activity.

Lennox and Coolidge (1949) reported that following operation there is a loss of sleep spindles. This was confirmed by Adler and Talbot (1951) who suggested that if sleep spindles persist, the operation has not been sufficiently extensive and is likely to be ineffective.

Bilateral topectomy with removal of areas 9, 10 and 46 produces similar effects although it does not affect the sleep spindles to the same degree.

Van der Drift and Magnus (1961) have observed that undercutting of areas 9 and 10 leads to the appearance of very slow polymorphic *delta* activity at 0·3—0·5 Hz, often limited to the frontal poles, which may persist unaltered for many years. It may prove difficult to distinguish from eye movement artefact and can be adequately recorded only if time constants of the order of 1 second are used.

ELECTROCONVULSIVE THERAPY

The EEG changes occurring during a major convulsion induced by electroconvulsive therapy (ECT) are similar to those in spontaneous attacks of grand mal (*see* page 74). A variable time after the convulsion, the EEG resumes its usual appearance. As successive treatments are administered, the generalized *delta* and *theta* activity—often frontally predominant—which follows the fit becomes more

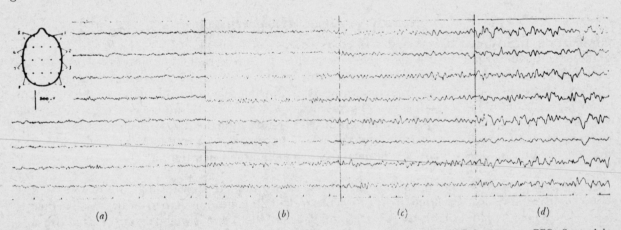

Figure 9.14—Endogenous depressive treated with electroconvulsive therapy (ECT). Woman aged 45 years. (a) Before treatment. EEG: Scanty alpha rhythm; low voltage fast activity. (b) Six hours after third ECT. EEG: Increased alpha rhythm in occipital regions; independent theta rhythm in posterior temporal regions. (c) Six hours after fifth ECT. EEG: Generalized higher voltage theta activity. (d) Six hours after seventh ECT. Patient mildly confused. EEG: Irregular bilateral delta activity occurring on a background of theta activity

persistent. In the average case, after three or four treatments spaced at intervals of 2–3 days, it fails to disappear completely between them. Subsequent treatments result in the slow activity becoming more widespread, of higher amplitude and of lower frequency while the *alpha* rhythm becomes disturbed and may disappear (*Figure 9.14*). Clinically, such EEG appearances are frequently associated with an obvious degree of confusion and memory disturbance but the EEG and clinical phenomena by no means run parallel.

There is much individual variation in the sensitivity of the EEG to ECT; in some patients the record may show little change after 10–12 convulsions; in others a considerable and persistent abnormality is evident after 2 or 3. The spacing of treatments also influences the severity of the EEG abnormalities. There is some evidence that when slow activity fails to persist, the outcome of treatment is likely to be unfavourable (Roth, 1951). After a variable period following the end of the course of treatment, the *delta* gives way to *theta* activity and the *alpha* rhythm emerges, being at first of low amplitude and decreased frequency until finally the EEG returns to its former state. The EEG changes are much less marked when unilateral ECT is used (Valentine, Keddie and Dunne, 1968) and although the fit that results is generally symmetrical the slow activity is frequently sufficiently more marked on the side to which the electrical current is applied, to allow this fact to be deduced from the EEG (Sutherland, Oliver and Knight, 1969).

It was shown by Roth (1951) that serial recordings made during barbiturate-induced sleep revealed changes in the EEG at an earlier stage of treatment than did routine recordings. He described a technique by which these changes could be quantified. The EEG is recorded 3–4 hours after treatment. Thiopentone sodium is given intravenously at the rate of 50 mg every 20 seconds until consciousness is lost. *Delta* activity limited to or of maximal amplitude in the frontal regions appears and becomes the dominant component until it is more or less suddenly replaced within 300 seconds by the fast activity typical of light barbiturate anaesthesia (*Figure 9.15*). The total period during which

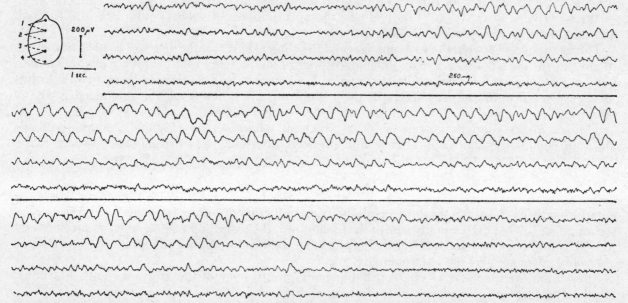

Figure 9.15—Delta *response to thiopentone narcosis 4 hours after third ECT. Man aged 45 years with endogenous depression. Total of 250 mg thiopentone sodium given at 150 mg/minute. EEG: Frontally predominant 2–2·5 Hz rhythmical* delta *discharge of 40 seconds duration, followed by period of relatively low voltage barbiturate fast activity*

the thiopentone-induced *delta* activity is dominant is expressed as a percentage of 300 seconds. This per cent time *delta* is always increased after the third treatment and often after the second. The percentage rises as a rule up to the eighth or ninth treatment and then tends to remain constant or to fall off. After termination of a course of 6–7 treatments, the per cent time *delta* begins to fall during the following week and reaches the pre-ECT level in 7–9 weeks. A per cent time *delta* over 55 per cent is usually accompanied clinically by confusion.

In cases of endogenous depression, the peak value of the per cent time *delta* shows little relationship to the result of the ECT assessed immediately following the course, when the great majority of patients show considerable improvement, but a significant relationship exists with the tendency to relapse within 6 months of treatment. Amongst 22 cases with values of per cent time *delta* below 40 per cent 11 relapsed at 3 months and 13 by 6 months; while of 19 cases with over 40 per cent, only 1 relapsed at 3 months and 2 by 6 months (Roth *et al.*, 1957). The technique may therefore be used to help decide whether a patient has had sufficient treatment.

In schizophrenia and the neuroses, including reactive depression, high peak values may be associated with little or no change in the clinical state and the method has no prognostic value in these conditions.

The sedation threshold (Shagass and Jones, 1958) usually tends to rise after the administration of ECT. A marked rise or a continuing rise with successive treatments suggests that the course will prove to be of little benefit. This finding is paralleled by the clinical observation that mounting anxiety during a course of ECT is associated with a poor outcome.

DRUGS

SEDATIVES AND TRANQUILLO-SEDATIVES

In ordinary dosage, sedatives such as chloral, paraldehyde and the various barbiturates lead to an increase in the amount of fast activity in the 20–30 Hz range often up to amplitudes of $100\mu V$. There is a very considerable individual variation in regard to the amount of fast activity produced by any one drug. Amylobarbitone is one of the more potent barbiturates and this accounts for its use by Shagass (1954) in measuring the sedation threshold. Chloral on the other hand produces relatively little fast activity and it is for this reason that it is sometimes preferred as an agent for inducing sleep in the EEG laboratory. In some individuals, therapeutic doses of sedatives also give rise to small amounts of diffuse *theta* and even *delta* activity.

The relationship between the EEG changes and the clinical effects of the drug are by no means close: in one patient the EEG may remain unchanged even in the presence of drowsiness while in another, obvious EEG changes have no parallel in the patient's clinical state. There is a tendency for all sedatives to aggravate epileptiform discharges. In the withdrawal phase following the prolonged intake of sedatives, the threshold to photic stimulation is reduced (Wulff, 1960).

The tranquillo-sedatives (anxiolytic drugs) such as meprobamate (Equanil) chlordiazepoxide (Librium) and diazepam (Valium) have similar effects, all giving rise to an increase in fast activity.

ANTICONVULSANTS

Apart from the barbiturates the anticonvulsant drugs in therapeutic doses have little or no effect upon the on-going EEG. This is equally true of the hydantoins, the oxazolidinediones and the succinimides as well as sulthiame and acetazolamide. In spite of its chemical similarity to barbiturates, primidone (Mysoline) does not give rise to fast activity.

Apart from the members of the oxazolidinedione group, none of the anticonvulsants has much effect on the form or incidence of epileptiform discharges.

CENTRAL ANAESTHETICS

The effects of thiopentone sodium given intravenously to produce anaesthesia have been considered on page 66. Other anaesthetic agents have similar EEG effects. Ether, nitrous oxide and cyclopropane, for example, all lead to the appearance of frontal fast activity—although this is often less prominent than in the case of thiopentone—with a diminution of *alpha* activity at the stage when speech becomes slurred. The fast activity becomes more widespread and of high amplitude and at the analgesia stage becomes intermixed with 3–7 Hz activity. As the level of anaesthesia deepens the EEG becomes dominated by slow activity which progressively increases in amplitude and decreases in frequency to 0·5–3 Hz. In deep anaesthesia, burst suppression occurs as with thiopentone sodium (Brazier 1955; Ellington 1968).

In anaesthesia the arousal response to stimulation is abolished; cortical evoked responses remain unaffected and may even be increased while evoked reticular potentials are reduced or absent. Such evidence indicates that anaesthetics owe their action to synaptic blocking in the reticular formation (Magoun 1962).

The use of the EEG to monitor anaesthesia has been described by Faulconer and Bickford (1960).

ANALGESICS AND NARCOTICS

The members of the analgesic and antipyretic group of drugs have little or no effect on the EEG in normal doses. Narcotics by mouth similarly have little effect unless they induce sleep.

NEUROLEPTICS (MAJOR TRANQUILLIZERS) AND ANTIDEPRESSANTS

In doses of 50 mg by mouth chlorpromazine (Largactil) may increase the amount of *alpha* activity if it is scanty but leads to a decrease when it is plentiful; some reduction in frequency may occur. There may be some decrease in fast activity and an increase in slow frequencies. With higher doses, especially when given intravenously some generalized *delta* activity may appear and the arousal response to afferent stimulation is likely to be reduced. Sometimes hypersynchronous high voltage discharges occur (Fink, 1965). Ulett, Heusler and Word (1965) have shown that when the drug is taken over a period, the changes are reversed within 10 weeks of its withdrawal.

Trifluoperazine (Stelazine), fluphenazine (Prolixin), thioridazine (Melleril), tetrabenazine (Nitoman), reserpine (Serpasil), the various butyrophenone compounds such as haloperidol (Serenace) and the group of tricyclic antidepressants such as imipramine (Tofranil) and amitriptyline (Tryptanol) all have effects similar to those of chlorpromazine. As with sedatives there is a very marked individual variation in the EEG response to these drugs. They all tend to potentiate epileptiform discharges.

LITHIUM CARBONATE

An intake of 1–2·5 g lithium carbonate daily was found to produce EEG changes in 60–70 per cent of patients (Platman and Fieve, 1969; Johnson, 1969). The *alpha* rhythm slowed but increased in amplitude and was accompanied by tremor and other evidence of toxicity.

STIMULANTS

Stimulants including the amphetamines, caffeine and ephedrine produce an 'arousal' effect with some reduction in *alpha* activity and an increase in low voltage fast activity.

HALLUCINOGENS

Hallucinogens have little or no effect upon the EEG although an 'arousal' response may occur.

MENTAL SUBNORMALITY (MENTAL DEFICIENCY)

SUBCULTURAL SUBNORMALITY

In subcultural subnormality the EEG patterns are similar to those of the general population with perhaps a somewhat higher incidence of non-specific abnormalities. In many of the pathological varieties of subnormality, the incidence of EEG abnormality is very much greater.

MONGOLISM (DOWN'S SYNDROME)

The majority of mongols have normal EEGs although Gregoriades and Pampiglione (1966) found a high incidence of infantile spasms and hypsarrhythmic EEG patterns in their series of mongol babies.

It is of interest, though, that if from a mongol population one selects those who additionally show evidence of emotional and behavioural problems, the incidence of abnormal EEGs is higher than in the non-disturbed mongols just as occurs when one selects from a general population those individuals with similar disturbances. In Menolascino's (1965) series the incidence of EEG abnormalities was 50 per cent in emotionally disturbed mongols compared with 13·4 per cent in the remainder of the group.

HYDROCEPHALUS

In hydrocephalus with subnormality, epileptiform activity is frequently present even in the absence of clinical seizures (Gibbs, Gibbs and Fois, 1955). In a series of 32 cases described by Fois, Gibbs and Gibbs (1958) aged from 7 weeks to 25 years, all with subnormality, the EEGs were abnormal in 16. Two cases showed focal spikes in routine recordings and a further 9 showed focal spikes or spike and slow wave discharges during sleep. In 21 of the patients the most striking abnormality was an asynchrony or independence of potentials recorded from the two hemispheres during sleep. K-complexes appeared independently on either side and sleep spindles and slow activity were also asynchronous. The authors attribute the asynchrony to 'breaking of the functional bridge' between the thalami due to ballooning of the ventricles. In fact, minor asymmetries of the kind described—particularly of sleep spindles—are not uncommon in normal children (*see Figure 4.12*).

MICROCEPHALY

Microcephaly is not a nosological entity and the term subsumes cases of varied aetiology including some examples of phenylketonuria. The incidence of epilepsy in microcephaly is high and it is not surprising that epileptiform discharges occur in the EEGs of two-thirds of cases. Hypsarrhythmic records may be seen. Others show a generalized excess of slow activity but normal records occur in about 25 per cent of cases. Fois and Rosenberg (1957) point out that in children with microcephaly low voltage records are very frequent. Such a finding is unusual in normal children and they suggest that it indicates 'decortication'. This theory obtains little neuropathological support.

GARGOYLISM

In the occasional cases of gargoylism in the literature in which EEGs have been recorded (Green, 1948; Jervis, 1950), these have been abnormal, dominated by high amplitude slow activity.

PORENCEPHALY AND PSEUDOPORENCEPHALY

In porencephaly and pseudoporencephaly focal abnormalities are frequent and usually provide good localization of the lesion. The focus may be of spikes, spikes and slow waves or slow activity. Localized attenuation of electrical activity is frequent. Generalized slow activity may occur and is sometimes paroxysmal. In a few cases the EEG is within normal limits (Naef, 1958).

AGENESIS OF THE CORPUS CALLOSUM

In agenesis of the corpus callosum both subnormality and epilepsy are commonly present; porencephaly may coexist. Few cases have been published with the EEG findings. Records usually show generalized paroxysms of spikes and slow waves with relatively normal interparoxysmal appearances. A lack of synchronization of the background potentials in the two occipital regions is claimed by Carpenter and Druckemiller (1953) but was not present in the case described by Lilienthal and Tarlau (1969).

Cerebro-oculo-renal Syndrome (Lowe's Syndrome)

In Lowe's syndrome mental subnormality is associated with hypotonia, cataracts and sometimes with glaucoma, hyperaminoaciduria and proteinuria. Poley and Dumermuth (1968) have described a rather characteristic EEG pattern. Generally in the first few months of life the EEG is normal but after the age of one year generalized fast activity at 25–32 Hz is present which is more marked posteriorly and tends to occur in high amplitude bursts. These features are accentuated during light and deep sleep.

Cerebral Palsy

In cerebral palsy the incidence of fits and of EEG abnormalities is appreciably higher in the spastic than in the athetoid group. In a series of 187 cases reported by Aird and Cohen (1950) fits occurred in two-thirds of the spastics and one-third of the athetoids; the incidence of EEG abnormalities was 88 per cent and 61 per cent respectively. The abnormal records showed epileptiform discharges which were focal in a large number of cases. The EEG is of little value in assessing whether or not a patient previously free from fits might develop them in the future. There is no definite correlation between the degree or quality of the EEG abnormality and the degree of subnormality.

Infantile Hemiplegia

Infantile hemiplegia, including examples of Sturge-Kalischer-Weber's syndrome (naevoid amentia) is another condition frequently associated with subnormality and epilepsy. There is a high incidence of EEG abnormalities. Although in some cases single or strictly unilateral spike foci, focal *delta* activity or an area of attenuation may be found (*Figure 9.16*), in others the abnormalities may be wide-spread. The EEG may be continuously abnormal with generalized spike or spike and slow wave

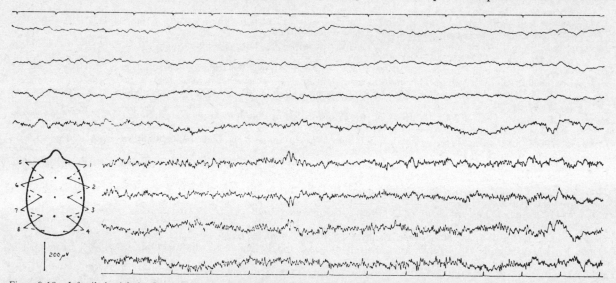

Figure 9.16—Infantile hemiplegia. Boy aged 5 years. Predominantly left-sided convulsions associated with acute febrile illness at 15 months, followed by hemiplegia and occasional further seizures. Severe behaviour disorder. EEG during sleep induced with 100 mg quinalbarbitone sodium (Seconal): Attenuation of all components over greater part of right hemisphere

discharges superimposed on a background of generalized irregular slow activity, so that no hint is provided that the lesion is unilateral. Sometimes multiple independent spike foci can be identified and mirror foci may also be discerned. In occasional cases the EEG may show no abnormality. Following hemispherectomy the improvement in the EEG and in the clinical state may be dramatic and all the epileptiform discharges may disappear. As a rule, the EEG over the missing hemisphere is of lower amplitude than that on the other side but occasionally no difference can be detected. The potentials recorded on this side originate in the remaining hemisphere and are conducted through the cerebrospinal fluid, skull and scalp. Cobb and Sears (1960) have shown that when the cerebrospinal fluid is replaced by air on the side of the hemispherectomy, larger voltage differences may be recorded on the same side with a bipolar technique.

OTHER DISEASES

Cerebral lipidosis (amaurotic family idiocy) is referred to on page 148, Schilder's disease on page 163, tuberous sclerosis on page 119 and phenylketonuria on page 99.

REFERENCES

Abbott, J. (1959). 'The EEG in Jakob-Creutzfeldt's Disease'. *Electroenceph. clin. Neurophysiol.* **11,** 184

Ackner, B. and Pampiglione, G. (1959). 'An Evaluation of the Sedation Threshold Test'. *J. psychosom. Res.*

Adams, A. (1959). 'Studies on the Flat Electroencephalogram in Man'. *Electroenceph. clin. Neurophysiol.* **11,** 35

Adams, R. D. (1966). 'Further Observations on Normal Pressure Hydrocephalus'. *Proc. R. Soc. Med.* **59,** 1135

— Fisher, C. M., Hakim, S., Ojemann, R. G. and Sweet, W. H. (1965). 'Symptomatic Occult Hydrocephalus with "Normal" Cerebrospinal-fluid Pressure'. *New Engl. J. Med.* **273,** 117

Adler, H. and Talbot, D. R. (1951). 'A Psychiatric, EEG and Psychological Study of Lobotomy in Chronic Schizophrenia'. *Dis. nerv. Syst.* **12,** 323

Aird, R. B. and Cohen, P. (1950). 'Electroencephalography in Cerebral Palsy'. *J. Pediat.* **37,** 448

Anderson, W. Mc. C., Dawson, J. and Margerison, J. H. (1964). 'Serial Biochemical, Clinical and Electroencephalographic Studies in Affective Illness'. *Clin. Sci.* **26,** 323

Arellano, A. P. (1951). Cit. by Schwab, R. S. *Electroencephalography in Clinical Practice*. p. 134. Philadelphia; Saunders

Arentsen, K. and Sindrup, E. (1963). 'Electroencephalographic Investigation of Alcoholics'. *Acta psychiat. scand.* **39,** 371

Bennett, A. E., Doi, L. T. and Mowery, G. L. (1956). 'The Value of Electroencephalography in Alcoholism'. *J. nerv. ment. Dis.* **124,** 27

Brazier, M. A. B. (1955). 'Studies of Electrical Activity of the Brain in Relation to Anesthesia'. In *Conference on Neuropharmacology,* p. 107. Ed. by H. A. Abramson. New York; Josiah Macy Jr. Foundation

Bruck, M. A. (1964). 'Synchrony and Voltage in the EEGs of Schizophrenics'. *Archs gen. Psychiat.* **10,** 454

— (1967). 'EEG-Synchrony and Voltage in Schizophrenia'. *Psychiat. Q.* **41,** 683

Caldwell, D. F. and Domino, E. F. (1967). 'Electroencephalographic and Eye Movement Patterns during Sleep in Chronic Schizophrenic Patients'. *Electroenceph. clin. Neurophysiol.* **22,** 414

Camp, W. A. and Wolff, H. G. (1961). 'Studies on Headache. Electroencephalographic Abnormalities in Patients with Vascular Headache of the Migraine Type'. *Archs Neurol.* **4,** 475

Carpenter, M. B. and Druckemiller, W. H. (1953). 'Agenesis of the Corpus Callosum Diagnosed During Life'. *Archs Neurol. Psychiat.* **69,** 305

Chamberlain, G. H. A. and Gordon-Russell, J. (1952). 'The EEGs of the Relatives of Schizophrenics'. *J. ment. Sci.* **98,** 654

— — (1953). 'The Myoclonic Threshold in Schizophrenia'. *Electroenceph. clin. Neurophysiol.* **5,** 169

Chandler, J. H. (1966). 'EEG in Prediction of Huntington's Chorea. An Eighteen Year Follow-Up'. *Electroenceph. clin. Neurophysiol.* **21,** 79

Cobb, W. and Sears, T. A. (1960). 'A Study of the Transmission of Potentials after Hemispherectomy'. *Electroenceph. clin. Neurophysiol.* **12,** 371

Cohn, R. (1958). 'On the Significance of Biocciptal Slow Wave Activity in the Electroencephalograms of Children'. *Electroenceph. clin. Neurophysiol.* **10,** 766

— and Nardini, J. E. (1958–59). 'The Correlation of Bilateral Occipital Slow Activity in the Human EEG with Certain Disorders of Behaviour'. *Am. J. Psychiat.* **115,** 44

Creak, M. and Pampiglione, G. (1969). 'Clinical and EEG Studies on a Group of 35 Psychotic Children'. *Devl. Med. Child Neurol.* **11,** 218

Crisp, A. H., Fenton, G. W. and Scotton, L. (1968). 'A Controlled Study of the EEG in Anorexia Nervosa'. *Br. J. Psychiat.* **114,** 1149

Critchley, M. (1962). 'Periodic Hypersomnia and Megaphagia'. *Brain* **85,** 627

Dalén, P. (1965). 'Family History, the Electroencephalogram and Perinatal Factors in Manic Conditions'. *Acta psychiat. scand.* **41,** 527

Davis, P. A. (1939–40). 'Evaluation of the Electroencephalogram of Schizophrenic Patients'. *Am. J. Psychiat.* **96,** 851

— (1941). 'The Electroencephalograms of Manic-depressive Patients'. *Am. J. Psychiat.* **98,** 430

— (1942–43). 'Comparative Study of the EEGs of Schizophrenic and Manic-depressive Patients'. *Am. J. Psychiat.* **99,** 210

Ditman, K. S. and Blinn, K. A. (1954–55). 'Sleep Levels in Enuresis'. *Am. J. Psychiat.* **111,** 913

Drift, J. H. A. Van der (1961). 'Ischaemic Cerebral Lesions'. *Angiology* **12,** 401

— and Magnus, O. (1961). 'The EEG after Selective Leucotomy'. In *Electroencephalography and Cerebral Tumours. Electroenceph. clin. Neurophysiol.* Suppl. **19,** 160

Driver, M. V. (1962). 'A Study of the Photoconvulsive Threshold'. *Electroenceph. clin. Neurophysiol.* **14,** 359

Elian, M. and Bornstein, B. (1969). 'The Kleine–Levin Syndrome with Intermittent Abnormality in the EEG'. *Electroenceph. clin. Neurophysiol.* **27,** 601

Ellingson, R. J. (1954–55). 'The Incidence of EEG Abnormality Among Patients with Mental Disorders of Apparently Non-organic Origin: A Critical Review'. *Am. J. Psychiat.* **111,** 263

— Wilcott, R. C., Sineps, J. G. and Dudek, J. J. (1957). 'EEG Frequency-pattern Variation and Intelligence. A Correlational Study'. *Electroenceph. clin. Neurophysiol.* **9,** 657

REFERENCES

Ellington, A. L. (1968). 'Electroencephalographic Pattern of Burst Suppression in a Case of Barbiturate Coma'. *Electroenceph. clin. Neurophysiol.* **25,** 491

Engel, G. L., Webb, J. P., Ferris, E. B., Romano, J., Ryder, H. and Blankenhorn, M. A. (1944). 'A Migraine-like Syndrome Complicating Decompression Sickness'. *War Med.* **5,** 304

Faulconer, A. and Bickford, R. G. (1960). 'Servoanesthesia'. In *Electroencephalography in Anesthesiology.* Springfield; Thomas

Feinberg, I., Koresko, R. L., Gottlieb, F. and Wender, P. H. (1964). 'Sleep Electroencephalographic and Eye-movement Patterns in Schizophrenic Patients'. *Compreh. Psychiat.* **5,** 44

Fenton, G. W., Hill, D. and Scotton, L. (1968). 'An EEG Measure of the Effect of Mood Change on the Thiopentone Tolerance of Depressed Patients'. *Br. J. Psychiat.* **114,** 1141

Fink, M. (1965). 'Quantitative EEG and Human Psychopharmacology'. In *Applications of Electroencephalography in Psychiatry.* p. 226. Ed. by W. P. Wilson. Durham, N. Carolina; Duke University Press

Finley, K. H. (1944). 'On the Occurrence of Rapid Frequency Potential Changes in the Human Electroencephalogram. *Am. J. Psychiat.* **101,** 194

Fois, A. and Rosenberg, C. M. (1957). 'The Electroencephalogram in Microcephaly'. *Neurology* **7,** 703

— Gibbs, E. L. and Gibbs, F. A. (1958). 'Bilaterally Independent Sleep Patterns in Hydrocephalus'. *Archs Neurol. Psychiat.* **79,** 264

Frey, T. S. and Sjögren, H. (1959). 'The Electroencephalogram in Elderly Persons Suffering from Neuropsychiatric Disorders'. *Acta psychiat., Kbh.* **34,** 438

Funkhouser, J. B. (1953). 'Electroencephalographic Studies in Alcoholism'. *Electroenceph. clin. Neurophysiol.* **5,** 130

Galbrecht, C. R., Caffey, E. M. and Goldman, D. (1968). 'Pentothal-Activated Changes in the EEG of Schizophrenic Patients: Response to Phenothiazine Therapy and Relationship to Selected Patient Variables'. *Compreh. Psychiat.* **9,** 482

Gastaut, H. (1966). 'New Developments in Clinical Electroencephalography'. In *Neurological Diagnostic Techniques,* p. 147. Ed. by W. S. Fields. Springfield; Thomas

— Dongier, S. and Dongier, M. (1960). 'Electroencephalography and Neuroses: Study of 250 Cases'. *Electroenceph. clin. Neurophysiol.* **12,** 233

Gibbs, F. A. and Gibbs, E. L. (1951). 'Electroencephalographic Evidence of Thalamic and Hypothalamic Epilepsy'. *Neurology* **1,** 136

— — (1963). 'Fourteen and Six per Second Positive Spikes'. *Electroenceph. clin. Neurophysiol.* **15,** 553

— — (1964). 'Six per Second Spike-and-Wave Discharge'. In *Atlas of Electroencephalography.* Vol. 3. p. 46 Reading Mass.; Addison-Wesley

— — and Fois, A. (1955). 'Osservazioni elettroencefalografiche nell'idrocefalia, microcefalia, oligofrenia fenilpiruvica'. *Riv. clin. Pediat.* 55, Suppl. 137, 155

— — and Lennox, W. G. (1943). 'Electroencephalographic Classification of Epileptic Patients and Control Subjects'. *Archs Neurol. Psychiat.* **50,** 11

Goldman, D. (1959). 'Specific Electroencephalographic Changes with Pentothal Activation in Psychotic States'. *Electroenceph. clin. Neurophysiol.* **11,** 657

Goldstein, L., Sugerman, A. A., Stolberg, H., Murphree, H. B. and Pfeiffer, C. C. (1965). 'Electro-cerebral Activity in Schizophrenics and Non-psychotic Subjects: Quantitative EEG Amplitude Analysis'. *Electroenceph. clin. Neurophysiol.* **19,** 350

Gordon, E. B. (1968). 'Serial EEG Studies in Presenile Dementia'. *Br. J. Psychiat.* **114,** 779

— and Sim, M. (1967). 'The EEG in Presenile Dementia'. *J. Neurol. Neurosurg. Psychiat.* **30,** 285

Green, M. A. (1948). 'Gargoylism (Lipochondrodystrophy)'. *J. Neuropath. exp. Neurol.* **7,** 399

Greenblatt, M., Levin, S. and di Cori, F. (1944). 'The Electroencephalogram Associated with Chronic Alcoholism, Alcoholic Psychosis and Alcoholic Convulsions'. *Archs Neurol. Psychiat.* **52,** 290

Gregoriades, A. and Pampiglione, G. (1966). 'Seizures in Children with Down's Syndrome (Mongolism)'. *Electroenceph. clin. Neurophysiol.* **21,** 307

Grossman, C. C. (1954). 'Laminar Cortical Blocking and its Relation to Episodic Aggressive Outbursts'. *Archs Neurol. Psychiat.* **71,** 576

— (1963). 'Maturational and Experimental Aspects of "Positive Bursts" '. *Electroenceph. clin. Neurophysiol.* **15,** 163

Hambert, G. and Torsten, S. (1964). 'The Electroencephalogram in the Klinefelter Syndrome'. *Acta psychiat. scand.* **40,** 28

Harding, G., Jeavons, P. M., Jenner, F. A., Drummond, P., Sheridan, M. and Howells, G. W. (1966). 'The Electroencephalogram in Three Cases of Periodic Psychosis'. *Electroenceph. clin. Neurophysiol.* **21,** 59

Henderson, D. K. (1939). *Psychopathic States.* New York; Norton

Hes, J. Ph. (1960). 'Manic Depressive Psychosis. A Case Report'. *Electroenceph. clin. Neurophysiol.* **12,** 193

Hill, D. (1948) 'Discussion on the Electroencephalogram in Organic Cerebral Disease'. *Proc. R. Soc. Med.* **41,** 242

— (1950). 'Electroencephalography as an Instrument of Research in Psychiatry'. In *Perspectives in Neuropsychiatry.* p. 47. Ed. by D. Richter. London; Lewis

— (1952). 'EEG in Episodic Psychiatric and Psychopathic Behaviour'. *Electroenceph. clin. Neurophysiol.* **4,** 419

— (1957). 'The Electroencephalogram in Schizophrenia'. In *Schizophrenia: Somatic Aspects.* p. 33. Ed. by D. Richter. Oxford; Pergamon

— and Watterson, D. (1942). 'Electroencephalographic Studies of Psychopathic Personalities'. *J. Neurol. Psychiat.* **5,** 47

Hoenig, J. and Leiberman, D. M. (1953). 'The Epileptic Threshold in Schizophrenia'. *J. Neurol. Neurosurg. Psychiat.* **16,** 30

Hockaday, J. M. and Whitty, C. W. M. (1969). 'Factors Determining the Electroencephalogram in Migraine: A Study of 560 Patients, According to Clinical Type of Migraine'. *Brain* **92,** 769

Hughes, J. R. (1960). 'The 14 and 7 per sec Positive Spikes—A Reappraisal Following a Frequency Count'. *Electroenceph. clin. Neurophysiol.* **12,** 495

— (1965). 'A Review of the Positive Spike Phenomenon'. In *Applications of Electroencephalography in Psychiatry,* p. 54. Ed. by W. P. Wilson. Durham N. C.; Duke University Press

— Gianturco, D. and Stein, W. (1961). 'Electro-clinical Correlations in the Positive Spike Phenomenon'. *Electroenceph. clin. Neurophysiol.* **13,** 599

197

— and Hendrix, D. E. (1968). 'Telemetered EEG from a Football Player in Action'. *Electroenceph. clin. Neurophysiol.* **24,** 183

Hurst, L. A., Mundy-Castle, A. C. and Beerstecher, D. M. (1954). 'The Electroencephalogram in Manic-depressive Psychosis'. *J. ment. Sci.* **100,** 220

Igert, C. and Lairy, G. C. (1962). 'Intérêt pronostique de l'EEG au cours de l'évolution des schizophrènes'. *Electroenceph. clin. Neurophysiol.* **14,** 183

Ingram, J. M. and McAdam, W. A. (1960). 'The Electroencephalogram, Obsessional Illness and Obsessional Personality'. *J. ment. Sci.* **106,** 686

Jervis, G. A. (1950). 'Gargoylism: Study of 10 Cases with Emphasis on the Formes Frustes'. *Archs Neurol. Psychiat.* **63,** 681

Johnson, G. (1969). 'Lithium and the EEG: An Analysis of Behavioural, Biochemical and Electrographic Changes'. *Electroenceph. clin. Neurophysiol.* **27,** 656

Kales, A., Jacobson, A., Paulson, M. J., Kales, J. D. and Walter, R. D. (1966a). 'Somnambulism: Psychophysiological Correlates'. *Archs gen. Psychiat.* **14,** 586

— — Kun, T., Klein, J., Heuser, G. and Paulson, M. J. (1966b). 'Somnambulism:Further All-night Studies'. *Electroenceph. clin. Neurophysiol.* **21,** 410

Kellaway, P., Crawley, J. W. and Kagawa, N. (1960). 'Paroxysmal Pain and Autonomic Disturbances of Cerebral Origin: A Specific Electro-clinical Syndrome'. *Epilepsia* **1,** 466

Kennard, M. A., Rabinovitch, M. S. and Fister, W. P. (1955). 'The Use of Frequency Analysis in the Interpretation of the EEGs of Patients with Psychological Disorders'. *Electroenceph. clin. Neurophysiol.* **7,** 29

Kiersey, D. K., Bickford, R. G. and Faulconer, A. (1951). 'Electroencephalographic Patterns Produced by Thiopental Sodium during Surgical Operations: Description and Classification'. *Br. J. Anaesth.* **23,** 141

Knott, J. R., Platt, E. B., Ashby, M. C. and Gottlieb, J. S. (1953). 'A Familial Evaluation of the Electroencephalogram of Patients with Primary Behaviour Disorder and Psychopathic Personality'. *Electroenceph. clin. Neurophysiol.* **5,** 363

Leffman, H. and Perlo, V. P. (1955). 'Metrazol and Combined Photic-metrazol Activated Electroencephalography in Epileptic, Schizophrenic, Psychoneurotic and Psychopathic Patients'. *Electroenceph. clin. Neurophysiol.* **7,** 61

Lennox, M. A. and Coolidge, J. (1949). 'Electroencephalographic Changes after Prefrontal Leucotomy'. *Archs Neurol. Psychiat.* **62,** 150

— Gibbs, E. L. and Gibbs, F. A. (1942). 'Twins, Brainwaves and Epilepsy'. *Archs Neurol. Psychiat.* **47,** 702

Lesse, S., Hoefer, P. F. A. and Austin, J. H. (1958). 'The Electroencephalogram in Diffuse Encephalopathies'. *Archs Neurol. Psychiat.* **79,** 359

Letemendia, F. and Pampiglione, G. (1958). 'Clinical and Electroencephalographic Observations in Alzheimer's Disease'. *J. Neurol. Neurosurg. Psychiat.* **21,** 167

Levin, S., Greenblatt, M., Healey, M. M. and Solomon, H. C. (1949–50). 'The Electroencephalographic Effects of Bilateral Frontal Leucotomy'. *Am. J. Psychiat.* **106,** 174

Levy, S. (1952). 'A Study of the Electroencephalogram as Related to Personality Structure in a Group of Inmates of a State Penitentiary'. *Electroenceph. clin. Neurophysiol.* **4,** 113

Liddell, D. W. (1958). 'Investigation of EEG Findings in Presenile Dementia'. *J. Neurol. Neurosurg. Psychiat.* **21,** 173

Lilienthal, E. and Tarlau, M. (1969). 'The EEG in Congenital Absence of the Corpus Callosum'. *Electroenceph. clin. Neurophysiol.* **26,** 635

Lombroso, C. T., Schwartz, I. H., Clark, D. M., Muench, H. and Barry, J. (1966). 'Ctenoids in Healthy Youths: Controlled Study of 14- and 6-per Second Positive Spiking'. *Neurology* **16,** 1152

Long, M. T. and Johnson, L. C. (1968). 'Fourteen- and Six-per-second Positive Spikes in a Nonclinical Male Population'. *Neurology* **18,** 714

Lundervold, A., Engeset, A. and Lönnum, A. (1962). 'The EEG in Cerebral Atrophy'. *Wld. Neurol.* **3,** 226

Lyketsos, G., Belinson, L. and Gibbs, F. A. (1953). 'Electroencephalograms of Nonepileptic Psychotic Patients Awake and Asleep'. *Archs Neurol. Psychiat.* **69,** 707

McAdam, W. and McClatchey, W. T. (1952). 'The Electroencephalogram in Aged Patients of a Mental Hospital'. *J. ment. Sci.* **98,** 711

Magoun, H. W. (1963). *The Waking Brain.* 2nd. Ed. Springfield; Thomas

Margerison, J. H., Anderson, W. Mc.C., Dawson, J. and Lettich, E. (1962). 'The Relationship between Sodium Metabolism, Verbal Output and the EEG in 21 Depressives'. *Electroenceph. clin. Neurophysiol.* **14,** 853

Mellbin, G. (1966). 'Neuropsychiatric Disorders in Sex Chromatin Negative Women'. *Br. J. Psychiat.* **112,** 145

Menolascino, F. J. (1965). 'Psychiatric Aspects of Mongolism'. *Am. J. ment. Defic.* **69,** 653

Mundy-Castle, A. C., Hurst, L. A., Beerstecher, D. M. and Prinsloo, T. (1954). 'The Electroencephalogram in the Senile Psychoses'. *Electroenceph. clin. Neurophysiol.* **6,** 245

Naef, R. W. (1958). 'Clinical Features of Porencephaly'. *Archs Neurol. Psychiat.* **80,** 133

Nevin, S. (1967). 'On Some Aspects of Cerebral Degeneration in Later Life'. *Proc. R. Soc. Med.* **60,** 517

Nielsen, J. (1969). 'Klinefelter's Syndrome and the XYY Syndrome'. *Acta psychiat. scand.* **45,** Suppl. 209, 144

— and Pedersen, E. (1969). 'Electro-Encephalographic Findings in Patients with Klinefelter's Syndrome and the XYY Syndrome'. *Acta neurol. scand.* **45,** 87

— and Tsuboi, T. (1969). 'Intelligence, EEG, Personality Deviation and Criminality in Patients with the XYY Syndrome'. *Br. J. Psychiat.* **115,** 965

Nuffield, E. J. A. (1961). 'Neuro-physiology and Behaviour Disorders in Epileptic Children'. *J. ment. Sci.* **107,** 438

Nymgaard, K. (1959). 'Studies on the Sedation Threshold'. *Archs gen. Psychiat.* **1,** 530

Obrist, W. D. (1954). 'The Electroencephalogram of Normal Aged Adults'. *Electroenceph. clin. Neurophysiol.* **6,** 235

Pacella, B. L., Polatin, P. and Nagler, S. H. (1944). 'Clinical and EEG Studies in Obsessive-compulsive States'. *Am. J. Psychiat.* **100,** 830

Palmer, D. M. and Rock, H. A. (1953). 'Brain Wave Patterns and "Crystallized Experiences" '. *Ohio St. med. J.* **49,** 804

Pasquelini, R. Q., Vidal, G. and Bur, G. E. (1957). 'Psychopathology of Klinefelter's Syndrome: Review of Thirty One Cases'. *Lancet* **2,** 164

Patterson, R. M., Bagchi, B. K. and Test, A. (1947–48). 'The Prediction of Huntington's Chorea. An Electroencephalographic and Genetic Study'. *Am. J. Psychiat.* **104,** 786

REFERENCES

Perris, C. (1966). 'A Study of Bipolar (Manic-Depressive) and Unipolar Recurrent Depressive Psychoses'. *Acta psychiat. scand.* **42,** Suppl. 194, 118

Pierce, C. M., Whitman, R. M., Maas, J. W. and Gay, M. L. (1961). 'Enuresis and Dreaming'. *Archs gen. Psychiat.* **4,** 166

Platman, S. R. and Fieve, R. R. (1969). 'The Effect of Lithium Carbonate on the Electroencephalogram of Patients with Affective Disorders'. *Br. J. Psychiat.* **115,** 1185

Poley, J. R. and Dumermuth, G. (1968). 'Cerebro-Oculo-Renal Syndrome (Lowe)'. In *Some Recent Advances in Inborn Errors of Metabolism*, p. 76. Ed. by K. S. Holt and V. P. Coffey. Edinburgh; Livingstone

Pollack, M., Jaffe, R., Woerner, M. G. and Klein, D. F. (1969). 'Fourteen and Six per Second Positive Spikes in Psychiatric Patients and their Sibs'. *Electroenceph. clin. Neurophysiol.* **27,** 669

Refsum, S., Presthus, J., Skulstad, Aa. and Östensjö, S. (1960). 'Clinical Correlates of the 14 and 6 per Second Positive Spikes'. *Acta psychiat. neurol. scand.* **35,** 330

Rey, J. H., Pond, D. A. and Evans, C. C. (1949). 'Clinical and Electroencephalographic Studies of Temporal Lobe Function'. *Proc. R. Soc. Med.* **42,** 891

Rockwell, F. V. and Simons, D. J. (1947). 'The Electroencephalogram and Personality Organization in the Obsessive-compulsive Reactions'. *Archs Neurol. Psychiat.* **57,** 71

Roth, M. (1951). 'Changes in the EEG under Barbiturate Anaesthesia Produced by Electro-convulsive Treatment and their Significance for the Theory of ECT Action'. *Electroenceph. clin. Neurophysiol.* **3,** 261

— Kay, D. W. K., Shaw, J. and Green, J. (1957). 'Prognosis and Pentothal Induced Electroencephalographic Changes in Electro-convulsive Treatment'. *Electroenceph. clin. Neurophysiol.* **9,** 225

Saul, L. J., Davis, H. and Davis, P. A. (1949). 'Psychologic Correlations with the Electroencephalogram'. *Psychosom. Med.* **11,** 361

Sayed, Z. A., Lewis, S. A. and Brittain, R. P. (1969). 'An Electroencephalographic and Psychiatric Study of Thirty-Two Insane Murderers'. *Br. J. Psychiat.* **115,** 1115

Schiff, S. K. (1965). 'The EEG, Eye Movements and Dreaming in Adult Enuresis'. *J. nerv. ment. Dis.* **140,** 397

Schneider, K. (1958). *Psychopathic Personalities.* Trans. by M. W. Hamilton. London; Cassell

Schwade, E. D. and Geiger, S. G. (1960). 'Severe Behaviour Disorders with Abnormal Electroencephalograms'. *Dis. nerv. Syst.* **21,** 1

Selby, G. and Lance, J. W. (1960). 'Observations on 500 Cases of Migraine and Allied Vascular Headaches'. *J. Neurol. Neurosurg. Psychiat.* **23,** 23

Shagass, C. (1954). 'The Sedation Threshold. A Method for Estimating Tension in Psychiatric Patients'. *Electroenceph. clin. Neurophysiol.* **6,** 221

— and Jones, A. L. (1958). 'A Neurophysiological Test for Psychiatric Diagnosis: Results in 750 Patients'. *Am. J. Psychiat.* **114,** 1002

Short, P. L. and Walter, W. G. (1954). 'The Relationship between Physiological Variables and Stereognosis'. *Electroenceph. clin. Neurophysiol.* **6,** 29

Silverman, D. (1967). 'Phantom Spike-Waves and the Fourteen and Six per Second Positive Spike Pattern: A Consideration of their Relationship'. *Electroenceph. clin. Neurophysiol.* **23,** 207

Slater, E. and Beard, A. W. (1963). 'The Schizophrenia-like Psychoses of Epilepsy. I: Psychiatric Aspects'. *Br. J. Psychiat.* **109,** 95

Small, J. G. (1968). 'The Six Per Second Spike and Wave—A Psychiatric Population Study'. *Electroenceph. clin. Neurophysiol.* **24,** 561

— and Stern, J. A. (1965). 'EEG Indicators of Prognosis in Acute Schizophrenia'. *Electroenceph. clin. Neurophysiol.* **18,** 526

— and Small, I. F. (1965). 'Re-evaluation of Clinical EEG Findings in Schizophrenia'. *Dis. nerv. Syst.* **26,** 345

— — (1967). 'A Survey of Enigmatic EEG Patterns in Psychiatric Practice'. *Electroenceph. clin. Neurophysiol.* **23,** 590

— Sharpley, P. and Small, I. F. (1968). 'Positive Spikes, Spike-Wave Phantoms and Psychomotor Variants: A Survey of these EEG Patterns in Psychiatric Patients'. *Archs gen. Psychiat.* **18,** 232

Smyth, V. O. G. and Winter, A. L. (1961). 'The EEG in Migraine'. *Excerpta med. International Congress Series No. 37,* 136

Spear, A. B. and Turton, E. C. (1953). 'EEG Findings in 100 Cases of Severe Enuresis'. *Electroenceph. clin. Neurophysiol.* **5,** 324

Stafford-Clark, D. (1959). 'The Foundations of Research in Psychiatry'. *Br. med. J.* **2,** 1199

— and Taylor, F. H. (1949). 'Clinical and Electroencephalographic Studies of Prisoners Charged with Murder'. *J. Neurol. Neurosurg. Psychiat.* **12,** 325

— Pond, D. and Doust, J. W. L. (1951). 'The Psychopath in Prison: A Preliminary Report of a Co-operative Research'. *Br. J. Delinq.* **2,** 117

Stewart, C. A. and Smith, I. M. (1959). 'The Alpha Rhythm, Imagery and Spatial and Verbal Abilities'. *Durham Res. Rev.* **2,** 2

Sugerman, A. A., Goldstein, L., Murphree, H. B., Pfeiffer, C. C. and Jenney, E. H. (1964). 'EEG and Behavioural Changes in Schizophrenia'. *Archs gen. Psychiat.* **10,** 340

Sutherland, E. M., Oliver, J. E. and Knight, D. R. (1969). 'EEG, Memory and Confusion in Dominant, Non-dominant and Bi-temporal E.C.T.' *Br. J. Psychiat.* **115,** 1059

Swain, J. M. (1959). 'Electroencephalographic Abnormalities in Presenile Atrophy'. *Neurology* **9,** 722

Thacore, V. R., Ahmed, M. and Oswald, I. (1969). 'The EEG in a Case of Periodic Hypersomnia'. *Electroenceph. clin. Neurophysiol.* **27,** 605

Tharp, B. R. (1967). 'The Six per Second Spike and Wave Complex (The Wave and Spike Phantom)'. *Electroenceph. clin. Neurophysiol.* **23,** 291

Thomas, J. E. and Klass, D. W. (1968). 'Six-per-second Spike-and-wave Pattern in the Electroencephalogram: A Reappraisal of its Clinical Significance'. *Neurology* **18,** 587

Ulett, G. A., Heusler, A. F. and Word, T. J. (1965). 'The Effect of Psychotropic Drugs on the EEG of the Chronic Psychotic Patient'. In *Applications of Electroencephalography in Psychiatry*, p. 241. Ed. by W. P. Wilson, Durham, N.C.; Duke University Press

— Gleser, G., Winokur, G. and Lawler, A. (1953). 'The EEG and Reaction to Photic Stimulation as an Index of Anxiety-proneness'. *Electroenceph. clin. Neurophysiol.* **5,** 23

199

Valentine, M., Keddie, K. M. G. and Dunne, D. (1968). 'A Comparison of Techniques in Electro-Convulsive Therapy'. *Br. J. Psychiat.* **114,** 989

Volavka, J., Matoušek, M. and Roubíček, J. (1966). 'EEG Frequency Analysis in Schizophrenia'. *Acta psychiat. scand.* **42,** 237

Walter, R. D., Colbert, E. G., Koegler, R. R., Palmer, J. O. and Bond, P. M. (1960). 'A Controlled Study of the Fourteen and Six-per-second EEG Pattern'. *Archs gen. Psychiat.* **2,** 559

Walter, W. G. (1953). *The Living Brain.* London; Duckworth

Weil, A. A. (1952). 'EEG Findings in a Certain Type of Psychosomatic Headache: Dysrhythmic Migraine'. *Electroenceph clin. Neurophysiol.* **4,** 181

— (1954). 'Depressive Reactions in Temporal Lobe Seizures'. *Electroenceph. clin. Neurophysiol.* **6,** 701

Weiner, H. and Schuster, D. B. (1956). 'The Electroencephalogram in Dementia. Some Preliminary Observations and Correlations'. *Electroenceph. clin. Neurophysiol.* **8,** 479

Wells, C. E. and Wolff, H. G. (1960). 'Electrographic Evidence of Impaired Brain Function in Chronically Anxious Patients'. *Science* **131,** 1671

White, P. T., DeMyer, W. and DeMyer, M. (1964). 'EEG Abnormalities in Early Childhood Schizophrenia: A Double-Blind Study of Psychiatrically Disturbed and Normal Children during Promazine Sedation'. *Am. J. Psychiat.* **120,** 950

Williams, D. (1941). 'The Significance of an Abnormal Electroencephalogram'. *J. Neurol. Psychiat.* **4,** 257

— (1969). 'Neural Factors Related to Aggression'. *Brain* **92,** 503

Wulff, M. H. (1960). 'The Barbiturate Withdrawal Syndrome: A Clinical and Electroencephalographic Study'. *Electroenceph. clin. Neurophysiol.* Suppl. **14,** 57

CHAPTER 10

SPECIAL TECHNIQUES

SENSORY EVOKED POTENTIALS

A following or paroxysmal response to photic stimulation is, of course, a series of evoked potentials, but the term has come to be used in a more restricted sense. When a precise stimulus, such as an auditory click or a flash of light is presented to a subject during recording, two kinds of evoked potential may occur in the EEG. These are the *non-specific* and *specific responses*. The non-specific response, which may well be the same for a variety of stimuli, is a small but fairly widespread transient discharge of greatest amplitude at the vertex. It may be associated with an immediate change in the on-going activity, such as a diminution of the *alpha* rhythm, if the stimulus has an element of novelty and arouses the subject's attention. This *alerting response* becomes progressively less marked if the same stimulus is repeated a number of times. During sleep, the non-specific response takes the form of a vertex sharp wave of a K-complex, sometimes followed by a train of faster waves (*see* page 65). The specific response occurs at a fairly constant latency after the stimulus and is maximal in the cortical area appropriate to the modality and laterality of stimulation.

Although some attention has been given to the non-specific responses in the past—for instance, to the V-wave in the alert state by Larsson (1956) and to the K-complex during sleep by Roth, Shaw and Green (1956)—more interest has been aroused by the specific responses, the latency, waveform and spatial distribution of which have been the objects of much research. Unfortunately, with the exception of the obvious responses that may be seen during photic stimulation at low flash rates, the majority of evoked potentials are too small to be clearly seen in the on-going EEG. The investigation of these potentials has therefore been dependent on the development of special techniques.

Photographic superimposition was the method first used (Dawson, 1947a) and it is not entirely outmoded by the advent of more sophisticated and expensive devices than a standard cathode ray oscilloscope and a plate camera. The principle is to trigger the sweep of the C.R.O. at each presentation of the stimulus so as to display a short sample of the EEG trace that follows. These are all superimposed on a single photograph, the brilliancy of the C.R.O. spot having been adjusted so that an individual trace is just visible on development of the film. One advantage of this method, not shared by all its successors, is that it gives some indication of the extent to which individual responses are scattered with respect to latency and waveform about their mean. A relatively small number (10–20) of stimulus presentations is usually adequate for the response to be seen. The main practical limitation of the method is that the response must have an amplitude comparable to or greater than that of the background activity if its presence is to be detected. In other words, the signal-to-noise ratio must not be less favourable than 1:1.

This limitation does not apply to average response computers (*averagers*) which are theoretically capable of detecting an evoked potential where the signal-to-noise ratio is as unfavourable as 1:100. These electronic devices in essence add up consecutive samples of the EEG trace following each stimulus presentation. The addition is done electrically by breaking each sample into perhaps a thousand intervals and consigning the value of the voltage in each interval to a particular storage element, *memory* or *address*. If the duration of each sample is 1 second, the voltage waveform over this interval would be sampled every millisecond and 1000 addresses would be required to store it in this *digital* form. As the stimuli are repeated, so the averager is triggered, either at the moment of each stimulus presentation or, preferably, a short time beforehand. Some indication of the level of the background activity is therefore obtained before the first component of the response. This interval can also be used for the insertion of a calibration signal. The evoked potential, so long as it follows the stimulus at a constant latency, and the calibration signal will accumulate in the *register* (the collective term for all the stores), whereas the summated on-going EEG activity, because it is randomly related in time to the stimuli, will fluctuate about zero. When the desired number of stimuli has been delivered, the voltages in the register are divided by the number of stimulus presentations and the average displayed on an oscilloscope screen.

The fidelity with which an average evoked potential is portrayed—assuming all the individual responses to be identical—depends on two circumstances. First, the relative amplitudes of the evoked potential and of the spontaneous EEG activity which, in this context, constitutes noise. If the latter is truly random, the signal-to-noise ratio is improved by a factor $\sqrt{N}$ where N is the number of responses averaged. Averaging 100 responses thus improves the signal-to-noise ratio by a factor of 10. The fidelity of the average evoked potential also depends on the *resolution* of the averager. This in turn is a function of the number of addresses available and of the relative durations of the sweep and the response. Clearly, the sweep duration must exceed the response duration if the whole of the response is to be accommodated. If the response duration is 400 ms and the averager has 1000 addresses, a sweep duration of 500 ms (2 addresses/ms) will give better fidelity than one of 1 second (1 address/ms). On the other hand, a sweep duration of 250 ms (4 addresses/ms) will give better fidelity still, but the latter part of the response will be lost. If averaging is to be performed in two or more channels simultaneously, the number of addresses is divided equally between them and the fidelity of each of the final output waveforms is correspondingly reduced.

There is no *a priori* reason to assume that the responses evoked by a long series of identical stimuli will themselves be identical. The effects of habituation, fatigue or drowsiness are known to alter the characteristics of some evoked responses. Such variations are completely concealed by an averager which displays but a single waveform at the end of each run. Apart from the obvious precaution of endeavouring to keep the subject at a constant level of awareness or alertness, it is useful to compare the average of, say, the first 20 responses with the average of the second 20. This can most easily be done with the aid of a storage oscilloscope which will hold a waveform almost indefinitely on the screen and allows any number of others to be added, either in superimposition or as a series of individual traces (*Figure 10.4a*). If the amplitude of the evoked potential is comparable to that of the spontaneous activity, a storage oscilloscope can be used to superimpose a number of individual responses in a manner analogous to photographic superimposition. It may then be possible to see not only whether responses are obtained, but also the extent to which these differ from one another.

Every experiment on averaging evoked potentials should begin with a dummy run in which the stimulator is set going but its output is not delivered to the subject. In this way, extracerebral potentials time-locked to the stimuli will summate and be evident in the average of the spontaneous EEG activity. It is also good practice to deliver the minimum number of stimuli consistent with achieving an acceptable signal-to-noise ratio. The larger the number of stimuli presented, the greater the possibility of some extraneous factor affecting the final result. Unless it is desired specifically to investigate the response to rhythmical stimulation, it is preferable to present the stimuli at random intervals. However, many workers compromise by using a low presentation rate of the order of 1 per second.

One of the main problems in evoked potential averaging is choosing the derivation(s) to be used. Because of the fairly wide spatial distribution of the non-specific response, it is not legitimate to assume that there is any site on the scalp that is entirely unaffected by it. Furthermore, there is the possibility, particularly with somatosensory stimulation, that the potential fields of the specific and non-specific responses will overlap. These factors undoubtedly contribute to the considerable variations in amplitude and waveform of the evoked potentials recorded in different laboratories. Some additional problems in evoked potential averaging are discussed by Barlow (1964), Cooper, Osselton and Shaw (1969), and Broughton, Meier-Ewert and Ebe (1969).

VISUALLY EVOKED POTENTIALS

Cobb and Dawson (1960) were the first to apply an averaging technique to the examination of visually evoked potentials. They found that the response was maximal at the midline, between the inion and a point some 6 cm anterior to it, and that it consisted basically of 4 components: a small positive and a small negative wave with latencies to the peak of 25–30 and 40–50 ms respectively, followed by larger positive and negative waves with latencies to the peak of 55–65 and 90–100 ms respectively. These components were followed by one or more oscillations of potential with a period of about 100 ms. They noted that the potential distributions of the initial and subsequent components were often different and that the amplitudes and latencies of the waves depended on the energy of the flash.

Subsequent investigators have, in general, confirmed these observations, although it is evident from a review of their findings (Jonkman, 1967) that very considerable variations in detail occur between different subjects and different laboratories. The number of variables is so great that it is essential at the present state of the art for each laboratory to establish a standard technique and to apply this to a range of normal subjects before attempting to apply it to clinical cases.

Some examples of the results obtained in a normal subject are shown in the following figures. The effect of deriving the evoked potential in two different ways from the right occipital electrode (O_2) is shown in *Figure 10.1a*. In the upper trace, the signal is derived between the occipital electrode and the chin; in the lower trace, it is derived between the right occipital and right parietal (P_4) electrodes. The traces were obtained simultaneously by averaging 256 responses to blue-white flashes at 1·5 f/s.

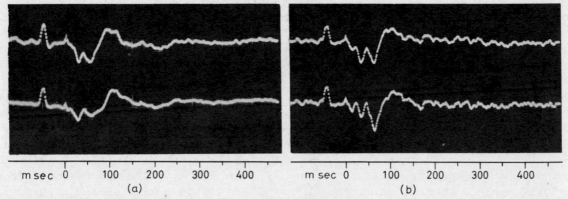

Figure 10.1—Visually evoked potentials. (a) Average of 256 responses to flashes at 1·5 f/s. Derivations: upper trace O_2 to chin; lower trace O_2 to P_4. (b) Average of 128 responses to flashes at 1·5 f/s. Derivations: respectively O_2 and O_1 to chin. Calibration 10μV. Sweep 640 ms. Negativity upwards

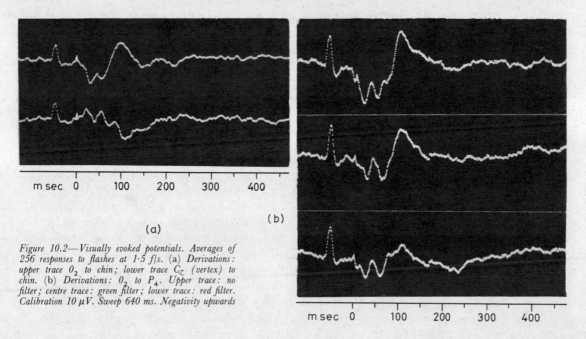

Figure 10.2—Visually evoked potentials. Averages of 256 responses to flashes at 1·5 f/s. (a) Derivations: upper trace O_2 to chin; lower trace C_z (vertex) to chin. (b) Derivations: O_2 to P_4. Upper trace: no filter; centre trace: green filter; lower trace: red filter. Calibration 10 μV. Sweep 640 ms. Negativity upwards

The sequence and latencies of the first three components (27, 37 and 53 ms) are substantially the same in the two traces, but the amplitudes and waveforms of the responses are appreciably different. In *Figure 10.1(b)* are shown the averages of 128 responses derived simultaneously from the right and left

203

occipital electrodes (O_2 and O_1) with respect to the chin. The waveforms are similar but the background activity is more evident because only half the previous number of responses were averaged. The higher voltage of the background activity could account for the difference between the initial components on the two sides. The average evoked potentials derived from the right occipital and vertex (C_Z) electrodes with respect to the chin are shown in *Figure 10.2a*. The vertex response, shown in the lower trace is compounded of delayed components from the specific response together with the non-specific response. The effects of green and red filters of comparable density on the evoked responses from the bipolar derivation O_2–P_4 are shown in *Figure 10.2b*.

The characteristics of visually evoked potentials in occipital, parietal and central areas in 100 normal subjects are well documented by Kooi and Bagchi (1964).

Visually Evoked Potentials in Clinical Disorders

Of all the possible ways in which visually evoked potentials might be considered abnormal, that of asymmetry between the two hemispheres is the most tangible. And of all the possible clinical phenomena which might be associated with such an asymmetry, that of homonymous hemianopic visual field defects is the most probable. Indeed, 75 per cent of Vaughan and Katzman's (1964) patients with field defects of this type gave responses in which some of the components were either of diminished amplitude or longer latency on the affected side. They found that the evoked responses were normal when more than 10 degrees of central vision remained intact. By using stimulus repetition rates of 3–10 f/s, Cohn (1963) was able to demonstrate a significant amplitude asymmetry in all patients with homonymous hemianopic field defects. The use of stimulus frequencies within the range customarily employed during conventional photic stimulation implies that some of the reported asymmetries would have been evident on inspection of the primary traces. Jonkman (1967), however, found that in patients with cerebral lesions the averaging of evoked responses at stimulus rates of less than 1 f/s gave a more reliable indication of the laterality of the cerebral pathology than using a higher flash rate and either averaging the responses or examining them in the primary trace; in fact, there was little to choose between the reliabilities of the last named two methods. Only a partial correspondence was found between asymmetry of evoked responses and asymmetry of the *alpha* rhythm at rest.

Of 19 patients with lateralized brain tumours examined by Jonkman, 17 showed asymmetrical visually evoked potentials, 9 of them having homonymous visual field defects. He found that strikingly asymmetrical responses occasionally occurred in patients with frontal and frontotemporal tumours and in some who showed only early clinical and EEG evidence of a space-occupying lesion. This important observation has been confirmed by Bergamini and Bergamasco (1967).

The findings in patients with cerebrovascular disorders appear to be similar to those in patients with cerebral tumours. Eight of the 17 such patients with asymmetrical responses examined by Jonkman had homonymous visual field defects. The asymmetry was sometimes most evident in the region maximally affected by the lesion, even when this was temporal rather than parieto-occipital in location. Four migrainous patients with consistently unilateral symptoms all showed asymmetrical responses between attacks.

Visually evoked potentials are modified, sometimes dramatically, by changes in the level of consciousness, although it must be borne in mind that the higher voltage and wider spatial distribution of the non-specific response in such circumstances may contribute to the changes described (Kooi, Bagchi and Jordan, 1964). Recording from normal subjects during overnight sleep, Corletto *et al.* (1967) found that the amplitude of visually evoked potentials increased as sleep deepened, but decreased during REM sleep to a level lower than that observed in the alert state. In coma or anaesthesia associated with generalized high voltage delta activity, the initial components of the response are either abolished or greatly delayed, but as *theta* and later *alpha* frequencies reappear during recovery, the response reverts to normal (Bergamini and Bergamasco, 1967).

Although there is some difference of opinion as to whether epileptics show anomalies in their visually evoked potentials, there is no doubt that those who are clinically photosensitive do so. Broughton, Meier-Ewert and Ebe (1969) compared both visual and somatosensory evoked responses in 10 photosensitive epileptics with those in an equal number of age- and sex-matched normal controls. The visually evoked potentials tended to be of higher voltage and wider distribution in the epileptics, the difference between the responses in the two groups being particularly marked at the vertex.

The somatosensory evoked potentials were more obviously different, those in the epileptics sometimes having components with amplitudes eight times as great as those in the controls. The authors infer from these findings that photosensitivity in epilepsy is a manifestation of a diffuse multi-modal alteration in cerebral excitability.

AUDITORY EVOKED POTENTIALS

An electrophysiological response to repetitive auditory stimulation can readily be detected by averaging from electrodes on the scalp, but it is very difficult to differentiate the specific response from other components. Recently, Vaughan and Ritter (1970) have shown that regular auditory stimuli give rise to an average evoked response the potential distribution of which over the scalp could be accounted for by a dipole layer source lying in a plane perpendicular to the surface of the skull and parallel to the orientation of the primary auditory cortex. Apart from its location, the response appears to be specific in that it is of higher amplitude over the contralateral hemisphere when monaural stimulation is employed.

Other audiogenic potentials comprise a non-specific response of cerebral origin and various potentials arising from the muscles of the neck and scalp. These myogenic potentials are most evident with high intensity click stimuli, but have also been shown to occur with brief pure-tone stimuli. Cody and co-workers (Bickford, Jacobson and Cody, 1964; Cody, Bickford and Klass, 1969) have given a great deal of attention to these 'artefacts' which they believe to arise from two sources:

(1) The *inion* or *sonomotor response*, which is mediated by the vestibular system, is best derived with respect to a reference on the nose or ear lobe. Its amplitude varies according to the degree of tension in the neck muscles, being diminished by relaxation and abolished by curarization. The latency to the first negative peak is about 15 ms. The stimuli employed by Cody, Bickford and Klass consisted of 10 ms bursts of a pure 1000 Hz tone. Their normal subjects required intensities of 60–110 dB above subjective threshold for the response to be elicited. Similar responses but of longer latency were evoked by repetitive light flashes and, in some subjects, by electrical stimulation of the median nerve.

(2) The *post-auricular response*, which is mediated by the cochlea, is best derived from an electrode in line with the roof of the external auditory meatus and about 1 cm behind the ear with respect to a reference electrode on the nose. Cody, Bickford and Klass found that its occurrence showed extreme intra- and inter-individual variability. Monaural stimulation sometimes gave a larger response on the ipsilateral side, sometimes on the contralateral side. Sometimes the laterality of the larger response would change at different intensities of stimulation and on different occasions. The latencies and configuration of the response also showed a wide variation. Using the same stimulus parameters as before, intensities of 30–110 dB above subjective threshold were necessary for the response to be elicited. It is thus clear that little significance can be attached to an asymmetry of evoked auditory potentials in the temporal and posterior temporal regions of the scalp.

Evoked Response Audiometry

The importance of detecting hearing loss in infants and in uncooperative brain-damaged children does not need to be stressed. A technique which requires minimal collaboration from the patient and can indeed be carried out during sleep, has obvious advantages over conventional methods. It is sometimes possible to demonstrate that commonplace sounds can be heard simply by presenting these during sleep. The consistent evocation of a V-wave or K-complex is evidence that the stimuli are being received if not perceived at a cortical level. However, habituation to repeated stimuli and the occurrence of apparently spontaneous discharges of an identical kind in the EEG, make even this simple evaluation difficult to achieve in practice (Taylor, 1964).

Much greater reliability can be placed on the results of averaging the non-specific vertex responses to repetitive pure-tone stimuli. These are delivered through calibrated earphones or a bone conduction transducer so that each ear can be tested separately. Each stimulus consists of a brief quantum of sound at a particular frequency, the waveform of the burst being suitably shaped to avoid the production of a click (Klig, Beitler and Stephenson, 1970). The duration of the stimulus is not critical: values in the range 30–200 ms can be used without any significant effect on the accuracy of the results.

Fifty to a hundred stimuli should be delivered at a rate of about one every 2 seconds. If a threshold is to be determined, the intensity of the groups of stimuli is progressively reduced, at first in 10 dB and then in 5 dB steps. The amplitude of the averaged response diminishes and its latency increases as the auditory threshold is approached. With practice, the results of evoked response audiometry in an alert co-operative subject should be within 10 dB of those obtained by the conventional method of testing. When the bone conduction threshold is being determined, a masking signal—random frequency noise—must be applied to the other ear.

In *Figure 10.3a* are shown auditory evoked potentials derived simultaneously from the temporal and vertex regions with respect to the chin. The second of these contains an obvious component of

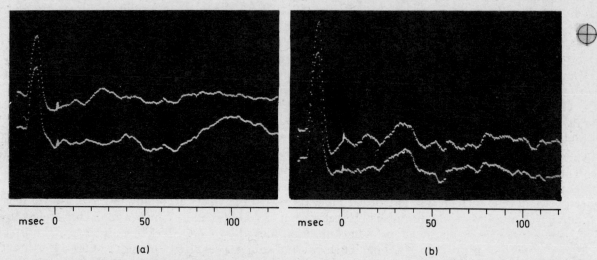

(a)   (b)

Figure 10.3—Auditory evoked potentials. Averages of responses to 1024 binaural clicks at 350 ms intervals. (a) Derivations: T_4 and C_z to chin respectively. (b) Derivations: T_4 and T_3 to chin respectively. Calibration 10 μV. Sweep 160 ms. Negativity upwards

the non-specific vertex response at about 100 ms. *Figure 10.3b* shows similar potentials derived simultaneously from each temporal region with respect to the same reference. The major specific component occurs at about 30 ms.

Additional precautions must be taken when evoked response audiometry is conducted during sleep. Cody, Klass and Bickford (1969) have shown that the latency of the non-specific response varies unpredictably during light sleep and that the investigation should be carried out only during slow wave sleep. The higher amplitude of the on-going activity and the occurrence of spontaneous K-complexes may necessitate the use of a greater number of stimuli. An estimate of the averaged amplitude of the spontaneous activity should be obtained by performing a dummy run in which the sound stimuli are not applied to the subject's ear.

SOMATOSENSORY EVOKED POTENTIALS

Cortical somatosensory potentials were first recorded from the scalp by Dawson (1947a) using a photographic superimposition technique. He subsequently extended his investigations with a specially designed electromechanical averager utilizing the summation principle (Dawson, 1954). Somatosensory evoked potentials have been studied by many workers since Dawson's original description; the account given by Giblin (1964) is particularly thorough.

The stimuli may be electrical or mechanical. The former may be delivered to digital nerve fibres in the fingers and toes, or to mixed nerves at more proximal sites—for instance, to the median, ulnar, anterior and posterior tibial nerves. The advantage of using the fingers is that the identities of the stimulated fibres are known (cutaneous and articular) and the incoming sensory nerve volley can easily be monitored proximally. Larger cortical potentials will be evoked if more than one finger is stimulated. A refinement of the method is to use a robust electromechanical transducer to deliver mechanical pulses to a finger (Sears, 1959). The largest sensory nerve volleys are initiated by tapping the nail.

206

The ideal position for the 'active' scalp electrode is overlying the area of the postcentral gyrus to which the region stimulated projects. If the hand is stimulated, the active electrode should be placed on the contralateral area of scalp 7 cm from the midline, as measured along a line joining a point on the mid-sagittal line, 2·5 cm behind the vertex, and the external auditory meatus (Giblin, 1964). The optimal position for recording the 'foot' response lies on the same transverse line close to the midline. The 'indifferent' electrode is customarily placed 7 cm anteriorly to the active electrode and about 7 cm from the midline.

When the median nerve is stimulated the earliest component of the somatosensory evoked potential has a latency of 16–20 ms (*Figure 10.4*). This value is in good agreement with observations on cells in the VPL 'hand' region of the thalamus which start to discharge 13–19 ms after such stimuli. It has

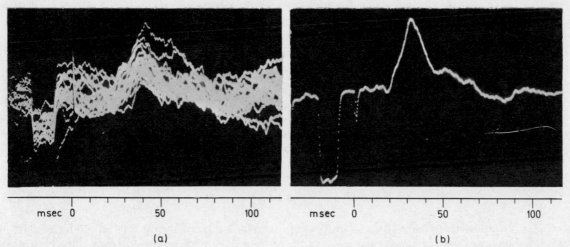

(a)   (b)

Figure 10.4—Somatosensory evoked potentials. (a) *Superimposition on storage oscilloscope of 20 responses to electrical stimuli of left median nerve at wrist.* (b) *Average of responses shown in* (a). *Calibration 10 μV. Sweep 160 ms. Positivity upwards. Derivation see* text

been found that if the active electrode is placed directly on the cerebral cortex within the 'hand' area, the initial wave is always positive (Giblin, 1964), as is also found in animal studies. This positivity is thought to reflect first, the arrival of impulses in the terminals of specific thalamocortical fibres and, secondly, the development of postsynaptic depolarization 'sinks' in relatively deep layers of cortex (*see* page 31). When scalp electrodes are used, however, the positivity may sometimes be preceded by a brief small negative potential. The discrepancy between the cortical and scalp potentials results from the fact that, compared with the cortical electrode, the scalp electrode is averaging activity over a larger area of cortex. If this larger area includes dipoles arranged obliquely, as in the fissures bordering the postcentral gyrus, then the average potential projected to the surface could well be negative (*see* pages 29–30).

In control subjects, the initial positive wave has a mean amplitude of 2·7 μV and never exceeds 8 μV (Halliday, 1967a); it is sometimes bifid and it reaches its maximum amplitude 28–36 ms after stimulation. As would be expected, the latency of the initial positive wave following stimulation of the lateral popliteal nerve is rather longer—around 36 ms (Dawson, 1947a). The positive wave is succeeded by a negative wave of rather variable amplitude and latency which signals excitation of superficial dendritic regions by polysynaptic intracortical routes (*see* page 31). This negative wave is itself followed by alternating positive and negative potentials for up to 0·5 second. In contrast to the early components of the somatosensory evoked potential the later waves, although sometimes large, are extremely inconsistent and consequently have not been studied in detail. This may well be due to their being mixed with components of the non-specific vertex response.

Somatosensory Evoked Potentials in Clinical Disorders

From a study of patients with different types of somatic sensory disturbance, Halliday and Wakefield (1963) and Giblin (1964) have concluded that only the dorsal column–medial lemniscal pathway contributes to the early (180 ms) components of the somatosensory evoked cortical potential. Damage within this system results in an increased latency, a reduced amplitude and an altered configuration of the evoked potential. In contrast, lesions involving the spinothalamic tracts but sparing the dorsal columns are without effect. This marked difference between the spinothalamic and dorsal column contributions to the somatosensory evoked potential can therefore be of some use in the delineation of focal lesions within the spinal cord and brainstem.

Another application of the somatosensory evoked potential technique is in the diagnosis of hysteria. Thus Alajouanine *et al.* (1958) and Halliday (1967b) found that the evoked responses were of normal amplitude in patients with hysterical hemianaesthesia. In this context, it is of interest that the responses are unchanged in normal subjects in whom local anaesthesia has been induced by hypnotic suggestion (Halliday and Mason, 1964). Normal responses are also found in patients with congenital indifference to pain (Halliday, 1967b).

Finally, there are two conditions in which the somatosensory responses are abnormally large. The most dramatic enhancement occurs in myoclonic epilepsy, particularly if the patient is jerking at the time of the recording (Halliday, 1966–67). These responses are commonly 5–10 times as large as in normal subjects; particularly large potentials can readily be detected without averaging and are usually accompanied by myoclonic jerks. In one patient in whom the brain was subsequently examined postmortem (Dawson, 1947b, 1950), the largest potentials were probably generated in the motor cortex rather than in the primary somatosensory area. A more modest increase in amplitude sometimes follows lesions of the brainstem; thus Halliday (1967b) observed enhanced potentials in about a quarter of such cases. This finding is of great interest and might conceivably be related to the postulated role of the reticular formation as a 'censor' for incoming information.

CONTINGENT NEGATIVE VARIATION

If a subject is presented with a warning stimulus followed by a second stimulus to which he is instructed to make a response, then a small electronegative potential can be recorded from the frontocentral region of the brain between the occurrence of the first stimulus and the operant response. This potential change, which is of the order of 20 μV in adults, can sometimes be seen in the primary trace but is best displayed by averaging about 10 trials. The phenomenon was first described by Walter *et al.* (1964) who named it the *contingent negative variation* (CNV). It is regarded as a measure of attention and expectancy and, for this reason, is also known as the *expectancy* or *E-wave*. *Figure 10.5a* from their original publication shows that presentation of either stimulus alone, or both in sequence at a fixed interval, evokes transient non-specific responses from the vertex. Only when the two stimuli are associated and the subject instructed to terminate the second by pressing a button does the CNV occur. Progressive extinction of the CNV occurs when the imperative stimulus is withdrawn and the operant response is no longer performed (*Figure 10.5b*). The CNV does not depend on the modality or intensity of the stimuli used, but its amplitude is positively related to the subject's degree of attention to the experimental situation. The CNV is thus augmented by incentive and diminished by distraction and fatigue. This may account for the fact that the CNV is either poorly developed or intermittent in children of less than 6 years of age (Cohen, Offner and Palmer, 1967). According to Low *et al.* (1966), the CNV in children from upwards of 13 years of age is indistinguishable from that of adults.

The technical aspects of averaging and recording the CNV are discussed by Bostem *et al.* (1969). They draw attention to the necessity of using a time constant of the order of 10 seconds if the form of the CNV is not to be distorted when the generally accepted inter-stimulus interval of about 1 second is used. An even longer time constant is preferable if rebound effects are to be studied (Timsit *et al.*, 1970).

One of the major complications in recording the CNV is the frequent occurrence of simultaneous eye movement potentials over the anterior part of the scalp. Vertical movements in particular give rise to a potential gradient between forehead and vertex which will contribute to the signal detected at the vertex with respect to a mastoid reference—the derivation most often used in CNV work. There is no completely satisfactory solution to this problem. Perhaps the best is to record the experimental data on magnetic tape, devoting at least one channel to monitoring eye movements, and then to eliminate from subsequent averaging any trial in which such a movement occurs. When averaging on-line, a co-operative subject can be instructed to fixate during the test procedure, but this does not

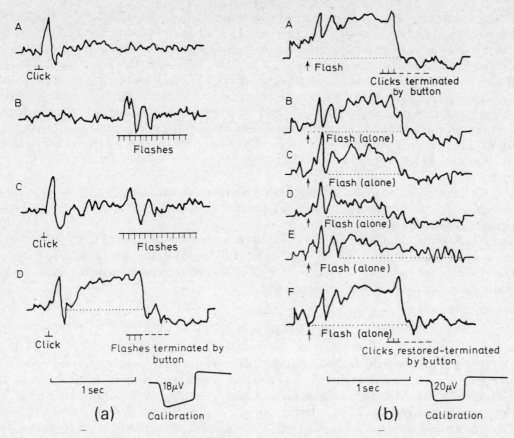

Figure 10.5—(a) Averages of responses to 12 presentations. A: response in frontovertical region to single click. B: response to multiple flashes at 15 f/s. C: response to click followed by flashes at fixed interval. D: as for C but flashes terminated by operant response of subject prior to which there is build-up of the CNV. (b) Averages of responses to 6 presentations. A: fully developed CNV between flash and clicks terminated by subject. B: CNV slightly attenuated in first 6 presentations after withdrawal of clicks. C, D and E: progressive diminution of CNV as the expectancy of reinforcement subsides. F: restoration of clicks quickly re-establishes CNV. Negativity upwards

(From Walter et al. (1964). 'Contingent negative variation: an electric sign of sensori-motor association and expectancy in the human brain.' Nature 203, 380, by courtesy of the Editor)

necessarily eliminate eye movement. An additional device is to derive eye movement potentials from a mid-frontal electrode and electrically to subtract an appropriate proportion of these from the signals derived from the vertex (McCallum and Walter, 1968). However, this method will not compensate for lateral eye movement potentials which may contaminate the mastoid reference. That the CNV cannot simply be ascribed to eye movement potentials has been convincingly demonstrated by its detection from epidural electrodes over the frontal cortex (Walter, 1968)—a location from which eye movement potentials are not recorded.

A further complication is engendered by the *Bereitschaftspotential* or *readiness potential* described by Kornhuber and Deecke (1965). This is a slowly increasing negative potential which occurs maximally in the central regions during the second or so prior to a limb movement. This inevitably contributes to the CNV which is recorded over a similar interval prior to the operant response.

A general review of the status of the CNV in brain research is given by Tecce (1971).

The CNV in Clinical Disorders

Investigation of the CNV in clinical cases has been concentrated largely on patients with psychiatric disorders. Groups of workers in Bristol and Liège have been pre-eminent in these studies. Walter and his colleagues were the first to demonstrate the slow development of the CNV in patients with anxiety, the ease with which the response could be diminished or eliminated by distraction—by presentation of irregular sound stimuli between trials—and the difficulty that was then experienced in re-establishing it (Walter, 1966; McCallum and Walter, 1968). Workers in Liège have examined groups of neurotic and psychotic patients and compared them with controls of comparable age (Timsit et al., 1970). Their groups comprised 70 neurotics (45 hysterics and 25 obsessionals), 45 psychotics (37 schizophrenics and 8 manic-depressives), and 45 controls. No significant differences were found between the distributions of CNV amplitudes in the 3 groups but, within the neurotic group, the hysterics were found to have more low voltage CNVs than the obsessionals. They also measured the prolongation of the CNV potential after the operant response—a rebound phenomenon which will be apparent only if the time constant of the recording system is 10 seconds or longer. They found that this revealed considerable differences between groups. In 9 out of 10 normal subjects the CNV extinguished immediately after the operant response, whereas 34 per cent of the neurotics and 91 per cent of the psychotics showed a prolongation of the negative potential by $1 \cdot 5$ second or longer. Of the psychotics, 56 per cent showed a prolongation in excess of $3 \cdot 5$ second in contrast to only $3 \cdot 5$ per cent of the normal and neurotic groups combined.

McCallum (1969) reported a comparison between groups of psychopaths, neurotics with anxiety, and controls in which the former had mean CNV amplitudes of only $8 \, \mu V$ and showed an appreciably lower degree of conditionability.

He and his colleagues (McCallum *et al.*, 1970) have reported anomalies of CNV in patients with a variety of organic brain lesions. Those with unilateral lesions generally showed a corresponding diminution or distortion of the CNV on the same side. A small number of patients with parkinsonism were found to have particularly low voltage responses.

OVERNIGHT SLEEP

It is more than 30 years since the first continuous EEG recordings were made during overnight sleep and attempts were made to detect the stage of sleep at which dreaming most consistently occurred (Loomis, Harvey and Hobart, 1937; Blake, Gerard and Kleitman, 1939; Knott, Henry and Hadley, 1939). However, it was not until 1955 that Aserinsky and Kleitman demonstrated the association between dreaming and *rapid eye movements* (REM) by awakening subjects at all stages of sleep and obtaining reports as to whether they had been dreaming at the time. Dement and Kleitman (1957) showed that there are cyclic variations in the depth of undisturbed overnight sleep and that these follow a fairly consistent pattern in normal subjects. Rapid eye movements were found to occur only in association with an EEG pattern characteristic of light sleep—namely, relatively low voltage arrhythmic activity with a complete absence of sleep spindles (*see* page 65). Much current research into overnight sleep is concerned with the proportions of time spent in the REM and non-REM stages and the ways in which these proportions vary in clinical disorders and in response to drugs.

APPARATUS AND TECHNIQUE

The acquisition of electrophysiological data continuously over many hours calls for some modification of conventional recording methods, if only to reduce the sheer bulk of the record obtained. It is customary to use fewer electrodes and hence fewer channels than in clinical EEG work, but the recording of additional variables, including eye movements, may require several channels extra to those used for the EEG. Where there are suitable facilities, it may be expedient to record from two or even three subjects simultaneously on a single 16-channel EEG machine. A slow paper speed can often be used for the greater part of the night. In some laboratories the data are recorded directly on to magnetic tape, the signals being monitored on a multi-channel cathode-ray oscilloscope. The data are subsequently played back, possibly at a higher tape speed, for analysis either visually or by computer (Johnson *et al.*, 1967; Itil *et al.*, 1969; Frost, 1970).

As the differentiation of sleep stages is dependent to a considerable extent on the ways in which the signals are derived, an international committee of the Association for the Psychophysiological Study of Sleep has made recommendations with regard to terminology, techniques and scoring methods (Rechtschaffen and Kales, 1968). Referring to the 10–20 system of electrode placement (Jasper, 1958), it is recommended that three common reference derivations should be made of the EEG: O_2, C_4 (or P_4) and F_4 all to A_1, or the corresponding derivations from the left side of the head. The use of a contralateral reference electrode maximizes the amplitudes of the signals obtained. The occipital derivation provides information about the *alpha* rhythm; the central or parietal derivation information about sleep spindles, V-waves and K-complexes (*see* page 65); the frontal derivation information about the slow activity of sleep. If one channel only is available for the EEG, then C_4 to A_1 or C_3 to A_2 is recommended. However, C_z to O_z (vertex to mid-occipital) is, in some circumstances, more informative. Disc electrodes attached to the scalp with collodion and with extra long leads are superior to any other type. The recording sensitivity should be selected in the range 200–50 μV/cm according to the amplitude of the signals obtained. The lower gain is necessary for children, in whom extremely high voltage *delta* activity may be seen in deep sleep.

The recommendation for the recording of eye movements is that at least two channels should be used. The signals should be derived from the following electrodes, each referred to the same reference electrode on an ear lobe or mastoid process: the first 1 cm above and medial to the outer canthus of one eye; the second 1 cm below and medial to the outer canthus of the other eye. Eye movements are normally conjugate so that the recommended derivations give rise to out-of-phase deflections for almost all such movements. This helps to distinguish them from most artefacts and from the slow EEG activity which may spread to all the electrodes during deep sleep. If only one channel is available, a bipolar derivation between the active electrodes specified above is adequate for recording the great majority of eye movements. A sensitivity of about 70 μV/cm and a time constant of about 0·3 second are suitable. Techniques for the more precise measurement of eye movements are described by Shackel (1967). If the subject finds collodion-attached electrodes uncomfortable near the eye, double-sided adhesive rings can be used instead.

It is recommended that the mental or submental EMG should also be recorded; this diminishes particularly during REM sleep. Disc electrodes should be attached with collodion to each side of the neck under the chin and a relatively high sensitivity of at least 20 μV/cm employed in amplifying the signal obtained between them. The EMG is composed essentially of high frequencies; a short time constant of 0·1 second or less and no high frequency attenuation should therefore be used (Jacobson *et al.*, 1965).

Many other measures of a subject's physiological state can be monitored on conventional EEG apparatus by the use of special transducers. During sleep, the ECG is most conveniently derived from

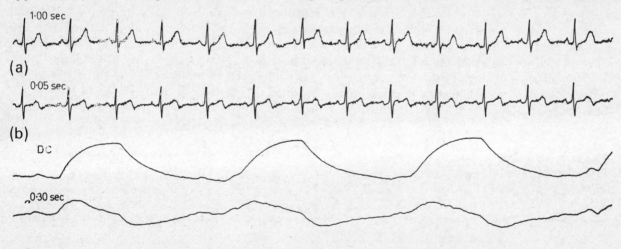

Figure 10.6—(a) *Recording of ECG from electrodes on upper arms with time constants of 1 s and 0·05 s respectively.* (b) *Recording of respiration from thermistor in nostril with time constants of infinity (d.c. setting) and 0·3 s respectively*

electrodes on the upper arms, the intrusion of muscle potentials then giving an indication of body movement. A short time constant can be used if only the heart rate is required; however, a value of about 1 second is necessary if the ECG waveform is to be faithfully reproduced (*Figure 10.6a*).

Respiration rate can be obtained either from one of a variety of thoracic strain gauges, or from a thermistor placed in front of the nose or mouth. This signal should be recorded with the maximum time constant available—preferably on a d.c. setting—if an indication of respiratory depth is required (*Figure 10.6b*).

It is impossible to obtain reliable indications of skin resistance and skin potential changes without the use of special electrodes and measuring devices (Venables and Martin, 1967).

Where only a few recording channels are available—possibly when the data are being recorded directly on to magnetic tape—some economy can be effected by combining two or more of the eye movement and other non-EEG signals in a single channel (Osselton, 1970).

SCORING OF SLEEP STAGES

The transition from wakefulness to deep sleep is a gradual process and it is impossible to define how the level of sleep at any one moment should be determined. It is therefore customary to divide a sleep record into epochs the duration of which might be anything from 10 seconds to 2 minutes depending on the method of analysis being used. Each epoch is then scored according to the stage of sleep which predominates during it. A very wide variety of criteria and of terms has been used to designate the different stages of sleep (Rechtshaffen and Kales, 1968), but it is now generally agreed that the following should be used:

Stage W (wakefulness)—for which the criteria are given on pages 52–54.

Stage 1 (drowsiness)—in which the EEG is of relatively low voltage and is composed of mixed *theta* and faster frequencies, often accompanied by slow eye movements.

Stage 2 (light sleep)—in which there are increased *theta* activity, V-waves, moderate voltage K-complexes and sleep spindles (*see* page 65).

Stage 3 (moderate sleep)—in which 20–60 per cent of the epoch is occupied by sequences of delta waves at 2 Hz or less. Classical K-complexes rather than V-waves tend to predominate during this stage.

Stage 4 (deep sleep)—in which more than 60 per cent of the epoch is occupied by slow activity at 2 Hz or less.

Stage REM—in which the EEG is similar to that of Stage 1 or early Stage 2 but in which sporadic irregular eye movements occur. Although there may be a temporary increase in the submental EMG during clusters of rapid eye movements, its general level is lower during REM sleep than in any other stage. This stage is also characterized by irregular heart and respiration rates and occasional twitching of limb and facial muscles. In these respects REM sleep represents a more active state than that of other sleep stages. On the other hand, the relative absence of the submental EMG and an elevated auditory threshold to arousal (Dement and Kleitman, 1957) suggest that it is a deeper stage than any other. For these conflicting reasons it is sometimes termed *paradoxical*.

Examples of the characteristic findings during the different stages of sleep are shown in *Figure 10.7*. The upper channel of each pair records eye movements plus electrically superimposed submental

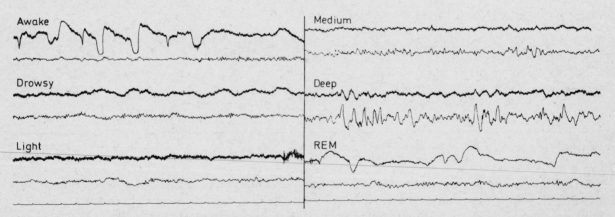

Figure 10.7—Stages of wakefulness and sleep. Upper channel of each pair: eye movements plus submental EMG; lower channel: EEG derived from C$_z$ to O$_z$ (vertex to mid-occipital). See text for details

EMG. The former signal is derived from an electrode 1 cm lateral to the outer canthus of one eye (black lead) and another about 1 cm directly below the margin of the other eye (white lead). This derivation maximizes the potential changes due to eye movements and minimizes contamination by the frontal slow activity of deep sleep. The lower channel of each pair records the EEG derived between vertex and mid-occipital electrodes.

Before attempting to score an overnight sleep record it is helpful to observe the range of phenomena which it contains. This is particularly true of children's records in which the slow activity present during drowsiness and deep sleep is often of very high voltage. If the record is to be scored in epochs, rather than a tabulation made of the durations of succeeding stages, then the epochs should be marked on the record at the first examination. This facilitates comparison between the scorings of independent observers and allows an estimate of inter-rater reliability to be made (Monroe, 1969).

Details of the method for scoring sleep stages are given by Rechtschaffen and Kales (1968). In view of the predominant interest of sleep researchers in the proportion of REM sleep, particular attention should be paid to the rules for scoring this stage. The essential criteria of REM sleep are defined as the character of the EEG, which must be of relatively low voltage, the concomitant absence or diminution of the submental EMG, and the presence of rapid eye movements. The latter are essentially episodic, the intervals between clusters possibly being as long as a few minutes. It has therefore been recommended that, provided the EEG and EMG remain appropriate to this stage, all such intervals should be included in the REM score. The periods before the first eye movement and after the last should also be included in the score for as long as the EEG and EMG criteria are fulfilled. Additional rules have to be applied if the period under consideration contains evidence of body movements. Such rules diminish but do not eliminate the subjective element in the scoring of sleep stages. The customary presentation of proportional sleep durations to an accuracy of one tenth of one per cent implies a degree of precision that is quite unrealistic.

Sleep in Normal Subjects

The overnight sleep profile for a normal adult male scored on the basis of a 2-minute epoch is shown in *Figure 10.8*. The descent into sleep is via consecutive stages whereas the emergence from deep

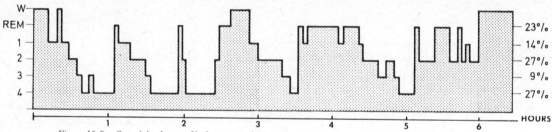

Figure 10.8—Overnight sleep profile for man aged 27 years with proportions of total sleep spent in different stages

sleep is usually by a jump to a much lighter level—a change which is often precipitated or accompanied by a body movement. It will be noted that the sleep changes follow a cyclic pattern the period of which is about 70 minutes in this subject. There is a preponderance of deep sleep during the early part of the night and a preponderance of REM sleep during the later part. The delay to the first REM episode after falling asleep is 55 minutes. These results were obtained on the second of two consecutive nights on which the subject slept in the EEG laboratory. As Agnew, Webb and Williams (1966) have shown, it is essential to allow at least one night for adaptation to laboratory surroundings. On the first night there is a significant reduction in the proportion of REM sleep and a longer delay to the first REM episode.

The characteristics of undisturbed overnight sleep in a group of 16 young men have been reported by Williams, Agnew and Webb (1964). They found that on three consecutive nights the proportion of REM sleep averaged over all subjects was 24·1 per cent, the range of individual variation being 14·4–29·9 per cent. There were similarly large individual differences in the proportions of time spent in the other sleep stages. In contrast, these proportions showed a considerable degree of consistency in a given subject from night to night. Very similar findings were obtained in a group of 16 young women (Williams, Agnew and Webb, 1966).

These findings are in keeping with an extensive study carried out by Feinberg, Koresko and Heller (1967) in which the characteristics of sleep on 4–5 consecutive nights were compared in groups of normal young adults (mean age 26·6 years), aged normal subjects (mean age 77·0 years) and aged subjects with chronic brain syndromes (mean age 77·7 years). Small numbers of children aged 6 and 10 years were also studied. Although the total sleep times for the young and the aged normal subjects were substantially the same, the latter spent a greater time in bed because of more frequent awakenings. On average, the young and aged normal subjects spent 25·0 and 22·8 per cent of their total sleep times in Stage REM. The average latencies to the first REM episode in the two groups were 66·9 and 57·9 minutes respectively. The proportions of REM sleep in the 6 and 10 year old groups of children were 29·8 and 25·3 per cent. In normal neonates the proportion is about 50 per cent (Parmelee *et al.*, 1968). There is thus a tendency for the proportion of REM sleep to fall with increasing age. The proportion of Stage 4 sleep also tends to diminish. A number of other sleep parameters were measured by Feinberg, Koresko and Heller and were found to show significant differences between the two normal groups.

Effects of Drugs

Oswald and his co-workers have shown that the pattern of overnight sleep is disturbed by a great variety of drugs. Paradoxically, the effects of CNS stimulants and depressants are often similar, taking the form of an initial reduction in the proportion of REM sleep, followed by a progressive return towards the normal baseline of 20–25 per cent if administration continues for a week or more and tolerance develops. Conversely, withdrawal results in an initial increase in the proportion of REM sleep (*REM rebound*), followed by a progressive return to the baseline. Both amphetamines (Oswald and Thacore, 1963) and barbiturates (Oswald and Priest, 1965) produce these effects which are shown diagrammatically in *Figure 10.9*. Barbiturates not only diminish the proportion of REM

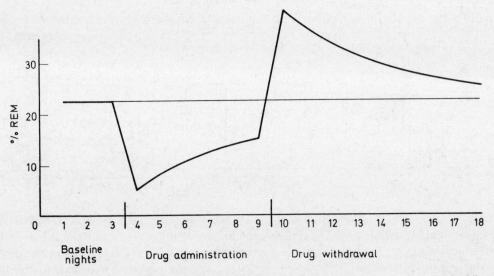

Figure 10.9—Diagrammatic representation of REM sleep variations in response to drug administration over 6 nights followed by withdrawal. (After Oswald, 1965)

sleep but also reduce the incidence of eye movements during this stage. Following withdrawal, both drugs produce an REM rebound, a temporary increase in the profusion of eye movements during REM episodes, and a reduction in the latency to the first REM episode. Premedication levels of REM sleep and normal REM latencies are not regained for several weeks. The delirium that may follow the sudden withdrawal of barbiturates and of alcohol is accompanied by a dramatic increase in the proportion of REM sleep (Evans 8 *et al.* 1966; Greenberg and Pearlman, 1967).

The phenomena of REM habituation and REM rebound also occur with many non-barbiturate hypnotics. Similar effects are produced by tricyclic antidepressant drugs, such as imipramine (Lewis and Oswald, 1969), some of which when taken in excess, may initially abolish REM sleep. In these circumstances, the REM rebound may not reach a maximum for several days after withdrawal—a delay which presumably relates to the rate of elimination of the drug from the brain. In therapeutic doses, these antidepressants and some of the monoamine oxidase inhibitors, such as phenelzine, do not produce a maximal depression of REM sleep until $1\frac{1}{2}$–3 weeks after the commencement of treatment. The clinical response is sometimes similarly delayed.

However, not all drugs that act on the CNS reduce the proportion of REM sleep: fenfluramine and iprindole have little immediate effect, while L-tryptophan and reserpine augment it (Oswald, 1969). These observations have given rise to the supposition that REM sleep is associated with restitutional processes in the brain. Increased cerebral blood flow and cerebral metabolic rate (Reivich *et al.* 1968) and a rise in brain temperature (Wurtz, 1967) during REM sleep in cats give some support to this hypothesis.

CLINICAL DISORDERS OF OVERNIGHT SLEEP

These have already been discussed under the following headings: narcolepsy and cataplexy (page 103); enuresis (page 170); somnambulism and nightmares (page 171); schizophrenia (page 185).

INTENSIVE CARE MONITORING

The growing practice of attempting to resuscitate patients who have sustained a severe cerebral insult has created an increasing demand for means of estimating the outcome. Since the EEG provides one of the few direct methods of assessing cortical function in coma, it has become an important criterion in the 'declaration of death', or of possible survival. It is therefore a surprising fact that few patient monitoring systems include facilities for the long-term recording of the EEG. While a minimum of two comprehensive EEG examinations are mandatory in circumstances where cerebral survival is in doubt, even in these cases it would be informative to know whether or not the EEG pattern had changed between examinations. Continuous magnetic tape recording of even a single channel from each patient in an intensive care unit and subsequent playback of the data at a much higher tape speed would permit a relatively rapid review of a patient's cerebral state from day to day. A continuous monitoring device utilizing a very slow chart recorder has been described by Prior, Maynard and Scott (1970). Chlorided silver disc electrodes attached to the scalp with collodion will provide reliable data over a period of several days with a minimum of attention.

Many of the problems encountered in an intensive care unit are common to recording anywhere other than in the EEG laboratory. The hazards of transporting the apparatus to the patient's bedside are compounded with those of working in a potentially hostile environment. The difficulties are greatest when the task is to demonstrate the presence or absence of electrocerebral activity: extraneous potentials from the surroundings, from the patient and from within the EEG machine itself all tend to obscure a genuinely apotential tracing.

Ideally, two technicians should work as a team whenever a seriously ill patient is examined outside the EEG laboratory, one dealing with the patient, the other with the apparatus. A clinical electro-encephalographer should also be on call to assess the clinical situation and to give an immediate report on the EEG findings. While one technician is applying the electrodes, the other should be checking over the EEG machine, particularly in regard to internal noise level and external interference. Calibration should be carried out at all the sensitivities available in the range 200–10 μV/cm and the noise level noted at the latter setting. This test should be performed without any significant high frequency attenuation.

The level of external interference can be estimated by connecting all channels across a 10,000 ohm resistor laid on the patient's bed. The unfavourable result of this test on one occasion is shown in *Figure 10.10a*; the high level of mains interference was confirmed when the patient was connected (*Figure 10.10b*). Application of a larger (ECG) electrode on the neck under the ear and using this as patient earth for both the EEG machine and cardiac monitor improved the situation to that of *Figure 10.10e*. Increasing the gain fivefold and introducing some high frequency attenuation revealed the

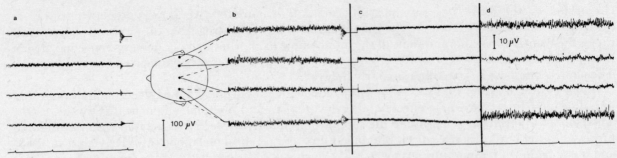

Figure 10.10—(a) *Dummy load test reveals noise and 50 Hz interference at gain of 50 μV/cm.* (b) *Confirmed by recording from patient.* (c) *Reduced by use of single lower resistance earthing electrode.* (d) *EEG and EMG activity revealed by eliminating 50 Hz interference with notch filter and increasing gain to 10 μV/cm*

existence of muscle potentials and a vestige of EEG signal of about 3 μV peak-to-peak (*Figure 10.10d*). If a notch filter at the supply frequency is available on the machine, it is perfectly legitimate to use it when mains interference cannot be eliminated by other means.

The most potent source of mains interference in an intensive care unit is likely to be an electric blanket or warming pad, but monitoring devices are occasionally troublesome. If these cannot be temporarily disconnected, it may be helpful to share a single common earth electrode on the patient—preferably on the head or neck—and to connect all mains-driven equipment to a single supply socket. External electrical interference may also arise from telephone and hospital call systems; chopper-type amplifiers are particularly susceptible (*Figure 10.11a*). (Dobbie, 1967). Some EEG machines also demodulate and record mains-borne radio-frequency signals from sources such as faulty diathermy

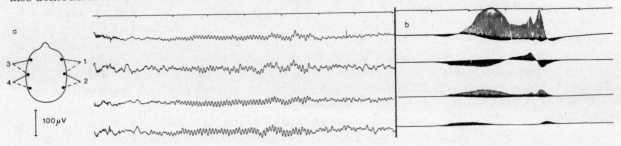

Figure 10.11—(a) *Rhythmical interference produced by hospital call system in chopper-type amplifiers.* (b) *Interference produced by mains-borne radio-frequency signal in push-pull type amplifiers*

equipment (*Figure 10.11b*). Interference of this type can be greatly reduced by the insertion of RF filters in the amplifier input circuits (Hospital Technical Memorandum, 1965). This may be a worthwhile investment if one particular machine is used for recordings outside the laboratory.

No specific recommendation can be made about the type of electrode that should be used, but chlorided silver discs attached with collodion or various types of needle electrodes all have their merits, the needles particularly in the speed with which they can be inserted. Outer surgical dressings should be removed and the scalp cleaned with alcohol. If time permits it is best to apply the full 10–20 placement of electrodes for a comprehensive examination, but this may be impossible if there are wounds on the scalp. The minimum requirements for an EEG examination to determine the presence or absence of electrocerebral activity have been laid down by the American EEG Society (Silverman *et al.*, 1969). These may be summarized as follows:

(1) Application of a minimum of 10 widely distributed electrodes to the scalp, plus an electrode on each ear, all of which should have contact resistances of not more than 5,000 ohms (10,000 ohms per pair).

(2) Use of bipolar derivations from pairs of widely spaced electrodes on the scalp and of common reference derivations with respect to either ear.

(3) Use of a sensitivity of up to 25 μV/cm and a time constant of up to 1 second, where possible, during part of the recording.

(4) Presentation of stimuli in a variety of modalities.

INTENSIVE CARE MONITORING

(5) Use of monitoring devices to detect the origin of possible extracerebral potentials.

(6) A recording time of 30 minutes on each of two occasions about 24 hours apart.

The simpler electrode array shown in *Figure 10.12a* allows a survey to be made which includes all the recommended types of derivation (*Figure 10.12b-d*). Where injuries make it impossible to place

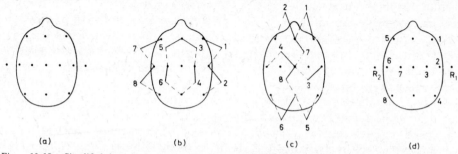

(a)   (b)   (c)   (d)

Figure 10.12—Simplified electrode placement and montages. Reference electrodes R_1 and R_2 on ears or mastoid processes

the electrodes equidistantly, a symmetrical placement should be devised which enables comparisons to be made between the two sides of the head. Common reference recording may be superior to bipolar in these circumstances.

Whether or not a record is of low voltage throughout, it is important to examine the background activity. This may necessitate increasing the gain to the order of $10\,\mu\text{V/cm}$. Failure to increase the gain sufficiently makes it more difficult to tell whether a record contains some traces of EEG activity or

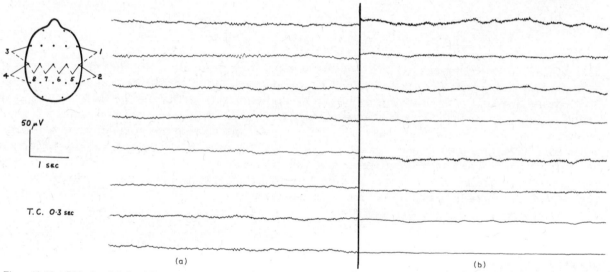

(a)   (b)

Figure 10.13—Difficulty of distinguishing very low voltage and apotential EEG records at gain of $25\,\mu\text{V/cm}$. (a) Shows traces of genuine EEG activity with some pulse artefacts in channels 1 and 3. (b) Shows no genuine EEG activity; potentials related to slow eye movements in channels 1, 3 and 5; traces of EMG activity in channels 1, 2, 3 and 5

whether it is truly apotential (*Figure 10.13*). Both low and high frequency attenuation may legitimately be introduced during parts of the recording if the signal-to-noise ratio is thereby improved.

A patient in coma should be tested for reactivity to light, sound, touch and 'painful' stimuli, but care must be exercised to prevent the stimulus introducing an artefact that might be mistaken for a cerebral response. Photic stimulation can give rise to three kinds of extracerebral potential. The 'spikes' which are recorded as a consequence of incomplete electrical screening of the stimulator can usually be differentiated from any cerebral response that occurs (*see* page 62), but those which arise because of photoelectric action at the surface of a chlorided silver electrode are less obvious. Thirdly, the presence of an electroretinogram can be demonstrated by averaging techniques for a considerable time after all spontaneous electrocerebral activity has ceased (Arfel, Albe-Fessard and Walter, 1968) and may occasionally be evident in the primary record from anteriorly placed electrodes when recording at very high gain.

Touch and pressure stimuli may be accompanied by an artefact induced by manual contact with the patient—in which case it is instantaneous—or may elicit a reflex movement which in turn produces an artefact in the tracing. Similar effects may be seen when there is movement of personnel in the vicinity of the patient and recording apparatus. These are due to disturbance of the electrostatic field and are particularly prone to occur if the electrode resistances are high.

The patient in an intensive care unit, as in other circumstances, is the most prolific source of extra-cerebral potentials, but these assume greater relative importance if the EEG itself is of very low voltage. The most intractable 'artefact' of all is pick-up of the ECG which is most severe when derivations are made from widely spaced electrodes. Repetitive artefacts may also occur synchronously with respiration, especially if this is assisted or performed artificially. Elimination of head movement does not necessarily eliminate this artefact, in which case, after discussion with the clinician in charge of the patient, it may be permissible to turn off the respirator for 10–15 seconds so that its contribution to the total recorded activity can be assessed. Other body movements may also induce artefacts. These can be monitored either by deriving an EMG from the part most often affected, or by recording from a judiciously placed strain gauge or accelerometer. It should not be necessary to stress that all such manoeuvres, together with alterations to the control settings on the EEG machine and the use of non-standard montages should be explicitly noted on the record at the time they are made.

A number of symposia have recently been held on the relevance of the EEG in defining death (Harvard Medical School, 1968; Gastaut, 1969; Driver *et al.*, 1969; Storm van Leeuwen *et al.*, 1969). There are also two books on the subject (Penin and Käufer, 1969; Juul-Jensen, 1970). The practical difficulties encountered in this kind of work are discussed by Montoya and Hill (1968) and, in children, by Pampiglione and Harden (1968).

SPECIAL ELECTRODES

The difficulty of detecting electrical activity from many important regions of the brain, because of their distance from electrodes on the scalp, has provided a stimulus for the development of special electrodes with which some of these regions can be approached from outside the skull. However, it should be appreciated that all such electrodes, because of their smaller contact area, have a higher resistance than conventional scalp electrodes and are therefore more prone to give rise to artefacts. When the contact area is particularly small—as with a needle or wire bared only at the tip—the metal-tissue interface no longer has the electrical property simply of resistance, but will behave approximately like a resistor in parallel with a capacitor. Consequently, the contact impedance will rise as the frequency falls and there may be attenuation of the slower EEG components. The effect can be offset to some extent by the use of a longer time constant in the EEG amplifiers, but this manoeuvre is feasible only if the electrode contact is stable.

Sphenoidal Needle Electrodes

An extremely important region of the brain in the pathogenesis of focal epilepsy is the antero-inferior portion of the temporal lobe, and it has been shown by Pampiglione and Kerridge (1956) that localized discharges can occur in this region that will escape detection by electrodes on the scalp. This was demonstrated by the bilateral insertion of what are generally known as sphenoidal needle electrodes. The electrode consists of a needle, about 6 cm in length, that is insulated by varnishing except at the tip and, most conveniently, has a flexible lead soldered to its proximal end. It is inserted perpendicularly to the surface, at a point approximately 2·5 cm anterior to the incisura intertragica, to pass below the zygomatic arch and through the mandibular notch until it comes into contact with the bone in the region of the foramen ovale at a depth of 4–5 cm. Although painful, this is a procedure that is tolerated without anaesthetic by most patients to whom it has been explained.

A development of this technique which is safer if a major seizure occurs with the electrodes *in situ*, is to use wires instead of needles (Rovit, Gloor and Henderson, 1960). These authors also describe the insertion of leads more anteriorly into the region of the pterygoid plate. These leads can be used in conjunction with sphenoidal electrodes in the more usual position and may provide additional information as to the location of discharges at the tip of the temporal lobe.

Nasopharyngeal Electrodes

The construction and method of insertion of nasopharyngeal electrodes are described by MacLean (1949) and Mavor and Hellen (1964). The latter authors use a 1·7 mm diameter silver rod insulated with varnish except at the bulbous tip. Bach-y-Rita *et al.* (1969) describe a more flexible electrode which consists of a No. 20 gauge silver wire threaded through No. 10 urethral catheter tubing. A bead is formed at the tip by looping the wire and filling with silver solder. One electrode is inserted up each nostril until the tip makes contact with the pharyngeal mucosa near the base of the sphenoidal bone. In this position the electrode records activity from the region of the uncus and anterior part of the hippocampal gyrus and possibly from the upper brain stem and hypothalamus.

A few laboratories use nasopharyngeal electrodes almost routinely, their insertion often being entrusted to the EEG technician, but the earlier types had a reputation, which was not entirely unjustified, for giving rise to artefacts. It is claimed that the more flexible electrode described by Bach-y-Rita *et al.* is greatly superior in this respect.

Nasopharyngeal electrodes are of greatest value in the investigation of patients with temporal lobe seizures in whom they may be used in conjunction with sphenoidal electrodes (Rovit, Gloor and Rasmussen, 1961).

Tympanic Electrodes

The construction and method of insertion through the external auditory canal of tympanic electrodes have been described by Arellano (1949). It would appear from illustrations in a subsequent paper (MacLean and Arellano, 1950) that the EEG activity recorded from the tympanic membrane is qualitatively and often quantitatively similar to that obtained from an electrode on the ear lobe.

Naso-Ethmoidal Electrodes

Lehtinen and Bergström (1970) have recently described the use of a commercially available flexible nasopharyngeal electrode to record from the inferior parts of the frontal lobes in the region of the ethmoid bone. Local anaesthesia is produced by a xylocain spray and the electrode is inserted upwards between the septum nasi and the conchae. Radiography shows that if these electrodes are inserted bilaterally their tips lie no more than 5 mm apart. A single electrode is therefore considered adequate. Examples are given of paroxysmal and slow wave activities which are largely confined to the inferior frontal regions and are not readily seen in derivations from electrodes on the scalp.

REFERENCES

Agnew, H. W., Webb, W. B. and Williams, R. L. (1966). 'The First Night Effect: an EEG Study of Sleep'. *Psychophysiol.* **2,** 263

Alajouanine, T., Scherrer, J., Barbizet, J., Calvet, J. and Verley, R. (1958). 'Potentiels evoqués corticaux chez les sujets atteints de troubles somesthésiques'. *Revue neurol.* **98,** 757

Arellano, Z., A. P. (1949). 'A Tympanic Lead'. *Electroenceph. clin. Neurophysiol.* **1,** 112

Arfel, G., Albe-Fessard, D. and Walter, S. (1968). 'Evoked Potentials in Coma'. *Electroenceph. clin. Neurophysiol.* **25,** 93

Aserinsky, E. and Kleitman, N. (1955). 'Two types of Ocular Motility Occurring in Sleep'. *J. appl. Physiol.* **8,** 1

Bach-y-Rita, G., Lion, J., Reynolds, J. and Ervin, F. R. (1969). 'An Improved Nasopharyngeal Lead'. *Electroenceph. clin. Neurophysiol.* **26,** 220

Barlow, J. S. (1964). 'Sensory Evoked Response in Man'. *Ann. N.Y. Acad. Sci.* **112,** 219

Bergamini, L. and Bergamasco, B. (1967). 'Possibility of the Clinical Use of Sensory Evoked Potentials Transcranially Recorded in Man'. *Electroenceph. clin. Neurophysiol.* Suppl. **26,** 114

Bickford, R. G., Jacobson, J. L. and Cody, D. T. R. (1964). 'Nature of Averaged Evoked Potentials to Sound and Other Stimuli in Man'. *Ann. N.Y. Acad. Sci.* **112,** 204

Blake, H., Gerard, R. W. and Kleitman, N. (1939). 'Factors Influencing Brain Potentials during Sleep'. *J. Neurophysiol.* **2,** 48

Bostem, F., Dongier, M., Low, M., McCallum, W. C. and Walter, W. G. (1969). 'Aspects Techniques.' In *Variations Contingentes Négatives*, p. 21. Ed. by J. Dargent and M. Dongier. Université de Liège

Broughton, R., Meier-Ewert, K.-H. and Ebe, M. (1969). 'Evoked Visual, Somato-sensory and Retinal Potentials in Photosensitive Epilepsy'. *Electroenceph. clin. Neurophysiol.* **27,** 373

Cobb, W. A. and Dawson, G. D. (1960). 'The Form and Latency in Man of the Occipital Potentials Evoked by Bright Flashes'. *J. Physiol.* **152,** 108

Cody, D. T. R., Klass, D. W. and Bickford, R. G. (1967). 'Cortical Audiometry: an Objective Method of Evaluating Auditory Acuity in Awake and Sleeping Man'. *Trans. Am. Acad. Ophthal. Oto-lar.* **71,** 81

— Bickford, R. G. and Klass, D. W. (1969). 'Averaged Evoked Myogenic Responses in Normal Man'. *Int. Audiol.* **8,** 391

— Klass, D. W. and Bickford, R. G. (1969). 'Cortical Audiometry: Test Problems and Sources of Error'. *Int. Audiol.* **8,** 337

Cohen, J., Offner, F. and Palmer, C. W. (1967). 'Development of the Contingent Negative Variation in Children.' *Electroenceph. clin. Neurophysiol.* **23**, 77

Cohn, R. (1963). 'Evoked Visual Cortical Responses in Homonymous Hemianopic Defects in Man'. *Electroenceph. clin. Neurophysiol.* **15**, 922

Cooper, R., Osselton, J. W. and Shaw, J. C. (1969). *EEG Technology*, p. 124. London; Butterworths

Corletto, F., Gentilomo, A., Rosadini, A., Rossi, G. F. and Zattoni, J. (1967). 'Visual Evoked Responses during Sleep in Man'. *Electroenceph. clin. Neurophysiol.* Suppl. **26**, 61

Dawson, G. D. (1947a). 'Cerebral Responses to Electrical Stimulation of Peripheral Nerve in Man'. *J. Neurol. Neurosurg. Psychiat.* **10**, 134

— (1947b). 'Investigations on a Patient Subject to Myoclonic Seizures after Sensory Stimulation'. *J. Neurol. Neurosurg. Psychiat.* **10**, 141

— (1950). 'Cerebral Responses to Nerve Stimulation in Man'. *Br. med. Bull.* **6**, 326

— (1954). 'A Summation Technique for the Detection of Small Evoked Potentials'. *Electroenceph. clin. Neurophysiol.* **6**, 65

Dement, W. and Kleitman, N. (1957). 'Cyclic Variations in EEG during Sleep and their Relation to Eye Movements, Body Motility and Dreaming'. *Electroenceph. clin. Neurophysiol.* **9**, 673

Dobbie, A. K. (1967). 'A Special Interference Problem with Chopper-Type Amplifiers'. *Wld. med. Electron.* **5**, 124

Driver, M. V., Poole, E. W., Crow, H. J., Winter, A. L., Harden, A. and Prior, P. F. (1969). 'The EEG in the Declaration of Death'. *Electroenceph. clin. Neurophysiol.* **27**, 332

Evans, J. I., Lewis, S. A., Gibb, I. A. M. and Cheetham, M. (1968). 'Sleep and Barbiturates: Some Experiments and Observations.' *Br. med. J.* **4**, 291

Feinberg, I., Koresko, R. L. and Heller, N. (1967). 'EEG Sleep Patterns as a Function of Normal and Pathological Aging in Man'. *J. psychiat. Res.* **5**, 107

Frost Jr., J. D. (1970). 'An Automatic Sleep Analyser'. *Electroenceph. clin. Neurophysiol.* **29**, 88

Gastaut, H. (1969). 'Recommandations provisoires de la Commission de la Société d'EEG et de Neurophysiologie Clinique de Langue Française chargée d'etudier Les Signes EEG de la "Mort Cérébrale" '. *Revue neurol.* **121**, 237

Giblin, D. R. (1964). 'Somatosensory Evoked Potential in Healthy Subjects and in Patients with Lesions of the Nervous System'. *Ann. N.Y. Acad. Sci.* **112**, 93

Greenberg, R. and Pearlman, C. (1967). 'Delirium Tremens and Dreaming.' *Am. J. Psychiat.* **124**, 133

Halliday, A. M. (1966–67). 'Cerebral Evoked Potentials in Familial Progressive Myoclonic Epilepsy'. *J. R. Coll. Physns, Lond.* **1**, 123

— (1967a). 'The Electrophysiological Study of Myoclonus in Man'. *Brain* **90**, 241

— (1967b). 'Changes in the Form of Cerebral Evoked Responses in Man Associated with Various Lesions of the Nervous System'. *Electroenceph. clin. Neurophysiol.* Suppl. **25**, 178

— and Wakefield, G. S. (1963). 'Cerebral Evoked Responses in Patients with Dissociated Sensory Loss'. *J. Neurol. Neurosurg. Psychiat.* **26**, 211

— and Mason, A. A. (1964). 'The Effect of Hypnotic Anaesthesia on Cortical Responses'. *J. Neurol. Neurosurg. Psychiat.* **27**, 300

Harvard Medical School (1968). 'Report of the *ad hoc* Committee to Examine the Definition of Brain Death'. *J. Am. med. Ass.* **205**, 337

Hospital Technical Memorandum No. 14 (1965). *Abatement of Electrical Interference.* London; H.M.S.O.

Itil, T. M., Shapiro, D. M., Fink, M. and Kassebaum, D. (1969). 'Digital Computer Classification of EEG Sleep Stages'. *Electroenceph. clin. Neurophysiol.* **27**, 76

Jacobson, A., Kales, A., Zweizig, J. R. and Kales, J. (1965). 'Special EEG and EMG Techniques for Sleep Research'. *Am. J. EEG Technol.* **5**, 5

Jasper, H. H. (1958). Report of the Committee on Methods of Clinical Examination in Electroencephalography. *Electroenceph. clin. Neurophysiol.* **10**, 370

Johnson, L. C., Nute, C., Austin, M. T. and Lubin, A. (1967). 'Spectral Analysis of the EEG during Waking and Sleeping'. *Electroenceph. clin. Neurophysiol.* **23**, 80

Jonkman, E. J. (1967). *The Average Cortical Response to Photic Stimulation.* Wassenaar; St. Ursula Kliniek

Juul-Jensen, P. (1970). *Criteria of Brain Death.* Copenhagen; Munksgaard

Klig, V., Beitler, S. and Stephenson, E. (1970). 'Sinusoidal Burst Generator for Auditory Evoked Response Research'. *IEEE Trans. biomed. Engng.* **17**, 74 (with corrections: *ibid* 1970, **17**, 269)

Knott, J. R., Henry, C. E. and Hadley, J. M. (1939). 'Brain Potentials during Sleep: a Comparative Study of the Dominant and Non-dominant Alpha Groups'. *J. exp. Psychol.* **24**, 157

Kooi, K. A. and Bagchi, B. K. (1964). 'Visual Evoked Responses in Man: Normative Data'. *Ann. N.Y. Acad. Sci.* **112**, 254

— — and Jordan, R. N. (1964). 'Observations on Photically Evoked Occipital and Vertex Waves during Sleep in Man'. *Ann. N.Y. Acad. Sci.* **112**, 270

Kornhuber, H. H. and Deecke, L. (1965). 'Hirnpotentialänderungen bei Willkürbewegungen und passiven Bewegungen des Menschen: Bereitschaftspotential und reafferente Potentiale.' *Pflügers Arch. ges. Physiol.* **284**, 1

Larsson, L. E. (1956). 'The Relation between the Startle Reaction and the Non-specific EEG Response to Sudden Stimuli with a Discussion on the Mechanism of Arousal'. *Electroenceph. clin. Neurophysiol.* **8**, 631

Lehtinen, L. O. J. and Bergström, L. (1970). 'Naso-Ethmoidal Electrode for Recording the Electrical Activity of the Inferior Surface of the Frontal Lobe'. *Electroenceph. clin. Neurophysiol.* **29**, 303

Lewis, S. A. and Oswald, I. (1969). 'Overdose of Tricyclic Anti-depressants and Deductions Concerning their Cerebral Action'. *Br. J. Psychiat.* **115**, 1403

Loomis, A. L., Harvey, E. N. and Hobart, G. E. (1937). 'Cerebral States during Sleep, as Studied by Human Brain Potentials'. *J. exp. Psychol.* **21**, 127

Low, M. D., Borda, R. P., Frost, J. D. and Kellaway, P. (1966). 'Surface Negative, Slow-potential Shift Associated with Conditioning in Man.' *Neurology* **16**, 771

McCallum, W. C. (1969). Contribution to discussion on 'Applications à la Pathologie'. In *Variations Contingentes Négatives*, p. 146. Ed. by J. Dargent and M. Dongier. Université de Liège

REFERENCES

— and Walter, W. G. (1968). 'The Effects of Attention and Distraction on the Contingent Negative Variation in Normal and Neurotic Subjects.' *Electroenceph. clin. Neurophysiol.* **25,** 319

— — Winter, A., Scotton, L. and Cummins, B. (1970). 'The Contingent Negative Variation in Cases of Known Brain Lesions'. *Electroenceph. clin. Neurophysiol.* **28,** 210

MacLean, P. D. (1949). 'A New Nasopharyngeal Lead'. *Electroenceph. clin. Neurophysiol.* **1,** 110

— and Arellano Z., A. P. (1950). 'Basal Lead Studies in Epileptic Automatisms'. *Electroenceph. clin. Neurophysiol.* **2,** 1

Mavor, H. and Hellen, M. K. (1964). 'Nasopharyngeal Electrode Recording'. *Am. J. EEG Technol.* **4,** 43

Monroe, L. J. (1969). 'Inter-rater Reliability and the Role of Experience in Scoring EEG Sleep Records: Phase 1'. *Psychophysiol.* **5,** 376

Montoya, M. L. and Hill, G. (1968). 'EEG Recording in Intensive Care Units'. *Am. J. EEG Technol.* **8,** 85; reprinted in *Proc. electrophysiol. Technol. Ass.* 1969, **16,** 3

Osselton, J. W. (1970). 'Techniques for Data Compression in the Recording and Analysis of Prolonged EEG and other Electrophysiological Signals'. *Am. J. EEG Technol.* **10,** 97; *Proc. electrophysiol. Technol. Ass.* **17,** 190

Oswald, I. (1965). 'Some Psychophysiological Features of Human Sleep'. In *Progress in Brain Research, Vol. 18* p. 160. *Sleep Mechanisms.* Ed. by K. Akert, C. Bally and J. P. Schade. Amsterdam, London, and New York; Elsevier.

— (1969). 'Human Brain Protein, Drugs and Dreams'. *Nature, Lond.* **223,** 893

— and Thacore, V. R. (1963). 'Amphetamine and Phenmetrazine Addiction: Physiological Abnormalities in the Abstinence Syndrome'. *Br. med. J.* **2,** 427

— and Priest, R. G. (1965). 'Five Weeks to Escape the Sleeping-Pill Habit'. *Br. med. J.* **2,** 1093

Pampiglione, G. and Kerridge, J. (1956). 'EEG Abnormalities from the Temporal Lobe Studied with Sphenoidal Electrodes'. *J. Neurol. Neurosurg. Psychiat.* **19,** 117

— and Harden, A. (1968). 'Resuscitation after Cardiocirculatory Arrest. Prognostic Evaluation of Early Electroencephalographic Findings'. *Lancet* **1,** 1261

Parmelee, A. H., Akiyama, Y., Schultz, M. A., Wenner, W. H., Schulte, F. J. and Stern, E. (1968). 'The Electroencephalogram in Active and Quiet Sleep in Infants'. In *Clinical Electroencephalography of Children,* p. 77. Ed. by P. Kellaway and I. Petersén. Stockholm; Almqvist and Wiksell

Penin, H. and Käufer, C. (Eds.) (1969). *Der Hirntod.* Stuttgart; Thieme

Prior, P. F., Maynard, D. and Scott, D. F. (1970). 'A New Device for Continuous Monitoring of Cerebral Activity: its Use Following Cerebral Anoxia'. *Electroenceph. clin. Neurophysiol.* **28,** 423

Rechtschaffen, A. and Kales, A. (Eds.) (1968). *A Manual of Standardized Terminology, Techniques and Scoring System for Sleep Stages of Human Subjects.* Washington D.C.; U.S. Government Printing Office, Public Health Service

Reivich, M., Isaacs, G., Evarts, E. and Kety, S. (1968). 'The Effect of Slow Wave Sleep and REM Sleep on Regional Cerebral Blood Flow in Cats'. *J. Neurochem.* **15,** 301

Roth, M., Shaw, J. and Green, J. (1956). 'The Form, Voltage Distribution and Physiological Significance of the K-Complex'. *Electroenceph. clin. Neurophysiol.* **8,** 385

Rovit, R. L., Gloor, P. and Henderson, L. R. (1960). 'Temporal Lobe Epilepsy—A Study using Multiple Basal Electrodes. I: Description of Method'. *Neurochirurgia* **3,** 6

— — and Rasmussen, T. (1961). 'Sphenoidal Electrodes in the Electrographic Study of Patients with Temporal Lobe Epilepsy—An Evaluation'. *J. Neurosurg.* **18,** 151

Sears, T. A. (1959). 'Action Potentials Evoked in Digital Nerves by Stimulation of Mechanoreceptors in the Human Finger'. *J. Physiol.* **148,** 30P

Shackel, B. (1967). 'Eye Movement Recording by Electro-oculography'. In *A Manual of Psychophysiological Methods,* p. 299. Ed. by P. H. Venables and I. Martin. Amsterdam; North-Holland

Silverman, D., Saunders, M. G., Schwab, R. S. and Masland, R. L. (1969). 'Cerebral Death and the Electroencephalogram'. *J. Am. med. Ass.* **209,** 1505

Storm van Leeuwen, W., Jonkman, E. J., Leenstra-Borsje, H., Boonstra, S., Blokzijl, E. J., Notermans, S. L. H and Visser, S. L. (1969). 'Symposium on the Significance of EEG for "Statement of Death" '. *Electroenceph. clin. Neurophysiol.* **27,** 214

Taylor, I. G. (1964). 'Examination of Children under Sleep using Electroencephalography'. In *Neurological Mechanisms of Hearing and Speech in Children.* Washington; Manchester University Press

Tecce, J. J. (1971). 'Contingent Negative Variation and Individual Differences: a New Approach to Brain Research.' *Archs gen. Psychiat.* **24,** 1

Timsit, M., Koninckx, N., Dargent, J., Fontaine, O. and Dongier, M. (1970). 'Variations Contingentes Négatives en Psychiatrie.' *Electroenceph. clin. Neurophysiol.* **28,** 41

Vaughan, H. G. and Katzman, R. (1964). 'Evoked Response in Visual Disorders'. *Ann. N.Y. Acad. Sci.* **112,** 305

— and Ritter, W. (1970). 'The Sources of Auditory Evoked Responses Recorded from the Human Scalp'. *Electroenceph. clin. Neurophysiol.* **28,** 360

Venables, P. H. and Martin, I. (1967). 'Skin Resistance and Skin Potential'. In *A Manual of Psychophysiological Methods,* p. 53. Ed. by P. H. Venables and I. Martin. Amsterdam; North-Holland

Walter, W. G. (1966). 'Electrophysiologic Contributions to Psychiatric Therapy.' In *Current Psychiatric Therapies.* Ed. by J. H. Masserman. New York; Grune & Stratton

— (1968). 'The Contingent Negative Variation: an Electrocortical Sign of Sensori-motor Reflex Association in Man'. *Prog. Brain Res.* **22,** 364

— Cooper, R., Aldridge, V. J., McCallum, W. C. and Winter, A. L. (1964). 'Contingent Negative Variation: an Electric Sign of Sensori-motor Association and Expectancy in the Human Brain.' *Nature, Lond.* **203,** 380

Williams, R. L., Agnew, H. W. and Webb, W. B. (1964). 'Sleep Patterns in Young Adults: an EEG Study'. *Electroenceph. clin. Neurophysiol.* **17,** 376

— — — (1966). 'Sleep Patterns in the Young Adult Female: an EEG Study'. *Electroenceph. clin. Neurophysiol.* **20,** 264

Wurtz, R. H. (1967). 'Physiological Correlates of Steady Potential Shifts during Sleep and Wakefulness. II: Brain Temperature, Blood Pressure and Potential Changes across the Ependyma'. *Electroenceph. clin. Neurophysiol.* **22,** 43

CHAPTER 11

THE VALUE AND LIMITATIONS OF ELECTROENCEPHALOGRAPHY

LIMITATIONS

The electrical potentials recorded in the form of an EEG are an expression of as yet ill-understood dynamic cerebral processes, some physiological and others pathological. Although clearly these discharges are dependent upon neural activity, they do not necessarily indicate the integrity or otherwise of the cerebral structure. This is well exemplified by those frequent cases with indisputable clinical evidence of cerebral destruction—and yet the EEG findings are within normal limits. In the case of head injuries, Williams' paradox—that a normal EEG indicates a poor prognosis—stresses the fact that total loss of neurones may have little or no effect upon the EEG patterns as recorded by our present techniques. Although many different disease processes produce EEG abnormalities the variety of these is restricted, for the EEG has a limited repertoire. Consequently, as a method of clinical investigation the EEG suffers the serious limitation of possessing little diagnostic specificity. So often a record can be declared abnormal—even grossly so—but at this point certainty must yield to speculation. Even if the clinical history of the patient limits the diagnostic possibilities, the selection and naming of a single condition as the cause of the particular EEG abnormality is seldom more than an inspired guess.

The EEG is particularly sensitive to such physiological variables as the level of awareness, the acid-base equilibrium and the blood sugar level. Variations in these may exert profound effects upon the EEG. If they are not appreciated, the real significance of the EEG changes will be overlooked and these may well be misinterpreted and regarded as evidence of disease. It is unfortunate that such physiological changes may give rise to EEG patterns indistinguishable from those resulting from pathological states. It is for such reasons as these that the contribution made by the EEG as a diagnostic aid in clinical medicine has been so limited. As a method of investigation, electroencephalography has failed to satisfy the expectations of its early days.

The criticism is sometimes made of electroencephalography that its approach is entirely empirical and that the interpretation of records is merely a question of approximate correlations (Hill, 1957). This cannot be denied; electroencephalography suffers all the limitations of any statistical method when it is applied to the individual patient, but as Pickering (1960) has pointed out, all medical diagnosis and prognosis is merely a matter of probability and fundamental understanding of the pathogenesis of disease is virtually non-existent. To criticize electroencephalography because it makes use of probabilities and because we do not understand the basic physiological mechanisms upon which the EEG potentials depend, is no more than one might say with justification about any branch of medicine or of the host of empirical investigations in everyday use. The Wassermann reaction is every bit as empirical as the EEG and even a chest radiograph merely provides a pattern of shadows with its attendant correlates. Electroencephalography differs only in that the probabilities involved are of a lower order than in most tests employed in other medical fields. It is this that limits the value of its application to clinical problems; in EEG reports the words 'certain' and 'diagnostic' have little or no place.

Incorrect Assumptions

It is not surprising that there should be disappointment at the failure of electroencephalography to fulfil its early expectations, but in large part these were engendered by a number of incorrect assumptions (Hill, 1957). The complex functional interrelationships of cortical and subcortical structures were not fully appreciated at the time these optimistic hopes were expressed, and the significance of the reticular activating system had not been realized. A belief in the autonomy of different regions of the brain proved to be an over-simplification and interpretations of records based on this view suffered in accuracy. It was some time before it was appreciated, for instance, that even though a localized cerebral lesion might exist, an associated focus of slow activity might be displaced at a considerable distance; and that a focal cortical lesion might give rise to a generalized EEG abnormality as in secondary subcortical epilepsy. It was also believed that certain EEG patterns had constant clinical concomitants. This was the basis of the Harvard studies of epilepsy (Gibbs, Gibbs and Lennox, 1938); 'wave and spike' activity was equated with petit mal and the '6 per second square-topped waves' with psychomotor epilepsy. As realization came that spike and wave activity occurred in patients whose attacks always took the form of grand mal and was occasionally found in individuals who never experienced any variety of epileptic attack whatsoever, this simple equation of electrical and clinical phenomena had to be abandoned. Nevertheless, a tendency of this kind is still apparent in reports emanating from many EEG laboratories. It is certainly difficult to avoid altogether for there is a not unnatural tendency to endeavour to make an EEG report as positive as possible with the intention, often belied in practice, of providing help to the referring clinician.

Abnormal Records of No Apparent Clinical Significance

A difficulty that some people experience in relation to electroencephalography is that a proportion of healthy subjects are described as having abnormal records. The objection is advanced that the classification of data leading to such a state of affairs is illogical and results in an impossible situation when dealing with practical problems (Bergman and Green, 1956–57). Certainly it may sometimes cloud the issue when considering individual clinical problems but it is not illogical. Very few problems in medicine are susceptible to precise and absolute decisions—again one must emphasize that it is so often a matter of probabilities. If a small percentage of subjects show EEG patterns differing from those of the great majority of the population, they can only be described as abnormal, even though the observation has little clinical significance.

Observer Reliability

Experienced electroencephalographers are well aware of the subjective element in EEG interpretation and it is therefore surprising that so few reliability studies have been made. The assessment of EEG findings should properly be divided into two stages: appraisal of the content of the record in purely electrical terms and their evaluation in the clinical context of a particular patient. While the second may rightly be influenced by many factors extraneous to the EEG itself, the first should be a more objective process the results of which should be reproducible from one occasion to another and from one assessor to another. Two small-scale studies by Woody undoubtedly question the validity of these assumptions.

In the first (Woody, 1966), a qualified electroencephalographer was given the EEGs of 15 boys with behaviour problems and those of 15 well-behaved boys as age-matched controls. He subsequently reassessed the records 8 months later. The records were scored on the basis of 12 factors, only one of which was interpretative in the sense that the record had to be classified as normal, borderline, slightly, moderately or markedly abnormal. While there was a high degree of consistency in measurements of the frequency of the dominant occipital activity and its responsiveness to eye opening, factors such as the measurement of the predominant frequency in other areas and estimates of the overall normality or otherwise of the records were not significantly related on the two occasions. Rather surprisingly, a multivariate factor 'general characteristics' was reliably re-evaluated for the experimental subjects but not for the controls.

In the second study (Woody, 1968), the EEGs of a further group of 15 boys with behaviour problems and those of 15 matched controls were presented to three qualified electroencephalographers independently. The author and assessors had a preliminary meeting for orientation and discussion of the rating scales which contained 30 factors. Results were expressed as 'coefficients of generalizability' (Cronbach, Rajaratnam and Gleser, 1963). These was excellent agreement on the evaluation of the records' general characteristics—which included factors for voltage distribution and lateral asymmetry —but poorer agreement on the characteristics of more specific features, such as those of the occipital activity, apart from its dominant frequency. An overall classification of the records into two broad categories—'normal or borderline' and 'abnormal'—showed agreement between pairs of assessors which varied from 60 to 80 per cent, but an agreement of only 53 per cent amongst all three assessors.

These studies are open to the criticism that they were conducted on only one and three electro-encephalographers respectively. Nevertheless, they suggest that even descriptive criteria are open to a considerable degree of personal interpretation and that estimates of intra- and inter-rater reliability should feature more prominently than they do at present in both clinical and research work in this field.

However, a lack of precision and objectivity is not unique to electroencephalography. The same difficulties arise with much less complex techniques, a number of which are far less objective than we have been led to believe. Acheson (1960) conducted an investigation into the reliability of ECG reports. The same observer was found to give different interpretations of the same series of ECGs in over 10 per cent of cases. When several observers were presented with the same series of records there was some measure of disagreement in about 40 per cent of cases. In occasional patients, a record regarded as normal by one observer would be reported upon as showing evidence of a myocardial infarct or of left ventricular hypertrophy by another. This is a salutary observation when one recalls that the ECG deals merely with the electrical potentials produced by a single syncytium and that from a practical point of view the problems are largely vectorial in character.

It is important to realize that other well-used and well-trusted methods of investigation have their limitations so that the complaints sometimes made against electroencephalography can be viewed in their proper perspective. Empiricism and its limitations must be recognized and acknowledged, whatever the discipline.

How can limitations such as those discussed in the introduction to Chapter 9 be minimized or avoided? Sufficient stress has perhaps already been laid on the substitution of planned serial studies in place of single 'routine' recordings. The use of special electrode placements and of unipolar as well as bipolar montages is to be encouraged, as is the discriminate use of provocation techniques. Never-theless it is not out of place to emphasize that, however good the standards of interpretation in any centre, their successful application depends on the quality of the records themselves and hence on the standards observed by the technicians who obtain them. The employment of precise but varied techniques, meticulously carried out, and a constant endeavour to obtain records free from undesirable artefacts are all-important. Is is equally essential that the technician be observant of clinical phenomena and alert to exploit unexpected occurrences. When provocation techniques are to be employed, especially those that may precipitate seizures, it is desirable that they should be carried out under medical supervision. For instance, the extent to which photic stimulation should be continued when it evokes a paroxysmal response, requires an immediate assessment of the information so far obtained and a decision as to whether further information of value is likely to be gained by prolonging the stimulation. Only by day to day co-operation between medical, technical and recording staff can the best use be made of whatever facilities are available.

It should not be necessary to emphasize that each EEG must be read in its proper context, in relation to a particular problem of an individual patient and that full clinical details should be available, including the results of other investigations. This implies that EEG interpretations should be carried out only by medical personnel who are in close touch with the clinical problem for which the patient has been referred; the issuing of brief factual reports by technicians to clinicians is greatly to be de-precated. The subjective element in interpretation must be appreciated and it should be realized that the rigid application of set 'criteria of normality' can prove misleading.

CLINICAL VALUE

What does the EEG have to offer to the clinician? The method must be applied with a full under-standing of its limitations and as Hill (1956) has pointed out, each EEG investigation should be re-garded and treated as a 'planned experiment'. As a rule, the value of a single recording is limited, particularly when interpretation has to be made with the aid of scanty clinical details. Most EEG departments spend far too much time endeavouring to provide a service, which in effect means supply-ing reports of little value on a variety of problems referred by clinicians who have little knowledge either of the indications for electroencephalography or of its limitations and to whose queries the EEG is often incapable of providing an answer. It would be far better if these requests were scrutinized carefully and a selection made of those cases in which the EEG has something positive to offer. These could be investigated thoroughly using appropriate ancillary techniques, a series of interrelated recordings being carried out which are planned to answer specific questions and chosen because they fall within the scope of the method.

Epilepsy

In primary subcortical epilepsy, electroencephalography is of relatively little value though the appearance of a spike and wave discharge may resolve doubts left by a poor witness' inadequate account of a petit mal attack. Its principal value is to distinguish those patients considered to have centrencephalic epilepsy, because their attacks take the form of grand mal unprefaced by any suggestion of an aura, but which in fact are initiated by a discharging cortical focus. Even in this group, difficulties may arise when the cortical discharge gives rise to secondary bilateral synchrony (*see* page 96). In cortical epilepsy, the EEG is of considerable value and frequently provides essential information unobtainable in any other way. Apart from the assistance provided in detecting and localizing a cortical epileptogenic lesion, the EEG may provide some indication of the extent of the lesion and in particular whether or not bilateral epileptogenic foci exist.

It is still not fully realized how varied the clinical phenomena accompanying psychomotor epilepsy can be and many cases still masquerade under other diagnostic labels, usually hysteria. The EEG frequently provides evidence that points to the true diagnosis.

There are other forms of attack—notably the episodes associated with spontaneous hypoglycaemia—which being rare, are likely to be regarded as hysterical; here again the EEG may provide a safeguard against such a mistake. In metabolic disturbances associated with hypopituitarism and Addison's disease, the bizarre behaviour which sometimes results, may lead to a misdiagnosis of a primary psychiatric disturbance and again the EEG may arouse the suspicion of error.

Intracranial Space-occupying Lesions

In cases of cerebral tumour, very careful EEG studies can provide good localization in a high percentage of cases, giving results comparable to those of air studies and carotid arteriography; but against this must be offset the occasional case with a well defined but utterly misleading focus, perhaps situated in the opposite hemisphere. In contradistinction to electroencephalography, both air studies and arteriography have the advantage of indicating effects produced directly by a tumour and although they sometimes prove unhelpful, they are unlikely to be actively misleading. Sometimes the EEG proves brilliantly successful and provides the first suggestion that a puzzling clinical picture may be the result of a space-occupying lesion. Subdural haematomas in elderly people often present with predominantly psychiatric disturbances and the EEG is very likely either to bring the correct diagnosis to mind or to provide sufficient moral support to encourage neurosurgical intervention. In the diagnosis of cerebral abscess, the EEG may be of considerable value, particularly when the condition arises as a complication of a general infection in a setting of clouding of consciousness.

Head Injuries and Cerebral Infections

In head injuries and in both bacterial and viral intracranial infections, the EEG is a useful aid to prognosis and may sometimes provide assistance in judging the efficacy and duration of treatment. It may provide an early indication of the onset of complications. This is true, too, of some of the encephalopathies, particularly that associated with liver disease, while in such conditions as subacute sclerosing panencephalitis, in which characteristic though not specific changes occur, the EEG has a high diagnostic value. In cerebrovascular disease serial EEG studies may again prove of prognostic value and may resolve doubts concerning the presence of a cerebral tumour.

Psychiatric Conditions

In psychiatric conditions, the practical value of the EEG is not very great, although in delirium, particularly those milder cases presenting with predominantly paranoid symptoms, it may provide a valuable indication of the true diagnosis. One useful role in elderly patients is to aid the differentiation of cases of pseudodementia from those with degenerative cerebral disease; the finding of a normal EEG when a diagnosis of arteriosclerotic or senile dementia has been made in a patient showing some degree of depression, suggests that the diagnosis should be re-scrutinized lest a reversible functional psychosis has been overlooked (Kiloh, 1961).

Limitations in Excluding Cerebral Disease

Many clinicians appear to believe that electroencephalographic examination can exclude the presence of organic disease. This belief is attested by the contents of so many EEG request forms. In fact, no method of investigation in which the correlations with disease processes are so low, can be relied upon in this way. It is probably true to say that a normal EEG can never be accepted as excluding any condition—even some attacks of epilepsy may be accompanied by normal records—though in a few conditions, such as cerebral abscess and subacute sclerosing panencephalitis, a tolerable degree of certainty can be attained. In many cases the probability of the suggested diagnosis being the correct one on clinical grounds is low—it represents little more than a nagging doubt in the mind of the clinician. Even so, in these cases the EEG is neither more nor less effective in aiding a decision than in cases where the probability of the suggested diagnosis being correct is high. The most that can be claimed in the case, say, of a suspected cerebral tumour, is that the finding of a normal EEG does diminish the probability of such a lesion being present, but it does not exclude it. To this extent, and only to this extent, may the finding of a normal EEG in such a case have some value.

Other Uses of the EEG

The EEG has proved useful in one or two surprising contexts. The development of compact evoked-response averagers has provided an accurate means of assessing deafness that is independent of the subject's co-operation (see page 205). Indeed, evoked-response audiometry during sleep is the best technique for measuring hearing loss in young children (Cody, Klass and Bickford, 1967).

The EEG has also been used to monitor variations in the level of anaesthesia and by using the integrated output of electrical energy from the cortex to activate a device controlling the amount of anaesthetic administered, the EEG may be employed to regulate its depth (Faulconer and Bickford, 1960). A more valuable use during operative procedures is to provide a rapid indication of whether the supply of blood to the brain is being maintained at an adequate level, particularly during operations in which whole body perfusion is being performed with an extracorporeal circulation (Martin, Faulconer and Bickford, 1959).

One of the commonest causes of coma nowadays is barbiturate poisoning; in a case of coma of unknown aetiology, this possibility can be entertained or excluded with a high degree of probability by the EEG (Cohn, Savage and Raines, 1950).

It is worth bearing in mind that electroencephalographic apparatus can be used to register other physiological variables than the electrical activity of the brain (Venables and Martin, 1967). One or more channels may be employed to record the ECG, respiratory rate, changes in skin conductance, the electromyogram or involuntary movements, simultaneously with the EEG. These techniques are of value in relating changes in the EEG to the autonomic changes induced by drugs or other stimuli. They have also been used in the study of epileptiform discharges (Johnson and Davidoff, 1964).

Forensic Psychiatry

In forensic psychiatry, electroencephalography with its shades of value and relatively low scale of probabilities finds little application. Curran (1952) discussed the cases of two murderers. In both of them, the EEGs showed quite obvious abnormalities—in one case spike and wave activity and in the other changes suggesting a localized brain lesion. There was no clinical evidence to support a diagnosis of epilepsy in the one or of a focal lesion in the other, and in neither case could the crimes be described as other than calculated and purposive. It was argued at both trials that the EEG abnormalities indicated the presence of 'brain pathology' relevant to the commission of the crimes. These arguments were discarded by both juries and at subsequent necropsy the brain in each case was considered to be normal. As Curran pointed out, the demonstration of an abnormal EEG in such a case cannot, particularly in the light of our present knowledge, be allowed to confer immunity on these individuals; otherwise the possession of an abnormal EEG might become a criminal asset.

Electroencephalography in Research

Although the application of the methods of electroencephalography has proved most valuable in neurophysiological research, the actual contribution of human electroencephalography to basic neurophysiological knowledge has been somewhat limited. It is not within the scope of the present volume to discuss in detail electroencephalography as a research method, but it would be wrong to omit some reference to its value in this field. Apart from its contributions to clinical research, reference to which has been made where appropriate in earlier chapters, wide use has been made of electroencephalography in the evaluation of the cerebral effects of drugs. A great deal of work has also been done on the relationships between behavioural and EEG changes both in animals and in man. (C.I.O.M.S., 1961; Glaser, 1963). But its greatest contribution has undoubtedly been the unravelling of the functions of the diffuse projection systems and the arousal mechanisms. (C.I.O.M.S., 1954; Evans and Mulholland, 1969.)

Future Developments

The future hopes of electroencephalography making greater and more valuable contributions in the field of clinical medicine may well lie in the development of more discriminative techniques based on a greater knowledge of the physiological basis of the EEG. So far techniques such as that used for establishing the photo-metrazol threshold (Gastaut, 1950) and the sedation threshold (Shagass, 1954) have proved interesting rather than useful, but they may be an indication of the pattern of investigation that will find more general application in the future. Methods derived from electroencephalography— electrocorticography and recording from chronically implanted electrodes within the brain—have already made contributions of interest and will continue to be used in the future.

The commercial availability of EEG apparatus for recording steady or very slowly changing differences of the order of microvolts has enabled others to follow up the pioneer work of Goldring and his colleagues in this field (O'Leary and Goldring, 1960). For instance, Cohn (1964) has shown that epileptiform and other paroxysmal discharges in the EEG are accompanied by steady potential shifts. The *contingent negative variation* of Walter *et al.* (1964) is essentially a very slow potential change which occurs in the interval between a warning stimulus and a second stimulus demanding an operant response (*see* page 208).

In the five years that have elapsed since the previous edition of this book, there has been a considerable increase in the number of EEG laboratories with access to general-purpose digital computers, as well as in the number of laboratories with their own special-purpose computers, such as averagers. There has been a corresponding increase in the output of publications on EEG analysis. The range and variety of computational methods used is outside the scope of this book, but a useful introduction to many of them can be obtained from Brazier (1961). However, there are two computer-dependent methods of presentation which give an added element of realism to the display of EEG data as potential fluctuations over the surface of the head. Both are developed from the method of contour mapping.

The chronotopograms of Rémond (1964a and b) give a continuous graphic display of how the potential gradient varies along a line of electrodes with the passage of time. It is a powerful method for examining the degree of synchronism between activities at different places on the head, particularly between activities in homologous regions on either side. The isometric projection technique of Harris, Melby and Bickford (1969) gives an apparent three-dimensional view on the screen of a cathode-ray oscilloscope of the potential field variations over a matrix of electrodes. This technique is the dynamic successor to the contour map, presenting EEG phenomena in an easily-understood spatio-temporal display. Both techniques, in so far as they allow the fluctuating potentials to be examined spatially and in detail with respect to time, overcome the lack of temporal resolution which is the major limitation of conventional EEG recorders.

Electroencephalography has had its period of youthful optimism and is now going through a period of scientific reappraisal. Its place in clinical medicine, although small, is secure and it remains to be seen whether some of the early hopes and predictions may yet be fulfilled.

REFERENCES

Acheson, R. M. (1960). 'Observer Error and Variation in the Interpretation of Electrocardiograms in an Epidemiological Study of Coronary Heart Disease'. *Br. J. prev. soc. Med.* **14,** 99

Bergman, P. S. and Green, M. A. (1956–57). 'The Use of Electroencephalography in Differentiating Psychogenic Disorders and Organic Brain Diseases'. *Am. J. Psychiat.* **113,** 27

Brazier, M. A. B. (Ed.) (1961). 'Computer Techniques in EEG Analysis'. *Electroenceph. clin. Neurophysiol.* Suppl. 20

C.I.O.M.S. (1954). *Brain Mechanisms and Consciousness.* Oxford; Blackwell

— (1961). *Brain Mechanisms and Learning.* Oxford; Blackwell

Cody, D. T. R., Klass, D. W. and Bickford, R. G. (1967). 'Cortical Audiometry: An Objective Method of Evaluating Auditory Acuity in Awake and Sleeping Man'. *Trans. Am. Acad. Ophthal. Oto-lar.* **71,** 81

Cohn, R. (1964). 'DC Recordings of Paroxysmal Disorders in Man'. *Electroenceph. clin. Neurophysiol.* **17,** 17

— Savage, C. and Raines, G. N. (1950). 'Barbiturate Intoxication: A Clinical Electroencephalographic Study'. *Ann. intern. Med.* **32,** 1049

Cronbach, L. J., Rajaratnam, N. and Gleser, G. C. (1963). 'Theory of Generalizability: a Liberalization of Reliability Theory'. *Br. J. statist. Psychol.* **16,** 137

Curran, D. (1952). 'Psychiatry Ltd'. *J. ment. Sci.* **98,** 373

Evans, C. R. and Mulholland, T. B. (Eds.) (1969). *Attention in Neurophysiology.* London; Butterworths

Faulconer, A. and Bickford, R. G. (1960). 'Servoanesthesia'. In *Electroencephalography in Anesthesiology.* Springfield; Thomas

Gastaut, H. (1950). 'Combined Photic and Metrazol Activation of the Brain'. *Electroenceph. clin. Neurophysiol.* **2,** 249

Gibbs, F. A., Gibbs, E. L. and Lennox, W. G. (1938). 'Cerebral Dysrhythmias of Epilepsy'. *Arch. Neurol. Psychiat.* **39,** 298

Glaser, G. H. (Ed.) (1963). *EEG and Behavior.* London and New York; Basic Books

Harris, J. A., Melby, G. M. and Bickford, R. G. (1969). 'Computer-Controlled Multidimensional Display Device for Investigation and Modeling of Physiologic Systems'. *Comput. biomed. Res.* **2,** 519

Hill, D. (1956). 'Clinical Applications of EEG in Psychiatry'. *J. ment. Sci.* **102,** 264

— (1957). 'Discussion on Changing Values in Electroencephalography'. *Proc. R. Soc. Med.* **50,** 899

Johnson, L. C. and Davidoff, R. A. (1964). 'Autonomic Changes during Paroxysmal EEG Activity'. *Electroenceph. clin. Neurophysiol.* **17,** 25

Kiloh, L. G. (1961). 'Pseudo-dementia'. *Acta psychiat. scand.* **37,** 336

Martin, J. T., Faulconer, A. and Bickford, R. G. (1959). 'Electroencephalography in Anesthesiology'. *Anesthesiology* **20,** 359

O'Leary, J. L. and Goldring, S. (1960). 'Slow Cortical Potentials: Their Origin and Contribution to Seizure Discharge'. *Epilepsia* **1,** 561

Pickering, G. W. (1960). 'Conclusion: The Physician'. In *Controlled Clinical Trials.* p. 163. Ed. by A. Hill. Oxford; Blackwell

Rémond, A. (1964a). 'Organization of Evoked Responses'. *Ann. N.Y. Acad. Sci.* **112,** 134

— (1964b). 'Topological Aspects of the Organization, Processing and Presentation of Data'. In *Symposium on the Analysis of Central Nervous System and Cardiovascular Data using Computer Methods.* Ed. by L. D. Proctor and W. R. Adey. Washington D.C.; NASA SP-72, 73

Shagass, C. (1954). 'The Sedation Threshold. A Method for Estimating Tension in Psychiatric Patients'. *Electroenceph. clin. Neurophysiol.* **6,** 221

Venables, P. H. and Martin, I. (Eds.) (1967). *A Manual of Psychophysiological Methods.* Amsterdam; North-Holland

Walter, W. G., Cooper, R., Aldridge, V. J., McCallum, W. C. and Winter, A. L. (1964). 'Contingent Negative Variation: An Electric Sign of Sensorimotor Association and Expectancy in the Human Brain'. *Nature, Lond.* **203,** 380

Woody, R. H. (1966). 'Intra-Judge Reliability in Clinical Electroencephalography'. *J. clin. Psychol.* **22,** 150

— (1968). 'Inter-Judge Reliability in Clinical Electroencephalography'. *J. clin. Psychol.* **24,** 251

INDEX

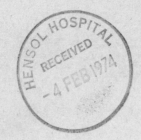